LOST DAUGHTERS

Lost Daughters

Recovered Memory Therapy
and the People It Hurts

Reinder Van Til

WILLIAM B. EERDMANS PUBLISHING COMPANY
GRAND RAPIDS, MICHIGAN / CAMBRIDGE, U.K.

Library of Congress Cataloging-in-Publication Data

Van Til, Reinder.

Lost daughters: recovered memory therapy and the people it hurts /
Reinder Van Til.

p.   cm.

Includes bibliographical references and index.

ISBN 0-8028-4272-0 (paper: alk. paper)

1. False memory syndrome.   2. False memory syndrome — Case studies.
I. Title.

RC455.2.F35V36   1997

616.85′82230651 — dc21   97-21298
                                                          CIP

For my daughter and my son . . .

"You shall know the truth,
and the truth shall set you free."

Contents

Foreword

If you want to write what is called a "non-fiction" best-seller, here is one formula: give a semi-fictional account of your life as a victim of abuse, preferably of the sexual sort. Blame Father-God or father — it does not make much difference which of them, and you get extra points for blurring the boundaries between them — or someone else "in power." Credit the therapist who helped you remember this autobiographical material, which you evidently had long suppressed. Toss in some psychotherapeutic jargon, giving your work a sort of scientific-sounding cast. Tell how you were messed up until you finally wrote this tell-all work that tells it like it is, or was, or as your therapist helped you think it was. Be lurid. If you can, suggest that the devil was responsible for it all, but secular versions of the drama are equally acceptable to much of the market. If you are generous or afraid of being found out, credit the ghostwriter who put it all together. Get ready for the celebrity promotion tour.

Lost Daughters will not be a best-seller — though, of course, the author and publisher and friends of either or of the approach, including this Foreworder, hope it will be a good- or even a better-seller. It does not lack all ingredients described in the formula a paragraph ago. There is an account of especially incestuous sexual abuses, or at least charges of such. God and father are here, though boundaries between the two are firm. Therapists and jargon get referred to, but often pejoratively. Seekers of the lurid will be disappointed, and the devil gets short shrift.

The problem for *Lost Daughters* on the celebrity circuit is that it goes against what is still the grain of the times, the common wisdom, and the fashions in law and therapy and personal relations. Or at least it appears

ix

in the earlier stages after a turn from the time in which almost all accusers and claimants to the victim- or abused-role were believed and their therapies and therapists given positive notice. Reinder Van Til both profits from and exemplifies a cultural shift in which what we at the Divinity School call "the hermeneutics of suspicion" or such public phrases as "keep your fingers crossed and your guard up" are more frequently to be brought into play.

These paragraphs and this whole book will be misread by anyone who thinks that sexual abuse, especially of incestuous sorts, does not occur or even that it is not common. Think again if you think that author Van Til wants to let off the hook anyone who abuses and whose offense is known only to God and the victim, or that he sees no potential in therapies or in laws protecting victims. But he is here to help readers find grounds for transcending the fashion, respecting the rights of more than the one who claims to have been abused, and a therapeutic and legal culture that brings automatic prejudice against fathers or whoever else represents power.

Van Til's own story, one that could have been a book-length "grabber," is briefly told, quickly finds company in the case stories of several others, and then gets set in an historical and cultural context. Depending upon several extensive book-length critiques of "Recovered Memory Therapy," he provides a framework for further inquiry, the reintroduction of common sense, and with it a sense of fairness directed to the (often falsely, it turns out) accused.

One thing that strikes the reader, or at least struck this historically minded reader, is the evidence of how swiftly cultural change can occur, and, speaking of victimage, how easily one can be victim of the moment. As Van Til gives an account of legislation passed in 1974 — so recently, says one part of me; how long ago! says another — and as he describes various moments in the development and critique of therapies, fashions, and laws, one can learn how quickly an approach to human understanding and interaction can come and crest and begin to go and then go.

So it is with the main theme of this work. When the public was being taught to presume that the accused were guilty unless proven innocent, and while certain understandings of human action were in favor — code name them "Recovered Memory Syndromes" and therapies — it was hard to hear more sides than one to a story. Especially when legal cases or autobiographical accounts were seasoned with scientific-sounding substantiations tied to patterns of science that quickly fell under a cloud or into disfavor, it was hard to raise questions without sounding medieval, unscientific, or repressive.

When reading the history of witchcraft or other crazes in late-medieval and early-modern times, we can see how they were tied to noncredible and obsolete worldviews. In the case of the long ago, it is easy to gain perspective on the passing moments. That is more difficult to do when dealing with one's own times, one's own stories. Yet, as we turn the pages, it is easy to see how "sixtyish" this or that therapeutic fad was, how dated to the seventies or eighties was another, how imprisoned we still may be by many currents in the nineties.

Some of the questioning of contentions for, say, Recovered Memory Therapy, occurs simply on the grounds on which it is supposed to occur in science. It gets tested and fails to meet tests. Its claims meet counterclaims, and the counterers often win. Most often an incident serves as a catalyst. Historians will certainly record such a moment in the case of the late Cardinal Joseph Bernardin. He was subjected to horrific embarrassment, predispositions to find him guilty, attacks by professional victims-rights groups, analysis by therapists, and exposure by the media in a certainly groundless case. His forgiving of a confessing and repentant maker-up-of-stories exemplified nobility in a trashy culture and serves as a model.

Several stories of other families add substance to Van Til's account and offer hope that the misuses of "Recovered Memory" and the thriving of ideologies like those that evidently attracted Van Til's own daughter will soon have had their day, and the craze will have passed.

Whenever accusations are made, the public in the time of legal trials, and the reader in the case of books, has to be wary. Could it possibly be, against all evidence, against all knowledge one has of a noble character like the Cardinal, that there might be something to the story? Could it be that, post–Recovered Memory Therapy prime, I, a reader, will be gulled into accepting too simply a story like Van Til's (and his former wife's) and others who claim to have been falsely accused and haunted by the accusations? There seems to be no way around the need to bracket suspicions and let trust grow as one follows a case. The context of a life lived, a witness made, an argument set forth, lead one to trust the present account, and thus to be ready for the context Van Til provides in his critiques of psychology-as-religion and certain therapies as being destructive.

Nothing in Van Til's book is to be read as the slightest legitimation of abuse or as a suggestion that victimage does not occur and is not a problem. But his writing can be of immense aid to those who believe, who know, that the time has come for more sides and claims than one to be heard if there is to be justice in a society most of whose members

FOREWORD

claim to be viewing human action in the light of divine intention and revelation. One hopes someday for a sequel, after the cultural moment passes and things get sorted out: *Found Daughters* and forgiven therapists and ideologues.

Martin E. Marty

Preface

This book is a combination of personal narratives and culture critique, so it can be read straight through or in fragments or combinations of ways. All the chapters bearing daughters' names as their titles (Kristin, Emily, etc.) are personal stories given to me either in interview form or written form (all the names of actual daughters have been changed). The intervening chapters contain my own critical reflections on the cultural problems named in the chapter titles, which have been in some way illustrated by the preceding narrative. In those chapters I have benefited greatly (indeed, borrowed shamelessly) from the work of professionals — memory scientists, psychological and sociological theorists, and investigative reporters — who have researched and published in the area of repressed memory and child sexual abuse hysteria during the past decade.

Thus, though my name is on the title page as the author, this book has many contributors, some more than they know. "Kristin," which is my personal story, and "Susan," Jane Doe's story, were originally published elsewhere and are used here, slightly edited, by permission. The other personal narratives are published here for the first time. I am deeply grateful to Roger and Liz, Leo and Katie, and Sherri Hauser-Hines for their patience with my less than stellar journalistic interviewing style and for their courage both in telling their stories and in standing up for the falsely accused for several years now. Sherri has told me her story in interviews and many personal conversations, but, because Sherri is such a fine writer, I asked for her own written account for use in this book. My sincerest thanks to all those who allowed me to retell their personal stories here.

I should emphasize at the outset what this book is *not* about. My principal subject is *false memories of* child abuse. It is not about child sexual abuse per se. I am assuming that it is a common human principle that all sexual abuse of children is terribly wrong. I am assuming as well that it was underreported during most of this century. Whether it has been overreported since the mid-1970s, I will leave it to the reader to infer. This book is also not about childhood *physical* abuse. Though I originally gave half a chapter to discussing the evolution of and differing views on the corporal punishment of children (the "caning" or "spanking" issue), my editor and I decided that the subject is so prickly that it might well blur the focus on the main issues of this book.

I must also emphasize that this book is not a scientific study, scholarly work, or research analysis. My reading on this subject has been wide, but also episodic and quirky. Many thoughts and quotations from experts in various fields found their way to me via photocopied newspaper and magazine articles (often clipped so as to destroy date and page numbers). I was happy to find a good many penetrating books on the subject, but I also encountered many ideas and thoughts in fragments and snippets of things from a wide variety of other published and unpublished sources. I have tried to be as careful as possible in attributing quotations and ideas to their precise source, but the whirlwind of publishing about this subject has tended to leave some of the fragments and snippets floating in the air.

For the critical analysis chapters, I am especially indebted to the following writers, some of whom have also inspired me personally, some of whom I have not met, only read: Mark Pendergrast for the best and most comprehensive study of "the problem," *Victims of Memory,* and for his warm collegiality; Elizabeth Loftus for her long-time brilliant research and public testimony on the limits and peculiarities of memory; Paul McHugh for his psychiatric wisdom and common sense and forthright public posture; Debbie Nathan for her sharp investigative reporting and profound analysis of child abuse hysteria in this country; Richard Ofshe for his unabashedly critical stance toward mind control and the recovered memory culture; Wendy Kaminer for her witty and incisive dissection of feminism and the recovery movement; Christina Hoff Sommers for her brave, insightful critique of "gender feminism"; and Frederick Crews for his penetrating "Freud-bashing" and the literary elegance he brings to the subject. Citations of these authors' works will be found often in the pages and notes of this book. Since I am merely a dabbler and dilettante in these professional areas, I have relied heavily on their ground-breaking and courageous work — courageous because it often flew in the face of the general mood of American liberal culture in the late eighties and early nineties. (The usual caveats and disclaimers about my responsibility for all errors and mistatements apply.)

A word of kudos and gratitude is especially due, I believe, the courageous women writers, psychologists, and educators who have persistently swum against the current of runaway child abuse hysteria: psychologist Loftus, investigative reporter Nathan, culture critic Kaminer, feminist critic Sommers, Carol Tavris for critiquing the bibles of the incest recovery movement, and Pamela Freyd for persistently showing the reality of the false memory syndrome. These women have continued their important analyses and critiques in the face of often vicious attacks and ostracization by the closing ranks of radical feminists and child protection advocates.

The title "Lost Daughters" came from Leo (of Chapter 3), who was one of the first to alert me to the enormous public scope of this problem. "The repressed memory enthusiasts think that we'll just eventually go away," said Leo. "We won't. We're not mere protesters — my God, we've lost our daughters."

CHAPTER 1

Kristin

Thanksgiving 1990

As the small knot of our family trudges happily through the forest preserve, sniffing the crisp air and rustling the leaves underfoot, my daughter Kristin, a twenty-year-old college junior, slips her hand in mine and proudly walks along that path holding hands with her dad as though she were five or six again. I remember what a doll she was at that age: how she'd run ahead along the trail, her natural curls bouncing on her neck, then come running back and pull me by the hand to where she'd squat down low and show me a chipmunk hole she'd discovered. I don't say anything now, not wanting to spoil the moment, but we both sense how sweet it is. It's one of those unmitigated joys of being a parent.

Later that weekend I stoke the fireplace and our little nuclear family — Joanne and I, forty-something mom and dad, Kristin, and Troy, our college freshman son — sit around the fireplace and read, sometimes aloud. It's a Thanksgiving re-creation of the days when both the kids were young and we spent those cold evenings reading by the warm fire. Kristin still wants to sit next to me, and she puts her head on my shoulder. It is a very satisfying feeling, my almost-grown-up daughter there beside me, smart, a strong personality, an accomplished musician. Indeed, both kids are bright and articulate, doing well at a good liberal arts college. Even though their mother and I are having a rough go at our relationship, these kids are all right. They're secure, confident, and feel warm in our love. Can anything be wrong with this picture?

Christmas 1990

Kristin announces during Christmas break that she has changed her college major from English to "gender studies," and she is toting around a book entitled *Intercourse* by Andrea Dworkin the way students at fundamentalist colleges carry around the Bible. Since being converted from my patriarchal upbringing by the early seventies, I have considered myself a card-carrying feminist. But I know that Andrea Dworkin is a radical-fringe lesbian feminist and that *Intercourse* is a man-hating tract the relentless message of which is that any heterosexual intimacy is innately violative of the woman, essentially a euphemism for rape. I sense trouble.

Joanne has been a feminist for more than twenty years, and we've always been a feminist household. So Kristin has grown up that way, comes by it honestly, and approaches life as any young feminist would. But this is the first indication I've seen of her embracing the radical fringe. College kids are like that, and her professor is probably encouraging it in the new "gender studies" course, but it's still troubling to me.

Later, a photocopied article about sexual violence appears on the dining room table, which is our family bulletin board. The writer makes some good, though exaggerated, points and several times criticizes "Western culture" for not only condoning but encouraging violence against women.

At dinner I mention the article.

"I like a lot of what it said," I begin, "but look, compared to other world cultures and societies — Mediterranean, African, Asian, say — Western culture has been a shining light in its respect for women's rights."

"How can you defend the pigs who perpetrate violence against women?" Kristin exclaims.

"I'm not defending anyone who — "

"You're trying to defend a culture that rapes one out of every four women?" Joanne shouts.

"Individual men rape individual women," I say evenly. "Cultures don't rape women."

Kristin seethes.

"A patriarchal, capitalist culture is at the core of rape," she says. "This writer is simply revealing men's abuse and their lies. But you just don't get it, do you?"

The air is hot with female wrath, and Troy and I listen open-mouthed to the ferocious response. You would have thought that I had just announced myself as an apologist for rape. The evening's donnybrook adds acid to my deteriorating relationship with my wife; even more worrisome, it also cuts me off from the affections of my daughter. The two of us have had stormy years during her adolescence, but that stemmed from the fact that we are so similar in personality: both sharp, argumentative, headstrong, and passionate. We have come through that period of conflict with our senses of humor intact and with an enduring love for each other.

But now, almost every time I open my mouth, Kristin simply glares at me. I've been ostracized by the female members of my family because I've had the effrontery to question the assumptions of a woman speaking about sexual violence. I realize that in less than a month I've changed in the eyes of my daughter from a warm, huggable, storybook dad into a middle-aged male pig.

I'm really quite appalled at the hostility of the reaction. Playing the devil's advocate has always been a necessary and respected part of argumentation in our home. So this is what I get for playing a little needed devil's advocate in this instance? It's bewildering. Later that evening, I tell Joanne that I don't deserve to be thrown onto her Jesse Helms junk pile just because I want some honesty out of the rhetoric. But Joanne isn't speaking to me.

January 1991

Kristin and I drive back to her school together at the end of the first week of January — mainly in silence. She has her headphones on almost the whole way, listening to tapes of Sinead O'Connor, the angry Irish singer.

Kristin breaks the silence. "I love Sinead's strength and openness," she says, punching the tape into the car stereo system. "And I love how she tweaks authority figures, the middle-aged white male establishment."

I know I'm in for some rhetoric now, but I hold my peace. She next plays the song "Sally" from a tape by Sade.

"The concept of prostitutes as the real heroines of our society is compelling, because they really *do* do our dirty work," she says.

Kristin has become chairwoman of the South Africa protest group on campus this year. I had actually been quite proud of her when she first joined the group; it was a good cause to stand behind. But after a couple of years of listening to her rhetoric, I realized that she knew very little about the South Africa situation. I knew that she was in it much more for the satisfaction she derived from being able to bug "the suits," as she and her friends referred to the board members and college authority figures.

After a rest stop, she wants to drive, so I can sit back and relax in the warm car and hark back to my college days of civil rights and antiwar protests, recalling how important and righteous it made us feel. Like we were, Kristin is just a kid of her times. And yet, as she drives fearlessly on the snow-covered roads, past semis in the unplowed left lane, with a spirit of resolve and no need of emotional input from her dad — she appears to be a grown-up woman. But such a seesaw of maturity and immaturity, such a battleground of emotions, and so full of dogmatic rhetoric. And now, stone quiet.

I start to reminisce aloud about our college protests concerning civil rights and the Vietnam war.

"Dad," she interrupts, "I don't want to hear about *your* student protest days. Maybe you want to relive your college days through me, but I just can't do that for you . . ."

"No, Kristin," I say, "I just want to connect with you." She has fallen silent again.

Out of the corner of my eye, I look at her beautiful profile now creased with a frown of anxiety as she listens to protest song lyrics. Some time earlier my wife had reluctantly revealed to me something that happened to Kristin during her recent study-abroad semester in Ecuador. She had developed a relationship with a young man in her exchange group that turned disastrous. During one of their evenings together, after some kissing and "making out," he wanted to have sex, but she declined. Not taking no for an answer, and not being able to persuade her into it, he eventually held her down and forced sex on her. It was an apparent textbook case of date rape.

I have brought it up with Kristin, asking whether she wanted to talk to me about this painful experience. But she has not chosen to do so. I'm not sure whether this is a measure of her alienation from me or simply the uncomfortable nature of the subject matter. I wonder whether the whole thing has contributed to her new hostility.

Standing outside her residence hall, with the north wind stiffening our hair and reddening our faces, we say our perfunctory good-byes and give each other a rather stiff-armed hug. I can't help wondering how long the growing-up process will require the two of us to be alienated from each other. Little do I know that this will prove to be the last time I will see my daughter face-to-face.

March 1991

My marriage, which blew a gasket at Christmas, threw a rod and lost all compression in January, and limped through February, now rattles to a halt.

The wheels have come off. Joanne, who is working toward her graduate psychology degree, is studying for her April comprehensive exams and says the tension in the air is making it impossible for her to concentrate. She asks me to move out. I agree. We have fought to a draw and are clearly heading in opposite directions. I realize that, in addition to everything else, our arguments over the new orthodoxies of feminism, catalyzed by Kristin's newfound dogmas and Joanne's deepening rhetoric, have further alienated us.

I take a small flat a few miles away in the city, leaving the house to Joanne. It seems logical, because my job will take me out of town much of the spring and she'll be home studying for exams. But it also means, of course, that I will not be around on the occasional weekends when the kids return from school. I immediately write them long letters and phone them about the breakup. They don't have much response — they have undoubtedly seen it coming — and yet I sense a quiet shock in their voices. Joanne and I have intentionally waited until they're both in college to make this break. But, good Lord, this sort of blow is *never* easy.

"We'll see each other during spring break," I tell them. And to Kristin, "I'll take you out to dinner for your birthday."

"It's a date," she says. "At least I'll get to see you — even if it's not at home. I've got something I need your advice on."

But a few weeks later, just before spring break is to begin, Kristin calls to say she cannot see me and we can't go out for dinner as planned.

"Why not?" I ask.

"I don't know, I can't tell you," she says. "I just can't see you right now."

It is all so mysterious that I call Joanne to see what she knows.

"I have an idea what it may be about, but I don't want to talk to you about it right now," she says.

"Does this have anything to do with the date-rape experience?" I ask.

"It may," Joanne replies mysteriously.

A week later I get a call from Joanne's therapist.

"You are not to see your daughter," she tells me. "This is per her request."

"Yes," I say, "I already know that."

Then she drops a bombshell: "I am authorizing Kristin's hospitalization because of suicidal tendencies."

"Suicidal — what do you mean, she's suicidal?" I gasp.

"Right now your daughter is a threat to her own life. I have had to exercise direct intervention."

It's shocking. Suddenly my daughter's mental health is in serious question, her life may be in danger, and nobody wants to talk to me, least of all Kristin. I scramble to discover what is going on. I finally pull out of Joanne that Kristin had begun seeing a college counselor months before, partly to cope with the aftereffects of the date-rape experience and partly because of a debilitating premenstrual syndrome that has brought on or exacerbated a general feeling of depression. For some weeks, Joanne tells me, Kristin has wanted to get on an antidepressant; Joanne has been steadfastly against it because of the drug's known side effects. But Kristin convinced her school counselor to refer her to a psychiatrist, who was willing to prescribe. Apparently the initial dosage was not right, however, and she has become suicidal. The hospital psychiatric ward is trying to get the dosage stabilized and keep her from hurting herself.

The next few weeks are harrowing for me. I'm out of town a good deal and out of the family loop. I am aware of an acquaintance's son who severely mutilated himself while taking the same antidepressant Kristin is now taking. I have read and seen other accounts of the drug's dangerous side effects, including the tendency, according to one report, to "make up one's own realities from hallucinations and fantasies."

Joanne herself is reluctant to talk to me, but I do get a few more details from her. Kristin has begun, with the aid of a therapist, to recall from the deep recesses of memory an experience of being sexually abused as a little girl. She spent time in day care with my sister back then, and she is now recalling, Joanne says, memories of being molested by her Uncle Jack. According to her newfound memory, he inserted tools such as screwdrivers and wrenches into her vagina.

I am devastated and sickened trying to imagine it; in fact, I *can't* imagine my brother-in-law Jack hurting my little girl in that way. But Joanne's view is different. As part of her course internship, she has counseled several women, ranging in age from eighteen to forty-five, all of whom claim they were sexually abused in childhood by men they knew or were related to.

"I'm rapidly coming to the conclusion that *all* women have been victimized growing up," she says. "In fact, as you know, I've been looking into the abyss of my own past." That means, she says, trying to pull up memories of her own father's abuse of *her*.

"I have no difficulty imagining what Jack did to Kristin," she concludes.

"Come on, this is nuts!" I protest. But Joanne isn't entertaining any other views.

June 1991

I have written and called Joanne, trying to establish some sort of reconciliation. I hope that we can start over as if from scratch, try to rediscover the chemistry we had, find what it was that we fell in love with. She does not respond.

Kristin dropped out of school when she was hospitalized. Now she is out of the hospital and living in an apartment on her own. She is also into individual and group therapy and drug treatment and psychiatric checkups at a tab of about $200 a week. Troy is back from college, and I learn that he is also "in therapy." In fact, everybody but me is in therapy.

When she finally does write me, Joanne says, "I'm on a painful path of growth toward becoming a more whole and independent person, but it won't make me better able to unite with you. I don't understand why you are the only one not seeing a therapist. How can you do the healing and stretching you need to do without help?"

In a later letter Joanne writes, "Kristin is really having a terrible time, really emotionally disabled. She's so skinny you might not recognize her. She's not the person I used to know. She has terrible memories during the day, and terrible nightmares at night. I'm enclosing an article on incest to give you some idea of what Kristin's going through."

I stare at the word *incest* sitting calmly there on the page.

Late July 1991

By this time no member of my family, not even Troy, will talk with me. Fridays, Joanne leaves the front porch door unlocked so that I can pick up my mail. I sneak up to the front door hoping that no neighbor will spot me and ask where I've been. I quickly grab my mail. Sometimes Forepaws the cat is on the porch and greets me. Nobody else does.

I do have a set of keys for the house, with Joanne's knowledge and assent, even though I know she is uncomfortable with the idea of me coming into the house. But I need to get into my former study for files and books from time to time, so I try to go there when I know no one else will be at home.

On one of these visits, something happens that reveals with terrible clarity why I have been the family pariah for these months. Not finding the book I need in my study, I go to look for it in the bedroom, where there are a couple more bookcases. In the bedroom I see, lying on a dresser, a letter that Joanne has written to me but obviously never sent. I instinctively know it is wrong to read something that has not yet been sent, and yet I have had zero communication from those I love, and I'm so hungry for some words that I read it anyway. Most of the sentiment in the letter does not come as a surprise to me. I have realized by now that Joanne does not want any relationship with me, that she resents me both personally and generically — as a man. I have heard her talk before about my being an instrument of her oppression, having controlled her life and selfhood, and being responsible during our marriage for her sense of "co-dependence." But toward the end of the letter there is a statement that shocks me out of my mind: "Now I know that you were betraying me during those years, betraying me with our own daughter. Our family life was a lie for all those years. I trusted you absolutely with Kristin and with all women and girls. I will never trust you again. I would never have believed this of you if I didn't see the evidence in Kristin."

There are no specifics, but in the context of loyalty and betrayal — and followed by talk of keeping me away from the children — the meaning is quite clear: I am being accused of the sexual abuse of my own daughter. I read those sentences over and over, but their meaning doesn't change. It is a horrible moment. A wave of panic and nausea breaks over me, a sense that I don't know — and have never known — who I am. Is it possible that some monster residing in me — part of a multiple personality, my evil alter ego perhaps — crept out of my bed and defiled my own daughter?

The letter goes on to say that Kristin has had "body memories" of my hand coming under the covers and turning her over, and then . . . apparently the memory goes blank. She is now in "recovered-memory therapy" in an effort to bring back the evil things she was a victim of.

When I come back to my senses, I know that I am not a multiple personality, that I have been conscious of my behaviors, and that I know the difference between right and wrong. And I know I have not touched any woman — let alone any young girl — in an unwanted way. I know that I have never touched my own daughter in any inappropriate or sexual way; I have never touched her in anything but a loving, fatherly way. Nothing even close to it ever came into my mind. Could she have translated reading stories to her in bed as a tot or some fatherly tickling and horseplay into sexual fantasies or fears? I agonize over the thought of it, the sudden revision of those wonderful early years.

I don't know where to turn. Any sexual-behavior issue, by its nature, taints the accused whether there is a shred of evidence for it or not. And I realize that you can't tell just anyone that you've been accused by your daughter of sexual abuse. For many people, such an accusation is as good as an indictment. So it's very difficult talking with even your best friend about such a thing. And the current psychotherapeutic mood and jargon adds the double whammy of declaring that any person who proclaims his innocence is simply "in denial." It is a wonderful catch-22 of the recovered-memory therapy community that denying anything is a symptom that you did it.

After two weeks of silence, the bitter lozenge of accusation that I have not revealed to anyone is still wormwood in my throat, and I finally decide I've got to tell someone. I go to my own family. My oldest sister is a liberal minister and a feminist, and she knows Kristin. She's been around the block a few times: she's worked in high schools, inner-city education programs, and prisons and has dealt with a number of "recovering" women. She says that Kristin may have had fantasies about marrying me when she was six or seven (the old Electra theme), and now at twenty-one, the most "confusing and chaotic time in a young woman's life," she is trying to deal with the guilt of that early passion to live with me and kill off her mother. Sis and I talk at length about some of her own Electra impulses and guilt feelings about our dad when she was Kristin's age. It's pretty Freudian, but it calms me down.

A bit reassured, I also have a couple of talks with Peter, the marriage counselor Joanne and I had seen before we split up.

"Child sexual abuse is absolutely the trendiest accusation that the so-called recovering culture comes up with these days," he says. (Indeed, in this summer of 1991, the tocsin of sexual abuse charges is in full voice and still peaking, and critics of recovered-memory therapy are almost unknown. Adult women recovering from childhood abuse have secured a large niche in the pantheon of the recovery movement; I have noticed that the better bookstores have whole sections dedicated to the subject.) Peter also encourages me to stop trying to make *sense* of this whole thing. "But," he says, "you have to confront your family before it self-destructs."

I call Joanne's therapist to see whether I can sit down and talk with her. I want to tell her what I've discovered and ask her to set up a meeting with all of us.

"I can't do that," she says. "As long as your wife is my client, I can't confer with you. And she'll have to agree to any joint session."

All I'm left with is my exasperation with the psychological system, which she doesn't want to hear.

September 1991

I write Joanne a long letter. "If this family is to make it past the summer," I conclude, "we have to deal with this right now." After two weeks, having heard nothing, I phone her.

"My therapist and I," she says, "don't think it's a good idea for you and me to have a session right now . . ."

"What do you mean 'it's not a good idea'?" I say. "This is not just about you and me. It's about our children and whether they'll have a future relationship with me."

"I *believe* Kristin, and you won't have a relationship with her," Joanne replies. "Anyway, it would just turn into a 'No, I didn't — Yes, you did' session."

"So you actually believe that I'm the kind of monster who could molest his own daughter . . . ?"

"I don't believe you're a monster. I believe you're simply a man who has done terrible things that your consciousness can't even face — so your conscious self is denying those things and burying them deep in your subconscious."

And that's that: a guilty verdict. I'm in denial, she declares, and adds a decisive *no* to any meeting to try to dispel this family demon. I slam the phone down into the receiver in frustration and beat on the wall of the phone booth. In the car, I pound the steering wheel with the heels of my hands. I curse Joanne, I curse God, and I especially curse the guild of psychotherapists as I drive over to O'Toole's Pub for an early start on an age-old kind of therapy.

After a few hours, I realize soddenly that I've been drinking with a vengeance. Back behind the wheel, I take out my rage on my car's accelerator, tires, and suspension system, screeching around entrance ramps and plowing down the freeway and the darkened streets with hate in my blurry eyes. It's a wonder I get home without killing myself or someone else.

A week later, I call Troy to see if he would like to spend a weekend with me, ride bikes, go to a ball game, whatever.

"No," he says, and adds enigmatically, "You know, children forgive their parents far too easily. I'm not going to fall into the forgiveness trap." And he rings off. (I do not realize it then, but I find out later that his lines come directly from *The Courage to Heal,* the bible of the incest recovery movement.) My son, who was always my buddy, has now also turned against me. Crying hot tears, I feel like he's kicking me when I'm down. The hurt and the anger are so sharp and so mixed together that all I can do is sob to myself in my empty apartment.

October 1991

During the next few weeks, I get several phone calls in which, as soon as I pick up to answer, somebody hangs up on the other end. Then, while I'm out of town on business, I get a message on my phone machine from Kristin.

"Dad," she says, very nervously, "I just want to tell you that you sexually abused me when I was a little girl. I want you to know that I will never forgive you, and you'll never see your grandchildren. I hope that you get help, because you're a very sick man."

The voice is so breathless, thin, and nervous sounding, so unlike Kristin's voice, that it seems like one of those kidnap messages, like someone is making her say it.

I cannot call her back because she has an unlisted number. Just to hear her voice, I keep the message on my machine for over a week, and every phrase becomes almost a litany. I finally erase it. It's breaking my heart.

November 1991

I move out of Chicago for good. I've been thinking about this move for years, and it's for professional rather than personal reasons. Even so, I call Peter and ask him if he thinks I'm running away from it all.

"No," he says, "you've made every effort to face your family and to get to the bottom of this. I think *they're* avoiding *you*."

So I leave town — with a bulging backpack of mixed emotions.

For the next year I am completely shut out by my family. But I begin to hear about other people who are in the same boat. One of the first articles I read is in, of all places, *Playboy* magazine. In an article entitled "Cry Incest," Debbie Nathan, a very good investigative journalist who attended a retreat for "survivors of abuse," exposes ideological therapists who are manufacturing memories of abuse for young women. In that article I learn for the first time about the False Memory Syndrome Foundation, a group started in Philadelphia by concerned parents who have been falsely accused of abuse by their adult children, almost always daughters.

I send for and receive the foundation's packet of information, and the similarity of my own story to the many stories I read there — some short, some long — is uncanny. One thing is true of all these accusing children: only after they are exposed to psychotherapy do they "recall" the incestuous abuse, and only after leaving their therapist are some able to recant and reunite with their parents, recognizing that their abuse was fabricated.

I hear other accounts. A friend's sister goes into severe depression after the breakup of her marriage and goes to a psychiatrist, who, after prescribing Prozac, urges her to dredge up memories of incestuous abuse from her childhood. In session after session the psychiatrist presses the abuse angle — even though it never happened. Finally, in exasperation, the woman seeks another therapist.

I watch TV newsmagazine programs exposing therapists who are coaching their clients into memories of ritual abuse (complete with filmed footage). A public radio program explores the "repressed memory" controversy and tells of an investigator who has been hired by some accused parents to look into their daughter's therapist. The detective, posing as a patient, describes to the therapist the most generic emotional complaints imaginable — depression, sleeplessness, fear of the unknown — and within two sessions the therapist tells her she's a victim of incest.

The information and the public exposure of these instances bolster me. The repressed-memory phenomenon, now nationwide in scope, is maddening. Yet the most astounding revelation in this whole sordid drama is yet to come, and it will come from where it all started — my own family.

October 1992

In the course of almost a year I have had only two phone conversations with Joanne — both about money. That's it. We're still married, though pursuing divorce, and we've been quite civil despite everything. I'm in Chicago for a week, so I risk asking her whether we can get together for dinner. Surprisingly, she agrees to it.

We decide to meet at our old favorite Italian restaurant, a tiny, quiet place with a good selection of pastas and wines. I'm there a little early, and I'm nervous, but I'm also eager to see Joanne because I want to hear about the kids. When she shows up, we formally shake hands, but that seems very wooden, and her vulnerable appearance inspires me to give her a hug. Joanne looks awful. Her face is pinched and anxious.

"I am just now getting out of a depression that has lasted for at least six months," she says after a little prompting. "Just after you moved, Kristin told me that she wanted nothing more to do with me. She would not say why — she just refused to let me contact her. A few months later, in February, Troy moved out. He also wouldn't say why, and he won't talk to me either. After I couldn't take the freeze-out anymore, I finally persuaded Kristin to agree to a session. We'd each have our therapist present, and we'd sit down and talk.

12

"It was a nightmare. One long tirade by Kristin. She accused *me* of abusing her along with you. She said you had raped her while I looked on and encouraged you. She said I had raped her with snakes; that I had threatened to slice into her baby brother, Troy, with a huge knife and that I had dismembered her cat with a knife, among many other acts smacking of animal sacrifice and satanic rituals. She went on and on, one thing after another, for more than an hour.

"I couldn't say anything to her. She was utterly convinced of the truth of what she was saying. When it was over, I stumbled out of that room shaking and sobbing, and when we got back to my therapist's office, the first thing she said to me was, 'I guess now you know what your husband felt like.'"

I am speechless. There is a brief sense of moral vindication, but it's in my mind only. My gut is turning over with the shock of the outrageous accusations. Joanne is weeping now and squeezing my hand. I feel the urge to embrace and comfort her, and yet I'm astonished that I'm hearing this for the first time right now, six months after it happened — six months in which I felt like the family's outcast.

Then she turns abruptly to me, staring into my eyes. "Tell me for sure that you didn't abuse her," she says. "You didn't, did you?"

I wearily shake my head as I look back at her. Her eyes are brimming with tears.

"I'm sorry I ever believed her," she says finally. "I'm just still so confused. How could this happen?"

The next day I run into Bob, an old friend of the family. While we exchange amenities, he looks at me oddly, and I think I know why.

"Can I buy you a drink?" he asks. "There's something I've wanted to talk to you about."

We go into a downtown bar, and after our drinks are set down, he leans forward and says, "I saw your daughter this summer . . . and, well, this is really bizarre, but . . ."

I'm pretty sure I know what he's wanted to bring up.

"Joyce and I were having coffee at a little sidewalk cafe, and I spotted Kristin drive by. She must have seen us too, because she did a quick U-turn right there on the street and parked the car. She popped out of the car, came right over to our table, and without so much as acknowledging me, said to Joyce, 'My parents sexually abused me when I was little, which I've recalled in therapy. I will never see them or speak to them again. I just wanted you to know.' It was a wooden little recitation, and she refused to look at me the whole time.

"Then, a few weeks later, we were at a music club where Troy is apparently a busboy. When he saw us, he came over almost immediately and gave us the same grim, hauntingly similar line: 'I was sexually abused by my parents, and I will never see them or talk to them again.' It was like he was assigned to make a pronouncement."

That hits me. Troy has progressed from a sympathizer with his sister to a believer in his own abuse. I tell Bob the whole story. He is incredulous, and we talk long and hard about what happened. He and his wife have known Joanne and me for twenty-five years, Kristin and Troy since they were infants.

"None of it's true, Bob," I say, realizing that I've been saying it for over a year now. In the end he can only wonder, taking my word for things because I'm his friend, hanging his head in heartfelt sadness over this poison that has devastated a family.

February 1994

It is now three years since I have seen my daughter, almost that long since I learned that she was accusing me of sexual abuse. Nationally, the cover has been torn off the "repressed-memory" racket in American psychotherapy. I have read and collected scores of articles and a dozen books on the subject. Feminists who consider any questioning of *any* "victimization" to be heresy have screamed foul, and the battle in the psychotherapeutic community has been joined.

Carol Tavris, social psychologist and author of *The Mismeasure of Woman,* in a telling *New York Times* article entitled "Beware the Incest-Survivor Machine" (3 January 1993), rips into the so-called bibles and rhetoric of the incest recovery movement, especially the symptoms of childhood abuse advanced by its gurus, which, she says, are generic enough to identify one as a "mere human being in the late twentieth century."

Wendy Kaminer, in an important essay entitled "Feminism's Identity Crisis" (*Atlantic,* October 1993), says, "It is heresy, in general, to question the testimony of self-proclaimed victims of date rape or harassment, as it is heresy in a twelve-step group to question claims of abuse. All claims of suffering are sacred and presumed to be absolutely true. It is a primary article of faith among many feminists that women don't lie about rape, ever; they lack the dishonesty gene." Kaminer goes on to say that "the marriage of feminism and the recovery movement is arguably the most disturbing (and potentially influential) development in the feminist movement today." Even more disturbing perhaps is her conclusion that "only five years ago [Andrea] Dworkin and [Catharine] McKinnon were leaders of a feminist fringe. Today, owing partly to the excesses of multiculturalism and the exaltation of victimization, they're leaders in the feminist mainstream."

"The U.S. appears to be witnessing its third great wave of hysteria," writes Richard Gardner, professor of child psychiatry at Columbia University, in *The Wall Street Journal,* citing the Salem witch trials and the McCarthy hearings as the other two. "Our current hysteria, which began in the early 1980s, is by far the worst with regard to the number of lives that have been destroyed and the families that have disintegrated."

The "repressed memory" controversy has become so big that it was featured in a *Time* magazine cover story ("Is Freud Dead?" 29 November 1993). "If penis envy made us look dumb, this will make us look totally gullible," says Paul McHugh, chair of the psychiatry department at Johns Hopkins University. "This is the biggest story in psychiatry in a decade. It is a disaster for orthodox psychotherapists who are doing good work." Says Richard Ofshe, social psychologist at the University of California, Berkeley, "Recovered-memory therapy will come to be recognized as the quackery of the 20th century."

Other articles and comments fill my files with the passing months. But the comfort and vindication I derive from them is hollow and short-lived. My children will probably never read a word of these pieces. I continue to grieve, sometimes quietly, sometimes with friends, about the damage that has been done.

Some of my friends have urged me to initiate a lawsuit against the therapist or therapists who have influenced my daughter to bring up these false memories of abuse, and I consider it. But will a lawsuit, I ask myself, bring my children back? Others caution that a lawsuit or any other kind of pursuit will only alienate my children from me further.

Meanwhile, Joanne and I have gotten a divorce — but are on the friendliest terms we've been on for over three years. We have a deep hurt and a sense of injustice in common, and we've had several long talks about our children in the past year. Joanne tells me that she has spent weekends alone looking at slides of the children when they were small. "Looking for the truth, I suppose," she says.

I have not seen Kristin in five years, Troy in four and a half. I've sent them letters — to the only addresses Joanne has for them — begging for some kind of reconciliation. I've sent gifts on their birthdays. There have been no replies to the letters, and the gifts have come back with no acknowledgment and no return address.

About nine months ago, Joanne wrote Kristin and Troy telling them to remove their belongings from the house, that she didn't want to see or hear from them until they were ready to talk about healing. While she was gone on vacation, they came and took all the personal stuff they wanted, plus they removed *all* the family photo albums and childhood memorabilia. Both have moved without leaving forwarding addresses, and both have unlisted phone numbers. They have cut off all contact. They are unreachable.

Joanne can't decide whether she's more devastated or furious. But her anger is definitely directed toward them; she has too much at stake in the psychotherapeutic community to rage against it. I have sent her copies of the false-memory articles and personal narratives that I have on file, but she lets me know that she doesn't really want to read them or hear about it. I tell her that I have contacted the False Memory Syndrome Foundation for assistance and information, but still she is uninterested. I have become frustrated by her unwillingness to acknowledge the culpability of the psychotherapeutic community.

Regarding my children, I now have only a sense of loss. I realize that Kristin and Troy have the pain of losing their parents just as profoundly as Joanne and I have the pain of losing our children. My rage is all toward the practice of "recovered-memory therapy." My children have been brainwashed by their so-called mental health care providers, a group with not only an agenda but, like pastors and priests, the power to inflict pain on impressionable people. Some of them have clearly seized on and exploited Kristin's depression and vulnerability for their own agenda and financial gain. I believe that Kristin and Troy have been hurt just as surely by these "health care professionals" as they would have been by recruitment into some radical and irrational cult. They have been led into some Waco or Jonestown of the mind.

*   *   *

In my dreams these days, or sometimes just riding in the car, with no warning, I get glimpses of Kristin as a little girl again. She's learning to read and she gets up close to my face with her sweet round cheeks and strawberry-blond curls and painstakingly mispronounces a new word. Or I see her triumphant and terrified face on her first solo bike trip around the block, me running behind, my hand at the ready, giggling. How she'd put her hand in mine and lean her head on my shoulder, all trusting. How she'd proudly tell her little friends, "That's my big daddy."

Remembering it, I laugh and cry all at once. My heart aches for that little girl . . . and for the woman she's become.

God, I want my children back. I miss them terribly.

CHAPTER 2

Recovered Memory Therapy

We must not be led astray by initial denials. If we keep firmly to what we have inferred, we shall in the end conquer every resistance by emphasizing the unshakeable nature of our convictions.

— *Sigmund Freud*

To treat for repressed memory without any attempt at external validation is malpractice, pure and simple.

— *Paul McHugh*

Stories remarkably similar to the narrative in the preceding chapter have been repeated many thousands of times throughout North America in the past several years. Adult women between college age and middle age have been retrieving, with the help of various psychotherapeutic techniques, memories of early childhood sexual abuse, memories they had never known they had of abuse they had never before suspected. Psychotherapy and a bulging shelf of incest recovery books have "facilitated" these women's newfound memories, and many of them in turn have denounced and rejected for life the alleged perpetrators of their early sexual abuse — usually their fathers (sometimes their mothers), grandfathers, uncles, or other family members.

Therapy based on the recovery of these "repressed memories of childhood sexual abuse" has precipitated a pitched battle within psychotherapeutic circles at the close of the twentieth century. A line is drawn in the sand: ranged on one side is a large cadre of therapists, from psychiatrists and highly educated psychologists to lay counselors and self-help gurus, from radical feminist social workers to pastors interested in family systems, all of whom claim to be helping adults recover their repressed memories of childhood sexual abuse and many of whom explore such ostensibly associated phenomena as multiple personality disorder and satanic ritual abuse. The therapists contend that uncovering these "memories" is the only way the victims will heal the malaise and depression that besets them.

On the other side of the line are the critics of recovered memory therapy (RMT), including psychiatrists, social scientists, and memory experts, as well as falsely accused family members and "retractors" (those who have gone through RMT, experienced its perils, and subsequently rejected it). They believe that RMT therapists are implanting in their clients memories of abuse that never actually took place, and they are attempting to warn the world of the damage RMT is doing in the name of treating emotional distress. They call it "false memory syndrome," and they sometimes compare it to a virus infecting the mental health care system of North America.

The problems resulting from the RMT controversy have reached epic proportions. It is a phenomenon that has not only rent the psychotherapeutic community but appears to have ramifications for our political and religious life as well. Even as the numbers swell of those adult women who, during therapy, report memories of abuse by their parents while they were growing up, the number of parents who say they have been falsely accused and the number of former patients who say they were misled by psychotherapy to falsely accuse their parents are also mounting. The False Memory Syndrome Foundation, founded in the spring of 1992 by parents claiming to have been falsely accused of sexual abuse by adult children in RMT, had by the spring of 1997 been contacted by 20,000 affected families. More than 400 accusing children have recanted earlier accusations. Accused parents have been involved in some 700 civil trials; more than 200 parents and children have initiated suits against therapists for malpractice. About 100 people have been incarcerated, most of them in a wave of hysterical prosecutions of daycare facility personnel during the late eighties; more than half of them are still in prison.[1]

I want to be clear at the outset that the issue we are looking at here

---

1. These figures were supplied in April 1997 by the False Memory Syndrome Foundation, 3401 Market St., Suite 130, Philadelphia, Pa. 19104-3315.

is not child abuse per se. I trust that any right-thinking individual in our culture would readily agree that the mistreatment, neglect, and active abuse — especially sexual abuse — of children is one of the most heinous of crimes. I further trust that few people can any longer escape an awareness that children are in fact being abused in our nation in substantial numbers. Our news media all too frequently report the sickening stories — Elisa Izquierdo, left by New York's social services with a drug-addicted mother who eventually smashed her against a wall and killed her, or Polly Klaas, abducted by a sociopath who sexually violated her before killing her. I do not wish in any way to overlook or underestimate the amount of real child abuse that occurs in this country, its horror, or its consequences for the children subjected to it or for society as a whole. Indeed, I know the evidence indicates that children are abused in far greater numbers than many — psychological professionals included — were prepared to say in the past. But, again, my focus in this book is not on the reality of child abuse in our society but rather on the ability of a therapeutic technique to uncover genuine instances of such abuse years after it is presumed to have occurred. The question is whether RMT provides a reliable means of identifying child molesters. Is it, as its proponents claim, a means for bringing peace and resolution into the lives of victims of abuse, or is it, as its critics claim, a means for inflicting its own kind of abuse on individuals and their families?

Because this issue involves the sexual abuse of children, it is quite natural that it should have become emotionally charged. It is a subject that seems to stir the passions, one way or the other, of nearly everyone who is drawn into it. Many people — mental health professionals and laypeople alike — are stung by their failure in the past to recognize the significance of the child abuse problem. They are now making a greater effort to hear the cries of the children, and many are convinced that the accusations of RMT patients must all be true. At the very least, they feel obligated to give them the benefit of the doubt. Other professionals see dangers in this new sensitivity. Clinical psychologist Michael Yapko has suggested that

> some therapists unquestioningly accept even the vaguest allegations of abuse, based on the most ephemeral dreams, impressionistic flashbacks, or suddenly revived but indistinct memories that have presumably been completely repressed for twenty or thirty years. . . . There is disturbing evidence that some therapists unintentionally insinuate into the minds of their clients memories of abuse that never happened. Therapists often find this hard to believe, because they underestimate the potent influence they can wield in the lives of clients and they certainly don't *feel* powerful,

20

pointing out that it is excruciatingly difficult to get their clients to make even the most meager changes.[2]

Growing numbers of accused parents, supported by growing numbers of researchers and professionals like Yapko, contend that the "memories" uncovered in RMT sessions are false and that the results of giving them the benefit of the doubt can be disastrous. Surveys conducted by critics of RMT indicate that *100 percent* of those claiming childhood abuse on the basis of repressed memories have either undergone RMT, been in a "survivors' group," or read one of the manuals of the recovered memory movement such as *The Courage to Heal.* The stakes of the debate are very high: personal anguish, shattered families, imprisonment. How valid are the claims of the accusers? What is RMT all about?

What Is Repressed Memory?

RMT has become the stuff of TV talk shows, movies, feature articles, and books. But where did this therapeutic technique originate? Does it have ties to established psychological practice, or is it an anomaly?

Few doubt that childhood sexual abuse was underreported before the 1970s or that it still is a problem today. Indeed, many North Americans have dark and humiliating memories of being abused, recollections that have stuck with them through childhood and adulthood. But, unlike the adults who have lived silently for years with such memories, most people who "recover" repressed memories with the help of RMT first entered therapy with no specific recollections of having been abused as children. Sometimes women coming in for psychological treatment (the overwhelming majority of RMT clients are women) have only an indistinct and confused feeling that something bad may have happened to them. Many are simply looking for help in dealing with depression, relationship problems, eating disorders, or an ill-defined anxiety. Some of those seeking help have read that the symptoms they exhibit may be signs of past child abuse and they want a therapist to confirm or dismiss the possibility. Few RMT therapists will fail to confirm such patients' suspicions; most are convinced that childhood sexual abuse is fairly common and that memories of such abuse are often repressed. Many interpret an individual's suspicion of abuse as a strong indication that such abuse did indeed take place.

2. Yapko, "The Seduction of Memory," *Networker,* September/October 1993, p. 33.

During therapy, under the influence of a number of therapeutic techniques, patients typically begin to "recall" vividly detailed encounters with abusers. Many are troubled by the fact that these new memories seem incompatible with their previous recollections of a happy or at least relatively benign childhood. Some note that the new memories seem to be qualitatively different from other memories in various ways. RMT therapists respond to these concerns with assurances that such reactions are common among victims of child abuse and that this is all in keeping with the nature of repressed memory. Encouraged to delve deeper into their subconscious, many patients begin to recall increasingly bizarre and horrific kinds of molestation and abuse — being forced to bear their father's babies, to sacrifice those infants in satanic rituals, to drink the blood of animals and babies, and the like. In such cases, growing numbers of therapists conclude that their patients are suffering from multiple personality disorder.

How credible are these recovered memories and these diagnoses? Is it really possible that a child could be subjected to repeated abuse and other outrageous practices and then remain completely unaware of it for years until therapy brings it back to the surface? RMT therapists believe that it is not only possible but common.

Proponents of RMT hold that when the mind — especially a young child's vulnerable mind — encounters a trauma too difficult to process, it develops a long-term coping strategy usually identified in the public debate as *repression:* it stuffs all memories of that frightful and threatening event down into some deep cellar of the unconscious, where it can linger intact for years or even decades until some experience, stimulus, or process calls it up. They believe that in some extreme cases, patients manage to repress memories of sexual abuse that occurred over a period of many years. They believe that even though these repressed memories remain quite invisible to the conscious mind, they nonetheless manage to invade the victim's life by way of the unconscious, producing various irrational or self-destructive behaviors. This is what leads the victim to seek out therapy.

Concerning the mechanism of repressed memory, Judith Alpert, professor of applied psychology at New York University says, "There is absolutely no question that some people have repressed some memories of early abuse that are just too painful to remember. In their 20s and 30s some event triggers early memories, and slowly they return. The event has been so overwhelming that the little girl who is being abused can't tolerate to be there in the moment so she leaves her body, dissociates, as if she is up on a bookshelf looking down on the little girl who is being abused. Over time, she pushes it deep down because she can't integrate the experience."[3] Along the same lines, Laura Davis asserts that "children actually forget the abuse happened; they store it away in a part of themselves that isn't available to their conscious minds. . . . Then ten or twenty years later, these repressed childhood memories surface, often creating havoc in their lives. . . . The process of recovering traumatic memories years after the original trauma is a well-documented psychological phenomenon."[4] Judith Lewis Herman, a nationally known practitioner of RMT affiliated with Harvard Medical School, outlines different degrees of repressed memory. Some adult women enter therapy with total and continuous memory of their abuse, she says; some have partial recollection and what she calls "delayed understanding" of their experiences; others have "profound amnesia" of the abuse. "There's something about traumatic memory," Herman asserts, "that seems to be both stored and retrieved abnormally, so that memories often intrude when they're not wanted, and are not accessible when you try to get them. That's the phenomenon. I think that's indisputable."[5]

But a majority of psychotherapists and experts in the workings of the mind are not at all convinced that the phenomenon of repressed memory is indisputable. Nor do memory researchers agree with Davis that the recovery of repressed memories is a well-documented phenomenon. And there is no published evidence to substantiate RMT therapists' claims that most incest survivors experience partial or full amnesia about the sexual trauma itself.

Many research psychologists are critical of the concept of repression in general, partly because it is associated with Freud, and much of Freudian theory is in disrepute today. Psychotherapists tend to give more credence to the possibility that memories of isolated incidents of trauma can be repressed and later recovered, but most would classify this as a very rare phenomenon. There is considerably less support outside the RMT community for the concept of "massive repression," however — that is, the repression of trauma experienced over long periods of time. Elizabeth Loftus, professor of psychology and adjunct professor of law at the University of Washington and leading memory researcher, says, "If repression is the avoidance in your conscious awareness of unpleasant experiences that come back to you, yes, I believe in repression. But if it is a blocking out of an endless stream of traumas that occur over and over

---

3. Alpert, quoted by Leon Jaroff in "Lies of the Mind," *Time*, 29 November 1993, p. 55.

4. Davis, *Allies in Healing: When the Person You Love Was Sexually Abused as a Child* (New York: HarperPerennial, 1991), p. 115.

5. Herman, quoted by Ellen K. Coughlin in "Recollections of Childhood Abuse," *Chronicle of Higher Education*, 27 January 1995, p. A8.

that leave a person with absolutely no awareness that these things happen, that make them behave in destructive ways and re-emerge decades later in some reliable form, I don't see any evidence for it. It flies in the face of everything we know about memory."[6] Researchers have been unable to locate any mechanism by which memories of dramatic and prolonged events such as long-term abuse could remain buried for decades and then abruptly pop into consciousness under the right circumstances. David S. Holmes of the University of Kansas has scrutinized sixty years of attempts to prove the existence of repression and has concluded that the concept has never been validated by experimental research: "Not only do these findings fail to provide support for the concept of repression, but they are the opposite to what would be predicted on the basis of repression."[7] The evidence suggests that people who experience traumatic events of the sort ostensibly uncovered in RMT therapy seldom forget them. Most victims of childhood abuse *never* forget the molestation, though fear or shame leads many to remain silent about the assaults for years or whole lifetimes. Studies of concentration camp survivors similarly indicate that most of them never forget the horrors. A small percentage of survivors manages to bury the memories — but not in a manner that could be classified as repression, because there is no evidence that the memories are buried intact or could in any way be effectively resurrected.

While there is virtually no support for the existence of massive repression outside the RMT community, proponents of RMT such as Ellen Bass, Laura Davis, Wendy Maltz, E. Sue Blume, Beverly Engel, and Renee Fredrickson contend that it is comparatively common.[8] Blume, for example, has said that it "is not unlikely that *more than half of all women* are survivors of childhood sexual trauma."[9] And some RMT proponents further claim that as many as 70 percent of those who have been abused have no conscious awareness of their childhood abuse.

6. Loftus, quoted by Leon Jaroff in "Lies of the Mind," p. 56.

7. Holmes, "The Evidence for Repression: An Examination of Sixty Years of Research," in Jerome Singer, *Repression and Dissociation* (Chicago: University of Chicago Press, 1990), p. 86.

8. Some of the more prominent books by RMT proponents are Ellen Bass and Laura Davis's *The Courage to Heal*, 3d ed. (New York: HarperPerennial, 1994), E. Sue Blume's *Secret Survivors: Uncovering Incest and Its After Effects in Women* (New York: Ballantine, 1991), Wendy Maltz's *The Sexual Healing Journey: A Guide for Survivors of Sexual Abuse* (New York: HarperCollins, 1992), Renee Fredrickson's *Repressed Memories: A Journey to Recovery from Sexual Abuse* (New York: Simon & Schuster, 1992), Beverly Engel's *Divorcing a Parent: Free Yourself from the Past and Live the Life You've Always Wanted* (New York: Fawcett, 1991), and Susan Forward and Craig Buck's *Toxic Parents: Overcoming Their Hurtful Legacy and Reclaiming Your Life* (New York: Bantam Books, 1989).

9. Blume, *Secret Survivors*, p. xxii.

In response to critics who question such numbers, many proponents of RMT cite a study conducted by Linda Meyer Williams of 129 women who had documented histories of sex abuse. Williams interviewed the women seventeen years after they had received hospital treatment for sexual assault in childhood. Of the 129 women interviewed, 38 percent said that they did not remember the instance of abuse that they had reported at the time of their initial treatment.[10] RMT proponents view this as compelling evidence that repression does occur in cases of childhood sexual abuse. But scholars have been quick to point out that such a conclusion cannot be safely drawn from the data. For one thing, Williams asked the respondents only about the one specific instance of abuse for which they had received treatment seventeen years earlier. Many of the women had simply forgotten that particular incident, although they had no trouble remembering a general pattern of abuse during childhood and so could not really be said to have *repressed* the memory as such. Only 12 percent of the women in the study said that they could not remember any abuse in childhood. Of that number, several were younger than five at the time of the treatment; most memory experts agree that most people have no reliable memories of things that happened to them before the age of five. Furthermore, Williams interviewed her subjects only once. When Donna Della Femina conducted a similar study, she interviewed her subjects twice and found that of those who said in the first interview that they had no memory of the previously documented abuse, 100 percent acknowledged in the second interview that they had not actually forgotten it but simply had not wanted to talk about it for some reason — they wanted to forget it and get on with their lives, they wanted to avoid hurting their parents, or the like.[11]

But if clients of RMT are not recovering repressed memories, what are they experiencing, and why do they come to be so convinced that they were abused as children? The answer appears to lie in the nature of memory.

What Is Memory?

We tend to think of memory as a more or less reliable mental recording of our experiences. Plato likened the mind to a wax tablet, the means by which

10. See Williams, "Recovered Memories of Abuse in Women with Documented Child Sexual Victimization Histories," *Journal of Traumatic Stress* 8 (1995): 649-73.

11. See Femina et al., "Child Abuse: Adolescent Records vs. Adult Recall," *Child Abuse and Neglect* 4 (1990): 227-31. See also Terence Campbell, "Response to Williams Study," *FMS [False Memory Syndrome] Foundation Newsletter* 3 (February 1994): 3-4; and Mark Pendergrast, *Victims of Memory*, 2d ed. (Hinesburg, VT: Upper Access, 1996), p. 86.

his culture recorded ideas for subsequent dissemination. Later ancient cultures compared the mind to a scroll. During the Industrial Revolution, the brain was thought of as a kind of machine and then later on as a kind of telephone switchboard. Freud, for his part, compared memory to a phonograph record on which was flawlessly recorded one's early and subconscious life. Later still, the model became a motion picture camera, a tape recorder, and a videocassette recorder. Today the reigning metaphor is the computer, precisely storing a host of facts and events for subsequent retrieval.

All of these models reflect the notion that human memory records events in an accurate and detailed fashion. But researchers tell us that this is a popular misconception. No one pretends to know exactly how human memory works, but it has at least become clear that it doesn't work like a mechanical recording device, preserving objectively accurate images of events. "The process is much more constructive," notes Elizabeth Loftus, arguably the country's leading memory researcher. "What we do when we remember is take bits and pieces of experiences, combine them together, and then essentially construct memory." Moreover, "we recast memories over and over again; otherwise, they deteriorate or disappear altogether." Memories fade unless we keep them alive by turning them over in our heads every so often — and every time we do that, we change them in subtle ways by adding new associations from our present experience and ways of thinking.

The findings of memory experts, notes Carol Tavris, support what poets and novelists have always known — "that memory is not a fixed thing, with its own special place or file drawer in the brain. . . . A 'memory' consists of fragments of the event, subsequent discussions and readings, other people's recollections and suggestions, and, perhaps most of all, present beliefs about the past." In addition, the brain never records every detail of any given experience; it captures only fragments, and in order to make sense of the recorded fragments, our memories automatically fill in gaps with assumptions about what was likely to have happened. In this way, memory becomes an interpretive process. "For an event to make it into long-term storage," says Tavris, "a person has to perceive it, encode it and *rehearse* it — tell about it — or it decays."[12] This process of interpretation and augmentation can help to produce false recollections as well as preserve genuine memories. If we go on a search for fragments of memory that we are told must exist — such as memories of abuse in childhood — we will

12. Tavris, "Beware the Incest-Survivor Machine," *New York Times Book Review*, 3 January 1993, p. 16.

likely begin by assembling fragments of genuine childhood memory and then throw into this mix ideas about abuse encountered in media reports, in the therapeutic context, and other sources. A continuing rehearsal of this mix of fragments can forge the disparate fragments into an apparently seamless whole, a narrative that over time comes to feel as real as any other childhood memory.

This is not easy for most people to accept. We all rely on our memories, and most of us feel that they serve us well. We can recall special events in our past with considerable clarity and are confident that these recollections are accurate. We share memories with others who experienced the same event, and we certainly seem to remember the same thing. But most of us are also familiar with the way in which people will correct one another as they recall common events — "No, that happened on Bob's birthday, not Susan's"; "No, it had to be 1973, not 1975, because Aunt Edna was still alive"; and so on. Research has shown that neither the vividness with which we recall details nor our confidence in the accuracy of our memories is necessarily related to their factual accuracy. As John Kihlstrom, a psychologist at the University of Arizona, says, "You just don't know what the truth is about something that may have happened decades ago. . . . Everything we know about memory of events says it is highly susceptible to reinvention."[13]

When the space shuttle *Challenger* exploded in 1986, Ulric Neisser and Nicole Harsch of Emory University asked forty-four students to record how and where they heard about the accident and to describe their emotional response to the news. A little more than two and a half years later, the researchers asked the same students the same questions. Most of the students described their memories of the event as "vivid," and yet not one of their recollections completely matched their original response, and more than a third of them were, in Neisser's words, "wildly inaccurate." But even more surprising than the significant changes in the details of their narratives was the subjects' confidence in their two-and-a-half-year-old memories. Many were astonished by what they had written down the day after the actual explosion and insisted that their present memory was correct, even when it was contradicted by the written record sitting in front of them. "This is my handwriting, so it must be right," said one student, "but I still remember everything happening the way I just told you. I can't

---

13. Kihlstrom, quoted by Daniel Goleman in "Childhood Trauma: Memory or Invention?" *New York Times*, 21 July 1992, pp. B5-B6. Kihlstrom had more to say along these lines in an unpublished paper entitled "The Recovery of Memory in the Laboratory and Clinic" written in April 1993.

help it." They simply could not believe that their new memories were mistaken. "As far as we can tell," Neisser concluded, "the original memories are just gone."[14]

Other studies have also looked into the ways in which our memories tend to change over time. Researcher Greg Markus interviewed about 1,700 high school seniors on cultural and political issues in 1973. Then in 1982 he reinterviewed the respondents and asked them to indicate how they had felt and responded in 1973. The results were striking: the subjects' 1982 recall of their 1973 attitudes was much more closely related to their attitudes in 1982 than to the attitudes they had actually expressed in 1973. "Retrospecting, they believed that their attitudes nine years earlier were very close to their current ones, much closer than they in fact were. This bias was so strong that an equation set up to predict subjects' recall of their 1973 attitudes gives almost all weight to their 1982 attitudes and virtually none at all to the attitudes they actually expressed in 1973 (with the important exception of their overall liberal versus conservative ratings)."[15]

Memory researchers refer to this phenomenon as "retrospective bias." Robin Dawes, a professor of psychology at Carnegie-Mellon University, says, "While memory from our experience is introspectively a process of 'dredging up' *what actually happened,* it is to a large extent determined by our current beliefs and feelings. This principle has been well established both in the psychological laboratory and in surveys. What we have at the time of recall is, after all, only our current state, which includes fragments ("memory traces") of our past experience; these fragments are biased by what we now believe (or feel) is true to an extent much greater than we know consciously."[16]

Our recall of our past is often organized in ways that "make sense" of the present — thus reinforcing our belief in the conclusions we have reached about how the past has determined the present. We quite literally "make up stories" about our lives, Dawes says, and "the fit between our memories and the stories enhances our belief in them. Often, however, it is the story that creates the memory, rather than vice versa." If we are invested in our current beliefs and perceptions, our memories will tend to suggest that they have not changed much over time, as the Markus study

14. Neisser and Harsch, "Phantom Flashbulbs: False Recollections of Hearing the News about Challenger," in *Affect and Accuracy in Recall: Studies in "Flashbulb" Memories,* ed. E. Winograd and Ulric Neisser (New York: Cambridge University Press, 1992), pp. 9-31.

15. Markus, quoted by Robin Dawes in "Biases of Retrospection," *Issues in Child Abuse Accusations* 1 (1989): 25.

16. Dawes, "Biases of Retrospection," p. 25.

indicates. If we are invested in a belief that we have changed significantly over time, our memories will tend to substantiate this perception regardless of the significance of the change. If we think we have changed for the better, for example, we will tend to remember the past (or our behavior or situation in the past) as worse than it was. "Certainly there have been times before a religious or psychiatric conversion," says Dawes, "when the individual was badly off (we all are at times), and memories of those times persist; recall can be organized around the traces of these memories. . . . Experimental evidence supports the contention that when we believe a change has occurred, we are apt to distort the past in the direction compatible with the change."[17]

Our memory is also distorted by present mood. It has been established experimentally that human memory of incidents experienced in a particular mood is more easily brought back by the re-creation of that mood. So our recall of events that occurred when we were in a bad mood — usually negative events — is facilitated by a current bad mood, and vice versa for good moods. One study published in 1987 focused on the relationship between current mood states and memory. Researchers examined two thousand people over a three-year period, classifying the subjects as depressives, remitted depressives, nondepressives, and predepressives. The results were consistent with the hypothesis that recollections of one's parents as rejecting and unloving are strongly influenced by current moods. "Whereas the currently depressed subjects recalled their parents as having been more rejecting and as having used more negative controls, the remitted depressives did not differ from the never depressed control group in their recall of parental behavior. Similarly, the subjects who were about to become depressed shortly after the initial testing did not differ from the control group in their recollections of the degree to which their parents used negative control methods."[18]

Thus, research indicates that how we feel about ourselves as adults colors the way we remember our past, including our childhood. This supports the commonsense notion that if we are confident and self-assured adults, we will tend to have a positive and cheerful view of our childhood, and if we feel emotionally distressed as adults, we will tend to have more negative recollections of childhood. It is important to note here that this principle does not provide any support for concluding that people who are emotionally distressed as adults necessarily had distressing childhoods. It

17. Dawes, "Biases of Retrospection," p. 26.
18. Dawes, "Biases of Retrospection," p. 27.

suggests only that distressed adults are inclined to *perceive* their childhoods as having been distressing.

Freud and Memories of Childhood Sexual Abuse

Proponents of RMT have cited the early writings of Freud in support of their beliefs. Especially relevant in this regard is his famous paper "The Etiology of Hysteria," in which he introduced his "seduction theory." Doctors had long been seeking the source of "hysteria" (a loosely defined psychological affliction encompassing a host of different symptoms almost always suffered by women). Addressing a conference of the Society for Psychiatry and Neurology in Vienna in 1896, Freud made the provocative assertion that "at the bottom of every case of hysteria there are *one or more occurrences of premature sexual experience.*"[19] He based this conclusion on a study of eighteen women whom he had diagnosed as suffering from hysteria. He reported that, using various techniques, he had managed to elicit memories of childhood sexual abuse from all eighteen of the subjects, and on the basis of this evidence he argued that all neuroses could be traced to forgotten infantile sexual trauma at the hands of older men, usually fathers. Privately he went on to assert that "in all cases, the *father,* not excluding my own, had to be accused of being perverse."[20]

Freud's Vienna contemporaries, most of whom characterized the "recollections" of hysterics as lies or fantasies, rejected his new theory. Richard von Krafft-Ebing, the august presider over the conference, dismissed Freud's ideas as "a scientific fairy tale." The pioneer of psychoanalysis was humiliated, and before long he, too, rejected his seduction theory on the grounds that it "broke down under its own improbability and the patients' contradictory stories."[21]

Freud apparently had reasons besides the opinions of his colleagues for backing away from his commitment to the seduction theory. Lawrence Wright notes that Freud's father died just a few months after he delivered his conference paper, and in his grief he realized that "it was absurd to classify this lighthearted sage as a child molester, even though his [Freud's]

19. Freud, "The Etiology of Hysteria," quoted by Richard Ofshe and Ethan Watters in *Making Monsters: False Memories, Psychotherapy, and Sexual Hysteria* (New York: Scribner's, 1994), p. 291.

20. Freud, *The Complete Letters of Sigmund Freud to Wilhelm Fliess, 1887-1904,* ed. Jeffrey Moussaieff Masson (Cambridge: Belknap Press, 1985), pp. 212-13.

21. Ofshe and Watters, *Making Monsters,* p. 290.

own siblings showed traces of hysteria. His beloved theory was at war with his sense of reality. In order to account for the common diagnosis of hysteria, child abuse would have to be practically universal, since only a portion of the cases would give rise to neurotic illness. 'Such widespread perversion against children is scarcely probable,' he realized."[22]

As he reconsidered his position, Freud began to take another look at his patients' accounts of their early abuse. In a letter to his friend Wilhelm Fliess, Freud wrote that one of his patients had described how the devil had pricked pins into her fingers and put a piece of candy on each drop of blood. "What would you say," Freud asked Fliess, "if I told you that my brand-new theory of the early etiology of hysteria was already well known and had been published a hundred times over, though several centuries ago?" Referring to the witch trials of Europe — and himself no believer in witches — Freud wondered, "Why did the devil who took possession of the poor things invariably abuse them sexually and in a loathsome manner? Why are their confessions under torture so like the communications made by my patients in psychological treatment?" As Wright puts it, "He had come to the same juncture that the profession he created would confront again a century later."[23]

In his small autobiography more than a quarter century later, Freud wrote,

> I must mention an error into which I fell for a while and which might well have had fatal consequences for the whole of my work. Under the pressure of the technical procedure which I used at the time, the majority of my patients reproduced from their childhood scenes in which they were sexually seduced by some grown-up person. With female patients the part of seducer was almost always assigned to their father. I believed these stories, and consequently supposed that I had discovered the root of the subsequent neurosis in these experiences of sexual seduction in childhood. My confidence was strengthened by a few cases in which relations of this kind with a father, uncle, or elder brother had continued up to an age at which memory was to be trusted. If the reader feels inclined to shake his head at my credulity, I cannot altogether blame him. . . . When, however, I was at last obliged to recognize that these scenes of seduction had never taken place, and that they were only fantasies which my patients had made up or which I myself had perhaps forced upon them, I was for some time completely at a loss. . . . When

22. Wright, *Remembering Satan* (New York: Vintage Books, 1995), p. 158.
23. Wright, *Remembering Satan*, p. 158.

I had pulled myself together, I was able to draw the right conclusions from my discovery: namely, that the neurotic symptoms were not related directly to actual events but to fantasies embodying wishes, and that as far as the neurosis was concerned psychical reality was of more importance than material reality. I do not believe even now that I forced the seduction-fantasies upon my patients, that I "suggested" them. I had in fact stumbled for the first time upon the *Oedipus complex,* which was later to assume such an overwhelming importance, but which I did not recognize as yet in its disguise of fantasy. . . . When the mistake had been cleared up, the path to the study of the sexual life of children lay open.[24]

He describes here the great turning point in his thinking and in the psychoanalytic movement he pioneered: the shift from thinking that hysteria grew out of real traumatic childhood sexual abuse to thinking that it grew out of repressed juvenile desires for sexual experiences with adults, usually their parents.

Thus, Freud's mature understanding of repression differs significantly from the concept of repressed memory common among proponents of RMT. As Wright explains,

Freud compared the function of repression to that of a watchman who stands guard between the large entrance hall of the unconscious mind and the small drawing room in which consciousness resides. The watchman is a censor, examining mental impulses to determine whether they will be allowed to enter further. "If they have already pushed their way forward to the threshold and have been turned back by the watchman, then they are inadmissible to consciousness; we speak of them as *repressed,*" Freud wrote. Such an impulse, for instance, might be the desire of a young girl for her father. The watchman would certainly frown on that; and although the image would be pushed back into the entrance hall, that doesn't mean that it is banished forever. Years, even decades, later, the forbidden desire might return, but this time in a clever and frightening disguise. . . . The shameful sexual desire of the young girl for her father is reexperienced as her father's desire for her; her fantasy of sexual union is recast as a remembered assault.[25]

Quite predictably, these later views are not popular with today's proponents of RMT. They are inclined to argue that Freud had it right

24. Freud, quoted by Wright in *Remembering Satan,* pp. 159-60.
25. Wright, *Remembering Satan,* pp. 160-161.

the first time, and some accuse him of having caved in to his mostly male professional colleagues who, they claim, saw in the theory an indictment of respectable family men, the good burghers of Vienna. In a book entitled *Assault on Truth*, Jeffrey Moussaieff Masson criticizes Freud at length on this point, arguing that by abandoning the seduction theory, Freud effectively buried the issue of child abuse for another three-quarters of a century.

But apologists for Freud's early views have to contend with some formidable evidence against their position. They may be operating on the assumption that Freud was a passive recipient of his patients' accounts of childhood abuse, but in fact Freud himself acknowledged having exerted considerable pressure on them to yield the stories and having encountered the "greatest reluctance" on their part in response to his coercion. "Before they come for analysis the patients know nothing about these scenes. . . . Patients are indignant as a rule if we warn them that such scenes are going to emerge. Only the strongest compulsion of the treatment can induce them to embark on a reproduction of them."[26] Elsewhere he says, "We must not be led astray by initial denials. If we keep firmly to what we have inferred, we shall in the end conquer every resistance by emphasizing the unshakeable nature of our convictions. . . . Moreover, the idea that one might, by one's insistence, cause a patient who is psychically normal to accuse himself falsely of sexual misdemeanors — such an idea may safely be disregarded as an imaginary danger."[27]

Thus, by Freud's own admission, he worked against the "greatest reluctance" of his patients, told them ahead of time what he was expecting, and used "most energetic pressure" to overcome "enormous resistance" on their part. His own description of his therapeutic techniques suggests that they were brutal and unyielding. And he later admitted his willingness to ignore patients' testimony that what they were visualizing did not feel like memory. Bluntly put, he bullied his patients into confirming the views he already held. Proponents of RMT have demonstrated an inclination to adopt not only Freud's early views but also the questionable techniques he used to substantiate those views.

26. Freud, *Standard Edition of the Complete Psychological Works of Sigmund Freud*, 24 vols., ed. James Strachey (London: Hogarth Press, 1953-1974), 3:204.

27. Freud, *Standard Edition*, 3:269. He also states that "one only succeeds in awakening the psychical trace of a precocious sexual event under the most energetic pressure of the analytical procedure, and against an enormous resistance" (*Standard Edition*, 3:153).

Symptoms of Repression

At about the same time Freud was promulgating his initial theory about the seduction of young girls, another pioneer in sexual theory was introducing *self*-abuse hysteria in North America. J. P. Kellogg, M.D., the cereal tycoon, dedicated himself to stamping out the great evil of masturbation. He lectured around the country and wrote several manuals for parents outlining the signs that their children might be masturbating. Among the symptoms on Kellogg's list were

- general debility, including exhaustion
- sudden change in disposition
- lassitude, dislike for play, and lifelessness
- sleeplessness
- nightmares
- failure of mental capacity
- untrustworthiness
- daydreaming
- bashfulness
- unnatural boldness
- confusion of ideas
- capricious appetite
- unchastity of speech, including fondness for obscene stories.[28]

Subsequent generations, less concerned about the dire consequences of masturbation, have been able to take a more cool-headed look at the list of symptoms and recognize that it is broad enough to apply to just about every adolescent who ever drew a breath. It is worthless as a diagnostic tool because it does not discriminate: it casts a net so broad as to cover everyone. Furthermore, most of the symptoms clearly admit of many different causes.

Unfortunately, as John Money notes, "Kellogg's list of suspicious signs has been given a new lease on life currently by the professional detectives of sexual child-abuse."[29] Proponents of RMT have developed similarly long lists of symptoms. The authors of *The Courage to Heal* tell their readers

---

28. Cited by Ross Legrand, Hollida Wakefield, and Ralph Underwager, "Alleged Behavioral Indicators of Sexual Abuse," *Issues in Child Abuse Accusations* 1 (Spring 1990): 4.

29. Money, quoted by Legrand, Wakefield, and Underwager in "Alleged Behavioral Indicators of Sexual Abuse," p. 5.

that if they can answer yes to the following questions, they may well be repressing memories of childhood incest:

- Do you feel powerless, like a victim?
- Do you feel different from other people?
- Do you feel that there's something wrong with you deep down inside? That if people really knew you, they'd leave?
- Do you feel that you're bad, dirty, or ashamed?
- Do you feel unable to protect yourself in dangerous situations?
- Do you find it hard to trust your intuition?
- Do you have trouble feeling motivated?
- Are you often immobilized?
- Are you afraid to succeed?
- Do you feel you have to be perfect?
- Do you have a hard time nurturing and taking care of yourself?
- Do you use work or achievements to compensate for inadequate feelings in other parts of your life?
- Do you feel confused much of the time?
- Do you experience a wide range of emotions or just a few?
- Do you have trouble expressing your feelings?[30]

Like Kellogg's list, this one is general enough so that most people will be able to see themselves in it. Who doesn't feel powerless now and then? Who doesn't feel different from other people on occasion? Who doesn't have trouble feeling motivated from time to time? And it is even more likely that people seeking out therapeutic help for anxiety or depression will report the broadly defined fears and inadequacies touched on in the questions. As Carol Tavris says, "The same list could be used to identify oneself as someone who loves too much, someone who suffers from self-defeating personality disorder, or a mere human being in the late 20th century. The list is general enough to include everybody at least sometimes. Nobody doesn't fit it. . . . To read these handbooks is to learn that almost any problem you have may be an indicator of abuse."[31]

Renee Fredrickson offers another list of what she characterizes as "common" warning signals of the presence of repressed memories of childhood trauma:

---

30. Bass and Davis, *The Courage to Heal,* p. 39.
31. Tavris, "Beware the Incest-Survivor Machine," p. 1.

- I showed no interest in sex until I was in my twenties.
- I am preoccupied with thoughts about sex.
- I have had a period of sexual promiscuity in my life.
- I often have nightmares.
- I have difficulty falling asleep or staying asleep.
- I remember vividly one or more nightmares from my childhood.
- There are certain things I seem to have a strange attraction or affection for.
- I am scared to be alone or to leave my house.
- I hate going to the dentist more than most people, and I neglect my teeth.
- Certain foods or tastes frighten or nauseate me.
- I do not take good care of my body.
- I identify with abuse victims in the media and often stories of abuse make me want to cry.
- I space out or daydream.
- Other people seem to have childhood memories at an earlier age than I do.[32]

Once again, this list contains some fairly vague and generic characteristics ("I do not take good care of my body," "I space out or daydream"). It also broadens the net by including symptoms at opposite ends of a spectrum — both attraction to sex and avoidance of sex are counted as symptoms, for example. We see this same kind of reaching in two directions in the way RMT therapists talk about their clients' awareness of past abuse. On the one hand, Beverly Engel asserts, in a manner typical of those in the RMT community, that "if you have any suspicions at all, if you have any memory, no matter how vague, it probably really happened. It is far more likely that you are blocking the memories, denying it happened." On the other hand, Fredrickson asserts in an equally typical fashion that "the existence of profound disbelief [that one was abused as a child] is an indication that the memories are real."[33] Clients who say they have no memories of abuse and reject the diagnosis of incest survivor are said to be "in denial." In effect, all women who enter RMT can be assured that they fit the profile of an incest survivor, because both having and not having memories of the abuse count as symptoms that it occurred. As television celebrity Roseanne told

32. Fredrickson, *Repressed Memories: A Journey to Recovery from Sexual Abuse* (New York: Fireside/Parkside, 1992), pp. 48-51.

33. Fredrickson, *Repressed Memories*, p. 171.

Oprah Winfrey's national audience, "When someone asks you, 'Were you sexually abused as a child?' there are only two answers: one of them is 'Yes,' and one of them is 'I don't know.' You can't say 'No.'"

In addition to the broad lists of symptoms that have appeared in various publications, two specific complaints are increasingly being linked to childhood sexual abuse: eating disorders and panic attacks.

In 1992, two nationally recognized experts on eating disorders, Harrison Pope and James Hudson of Harvard Medical School, published the results of an extensive study showing that the incidence of past sexual abuse among people with eating disorders is no different from that in the general population.[34] Despite these findings, however, many RMT therapists continue to tell their clients that as many as 85 to 90 percent of adults suffering from bulimia, anorexia nervosa, and obesity were sexually abused as children. It is possible that the people who came up with these figures made a common error in reasoning. They may have determined that 90 percent of their clients with repressed memories of childhood abuse also had eating disorders and incorrectly reasoned that therefore 90 percent of people with eating disorders had repressed memories. This would be like hearing that 60 percent of people who die in traffic accidents were not wearing seat belts and concluding that 60 percent of all people who do not wear seat belts will wind up dying in a car crash. But whatever the source of the high correlation between eating disorders and repressed memories cited by the RMT community, the figures are increasingly being cited outside that community, in the two hundred or so eating disorder clinics in the United States. On the basis of this misinformation, therapists in these clinics are encouraging yet greater numbers of people to seek out additional therapy in search of repressed memories.

RMT therapists are also claiming a high correlation between panic disorder and repressed memories. The symptoms of panic attacks include inordinate sweating, rapid heartbeat, constricted throat, and the sensation of a heavy weight on one's chest. RMT literature characterizes these symptoms as "body memories" — instances of the body reproducing responses to past abuse after the conscious mind has repressed memories of the incidents. A constricted throat, for instance, is interpreted as a body memory of an assault involving oral sex. Studies of panic disorder indicate that nothing this simple is likely to cause the attacks. The symptoms are typically understood to be expressions of an individual's inability to deal

34. Pope and Hudson, "Is Childhood Sexual Abuse a Risk Factor for Bulimia Nervosa?" *American Journal of Psychiatry,* April 1992, p. 460.

adequately with accumulated mental, emotional, and physical stress, not reactions to traumatic experiences in the distant past.

Techniques of RMT

RMT therapists use a variety of techniques in their efforts to recover their clients' repressed memories, including "guided imagery," abreaction (reliving traumatic experiences), hypnosis, investigation of body memories, and the use of sodium amytal (the so-called truth serum). Renee Fredrickson has also advocated the use of dream interpretation and free association. With the exception of body memories (which are broadly dismissed outside of RMT circles as pseudoscience), these are all familiar and accepted tools in the larger therapeutic community. But critics charge that, given the way these techniques are typically employed in the context of RMT, they are far more likely to produce false memories than to recover genuine memories. Part of the problem is that many RMT therapists receive no formal training in the proper use of the techniques and hence may lack the critical skills to assess the validity of the "memories" that are recovered with their help. A larger problem is that most RMT therapists are ideologically predisposed to reject the possibility that these techniques could produce false memories, whatever the evidence to the contrary. They feel a moral obligation to "believe the victim," and they do not consider it credible that anyone can recover false memories of abuse. In essence, they repudiate the sort of critical objectivity that is essential to the proper use of the various techniques.

Dream Analysis

People have been fascinated with the significance of dreams throughout human history. The ancient Egyptians were very serious about interpreting dreams, as were both the Hebrews and early Christians of the Bible. Dream analysis has been a staple of many kinds of psychotherapy since Freud.

There is no real consensus about the precise significance of dreams, although many theorists maintain that there is a continuity between our waking life and dreaming life, that in one way or another we tend to process or deal in our dreams with things that concern or preoccupy us when we are awake. This being the case, it would not be surprising that an individual in RMT therapy, reading about child abuse and in other ways reflecting on the problem, would process these waking experiences in dream images of abuse. But to take these dreams — without any other corroborating evidence — as proof that the dreamer actually suffered child abuse is both simplistic and dangerous. Yet there are indications that dreams are interpreted in precisely this manner in RMT therapy. For an example of this sort of literal interpretation of one aspect of a dream, see Chapter 9.

Guided Imagery

Guided imagery is widely used in a variety of therapeutic and quasi-therapeutic contexts principally as a relaxation technique. It involves visualizing and concentrating on specific images in order to attain various goals. In therapeutic contexts, the therapist will typically tell the client to close his eyes, take a few deep breaths, and focus on a mental image — a still pool of water, say, or a beautiful polished stone — in order to attain a state of increased relaxation. The technique is sometimes used in the medical community as a diagnostic tool: a patient is told to allow her mind to present her with a picture that represents her illness and then is guided in imaginary dialogue with the image. This dialogue can provide the guide with insights into the patient's hopes and fears concerning the illness and possible treatments; some diagnosticians maintain that it can also provide insights into the nature of the illness not offered by more traditional techniques.

Some RMT therapists use guided imagery to "recover" memories of abuse. For example, the therapist may ask the client to visualize a safe place in her mind as a room with a window through which to view scenes of childhood — including scenes of abuse. The client is told that initially the recovered imagery may seem like fantasies, but focus and discipline will establish the fact that they are actually flashbacks to events in her past. Some therapists encourage clients to view these scenes of abuse as if they were recorded on video, freezing various frames, rewinding the tape, fast forwarding it, and so forth.

Whatever the value of guided imagery in other therapeutic contexts, it does not appear to be a trustworthy means of recovering memories. It involves an authoritative therapist directing a suggestible client to focus on images of abuse and revisit them repeatedly until they become vivid and detailed. This is precisely the sort of method that memory researchers have used to implant false memories in test subjects.

Hypnosis

When guided imagery is used as a technique to recover repressed memory in the manner described above, it is basically serving as a kind of hypnosis. Long caricatured in popular representations, hypnosis is essentially a state of deep relaxation in which a subject is unusually open to the suggestions of a hypnotist. Not all people can be hypnotized. The best candidates tend to be trusting, imaginative, and hungry for approval from authority figures. Research suggests that somewhere between 10 and 30 percent of the general population falls into this category.

The hypnotic state covers a spectrum from mild relaxation to a deep trance in which the subject is effectively aware of and responsive to only the hypnotist. The hypnotist's suggestions to a subject in a deep trance can produce physiological responses that would not occur outside the trance state; for example, the hypnotist can induce temporary blindness, paralysis, sensations of heat and numbness, rigidity of limbs, and so on. The hypnotist can also make suggestions that will alter some subjects' behavior outside the hypnotic state — suggestions that help curb a desire for cigarettes or food, for instance, or that reduce pain or anxiety associated with medical procedures. The hypnotist can also effect other cognitive changes in a suggestible subject, such as inducing hallucinations and selective amnesia. And hypnosis has long been used as a means to recover faded or repressed memories.

The relationship between hypnosis and memory is somewhat controversial. Freud was initially enthusiastic about using hypnosis to recover memory, but over time he became disenchanted with it because he found that many of his patients were not adequately suggestible, and he abandoned it in favor of free association. Others have found that there is reason to question the accuracy of the memories recovered through hypnosis. Among the findings of an extensive study of hypnosis and brainwashing conducted by the U.S. government during the 1950s was the fact that it was possible to implant false memories with hypnosis. One of the few points regarding hypnosis and memory about which there is a general consensus is that hypnosis does serve to powerfully increase people's *confidence* in what they recall regardless of whether it increases their ability to remember actual events.

RMT therapists who use hypnosis typically undertake a process of hypnotic regression, leading the subject back in time to relive incidents of abuse in childhood. As a practical matter, it is seldom possible to verify the accuracy of the "memories" recovered in this way. But since both the therapist and the subject are looking for memories of abuse and fully expect to find them, they are overwhelmingly inclined to accept any such experiences as genuine recollections of past events. As in the case of guided imagery, we have here a situation in which a highly suggestible individual is being led by an interested party toward a preselected goal. Even if neither of the parties sets out to produce false memories, their expectations and predispositions may powerfully affect the outcome. Michael Yapko has written of his experience with therapists who are willing to make diagnoses on the thinnest of evidence and to advocate the use of hypnotism without any clear understanding of how it works or what it involves:

> Recently, a woman called me to ask if I would hypnotize her in order to determine whether she had been molested as a child. She told me that she felt chronic low self-esteem and had recently phoned another therapist to make a first appointment. The therapist, *never having met her,* said on the telephone that her problem with self-esteem meant that she must have been abused as a child, and she should be hypnotized to "recover" her repressed memories. This therapist obviously viewed hypnosis as a kind of truth serum or magical lie detector that could reliably uncover long-buried memories that, camera-like, had recorded the exact, objective and complete truth of her past events.
>
> Even more shocking than such ignorance about hypnosis and suggestion, however, is the thought that a therapist working with as sensitive and potentially devastating material as child abuse would make an off-the-cuff diagnosis to a complete stranger and then be willing to dump her in someone else's office for a hit-and-run session involving investigative hypnosis. It is hard to imagine a more egregious disregard for good clinical judgment and ethical standards of practice. And yet, every day I get at least one phone call from a therapist asking me to spend a session hypnotizing a client to find out whether there was childhood abuse or not, as if the procedure of uncovering child abuse were as expeditious and unproblematic as getting dental x-rays.

When Yapko called this woman's therapist to check out the story, the therapist readily admitted to having arrived at the diagnosis of childhood sex abuse on the basis of a single phone conversation — and she couldn't understand why he was upset about it.[35]

In 1992, Yapko conducted a survey of nearly a thousand therapists regarding memory and suggestibility. The average age of the respondents

35. Yapko, "The Seduction of Memory," p. 34.

was 44, their education level averaged slightly beyond master's level, and their average time in practice was more than eleven years. He found that "many had little or no formal knowledge of the role and power of suggestion in therapy, or of the accumulated research data about memory. They held surprisingly naive and outmoded views about the mind's capacity to remember." Of the respondents, 45 percent agreed that the mind is like a computer, accurately storing events as they occur; 43 percent agreed that if someone doesn't remember much about his or her childhood, it is most likely because it was somehow traumatic; 75 percent said that hypnosis is a valuable tool for facilitating accurate recall when memories are not forthcoming; and 54 percent agreed that hypnosis could be used to recover accurate and detailed memories as far back as birth. There is no generally accepted research to support any of these positions. In general, Yapko's findings led him to conclude that many of the individuals he interviewed were conducting therapy based on significant misconceptions about how the mind works. "Furthermore, almost all respondents confessed their inability to separate truth from fiction in their clients' reports of abuse. Unfortunately, most of the surveyed clinicians also indicated that precisely *because* they had no way of distinguishing false from true memories of abuse, they were inclined to accept noncritically whatever story the client told."[36]

Abreaction

Many RMT therapists endorse abreaction (often referred to as "working through the pain" or something similar) as a necessary step toward healing for those who have suffered childhood sexual abuse. The idea is that in order to overcome the fear and pain associated with the abuse, the client must face it head on. Once the memories of the abuse have been "recovered" with the help of the techniques mentioned above, the client must relive the trauma with the same levels of fear, anxiety, and emotional pain she felt during the initial assault. Some therapists encourage their clients to act out the scenes physically, wrestling on the floor with an image of the abuser and striking back at the abuser by punching pillows, shouting denunciations, and the like.

The therapeutic community is divided over the value of cathartic

36. Yapko, quoted by Lois Blinkhorn in "Sexual Abuse Cases on Trial," *Milwaukee Sentinel,* 10 July 1994.

techniques of this sort. There does seem to be evidence that they are effective in at least some cases, although the specific means by which they produce relief remains in dispute. Some evidence suggests that any sort of strong emotional discharge produces relief, regardless of whether it is grounded in actual memories. Apart from its therapeutic benefits, however, it seems only reasonable to suppose that abreaction as it is typically practiced in RMT would serve to reinforce perceived memories of abuse recovered by other means, since it involves the client's reliving the event in a highly emotional and suggestible state.

*　　*　　*

We have seen how proponents of RMT identify large numbers of people as possible victims of childhood abuse by drawing up long lists of symptoms that effectively apply to just about everyone in our culture. We have seen how RMT therapists have a tendency to confirm their initial diagnosis by misusing established therapeutic techniques and misinterpreting their results. The question remains, though, how they manage to be so effective in convincing clients that they were abused as children. Why do people who entered therapy with no memories of past abuse become convinced, after only a few sessions, that they were in fact abused — convinced enough to overturn their lives, tear apart their families, and in some cases initiate legal action against the presumed offenders? There is no single explanation for this phenomenon, but one factor that is clearly important is the power of suggestion, to which we are all susceptible.

The Power of Suggestion

Maryanne Garry and Elizabeth Loftus tell the true story of a Texas woman named Sally who awoke one night with a gun to her head, held by a masked man who then raped her and her daughter. The next day, after calling her coworker Lois Von Williams to tell her she was not coming in to work, Sally was convinced by her boyfriend that the rapist's elaborate effort to conceal his identity meant that he must be someone she knew. The boyfriend kept saying that she must have seen him somewhere — in the street, in church, at a party, whatever. After a while, Sally found that she was able to put a face on her attacker: it was Clarence Von Williams, the husband of her coworker Lois, a man whom she had just met at a party a few weeks earlier. She accused Von Williams, and he was arrested.

Over time, Sally became more and more convinced that Von Williams was the one who had attacked her, and she positively identified him at the trial. Despite the absence of any corroborating evidence, the jury found Von Williams guilty of aggravated rape, and he was sentenced to fifty years in prison. A couple of months later, another man, Jon Simonis, was arrested for an unrelated crime, and he eventually confessed to more than seventy crimes, including the crimes against Sally and her daughter for which Von Williams had been convicted. After seeing Simonis's videotaped confession, the prosecutors overturned Von Williams's conviction and freed him.

But when Sally looked at the same videotape, she refused to believe that Simonis was the man who had attacked her and her daughter, even though his confession included details that only a person who was actually there could have known. Why was Sally so convinced that Von Williams was the rapist? Because she was susceptible to suggestions. Her memory was gradually colored by a variety of sources. It began when she made her original phone call to her coworker Lois Von Williams. Next, the repeated suggestion and sincere belief that Sally must have known her attacker came from someone she trusted, her boyfriend. She solidified the false memory in her consciousness when she put Clarence Von Williams's face with the attacker in her mind's eye and thus identified him as the rapist.

"Sally's repeated denials in the face of the real criminal's confessions indicate a sincere belief in a false memory," say Garry and Loftus. "For researchers interested in false memories, Sally provides an anecdote more powerful than any laboratory researcher could hope to develop artificially. This false memory was not brought about by hypnosis, often colloquially associated with 'the power of suggestion.' Cognitive psychologists know that the power of suggestion has a power all its own."[37]

As Garry and Loftus show, the power of suggestion is related to another phenomenon in psychology, about which a growing body of research has accumulated since the mid-1970s, known as the "misinformation effect": "The misinformation effect is an umbrella category of phenomena in which subjects who are misled about previously witnessed events often integrate that inaccurate postevent information into their accounts of the event."[38] Almost nobody would argue with the claim that extraneous information after the fact can bias a person's memory of an incident. But RMT proponents contend that only small details of memory can be affected

---

37. Garry and Loftus, "Pseudomemories without Hypnosis," *International Journal of Clinical and Experimental Hypnosis* 42 (October 1994): 364.

38. Garry and Loftus, "Pseudomemories without Hypnosis," pp. 364-65.

in this way, that there is no proof that the memory of significant events can be altered, that memories of real traumatic events can be significantly revised, or that whole narratives of things that never occurred can be implanted in human memory. Loftus disagrees, citing many studies showing that people can be led to believe that they have witnessed something they did not. For example, Robert S. Pynoos and Kathi Nader studied the aftermath of an incident in California in which a sniper shot a high-powered rifle into an elementary school playground, killing one child and one adult, injuring several children, and pinning down many more under gunfire — in other words, subjecting all those involved to significant trauma. The researchers not only received wildly differing accounts of the incident from the actual eyewitnesses but also found that many children who for one reason or another were not at the school that day nonetheless reported vividly detailed memories of the shooting. They had apparently assembled "memories" of the event from bits and pieces of the stories of schoolmates who had actually experienced the trauma.[39]

Another well-known and well-regarded researcher, S. J. Ceci, managed to convince the majority of children in a study that at some point in their past they had gotten their hand caught in a mousetrap and had had to go to the hospital to get the trap removed. He did this simply by inducing the children to repeatedly think about the event and then questioning them about it.[40] In other experimentation, Nick Spanos developed somewhat similar results with adult volunteers. Using hypnotic suggestion, he induced some of his subjects to "remember" that they had been abused as children in a previous life.[41] These and other experiments have shown that memory is reconstructive, and — at least for those who discount the validity of past-life experience — they establish that false recollections can be induced by hypnotic suggestion.

Many involved with RMT contend that recovered memories must be genuine because many of them are so richly and vividly detailed. "I find it highly unlikely that someone who can remember what pattern was on the wallpaper and that a duck was quacking outside the bedroom window where

39. Pynoos and Nader, "Children's Memory and Proximity to Violence," *Journal of American Academy of Child and Adolescent Psychiatry* 28 (1989): 236-41.

40. See S. J. Ceci, E. F. Loftus, M. D. Leichtman, and M. Bruck, "The Possible Role of Source Misattributions in the Creation of False Beliefs among Preschoolers," *International Journal of Clinical and Experimental Hypnosis* 42 (1994): 304-20, and S. J. Ceci, M. L. C. Huffman, and E. F. Loftus, "Repeatedly Thinking about a Non-event: Source Misattributions among Preschoolers," *Consciousness and Cognition* 3 (1994): 388-407.

41. Spanos et al., "Secondary Identity Enactments during Hypnotic Past-Life Regression: A Sociocognitive Perspective," *Journal of Personality and Social Psychology* 61 (1991): 308-20.

she was molested by her father when she was four years old is making it up," said Jill Otey, a Portland attorney whose office specializes in women remembering childhood abuse. "Why in the hell would your mind do this?"[42] But research has shown that false memories are often characterized by just this sort of detail. In an experiment that has become somewhat famous, Elizabeth Loftus and James A. Coan told a number of subjects, in a range of ages, a fictional story about their having been lost in a mall during childhood. With little effort, the researchers were able to develop in these subjects a false memory of the event that in many cases was richly detailed. The subjects supplied elaborate descriptions of the mall itself, of a man who came to their rescue (including the pattern on the shirt he was wearing), and so forth. When later told that the memory was false, a good 25 to 30 percent refused to believe it. They tended to cling most strongly to the specific details they had added to the bare bones of the story supplied by the researchers.[43]

Suggestion is a powerful distorter of fact. The famous child psychologist Jean Piaget wrote that for years he delighted in recounting his earliest memory:

> I can still see, most clearly, the following scene. . . . I was sitting in my pram, which my nurse was pushing in the Champs Elysees, when a man tried to kidnap me. I was held in by the strap fastened around me while my nurse bravely tried to stand between me and the thief. She received various scratches, and I can still see vaguely those on her face. Then a crowd gathered, a policeman with a short cloak and a white baton came up, and the man took to his heels. I can still see the whole scene, and can even place it near the tube station. When I was about fifteen, my parents received a letter from my former nurse saying that she had been converted to the Salvation Army. She wanted to confess her past faults, and in particular to return the watch she had been given as a reward on this occasion. She had made up the whole story, faking the scratches. I, therefore, must have heard, as a child, the account of this story, which my parents believed, and projected it into the past in the form of a visual memory.[44]

The fascinating thing about Piaget's "memory" is that, even after he knew the incident had been made up, indeed even when he was an old

---

42. Otey, quoted by Anastasia Toufexis in "When Can Memories Be Trusted?" *Time*, 28 October 1991, p. 86.

43. For a description of the experiment, see the *Harvard Mental Health Letter* 9 (March 1993): 5.

44. Piaget, *Plays, Dreams, and Imitation in Childhood*, cited by Elizabeth Loftus and Katherine Ketcham in *Witness for the Defense* (New York: St. Martin's Press, 1991), pp. 17-19.

man, he could "still see, most clearly" in his mind's eye the kidnapping attempt that he knew had never taken place. How many of us "remember" family events or bits of personal history simply because they were rehearsed in our families so often? Memory is largely a matter of rehearsal: we tend to lose memories that we don't refresh through repetition. And, as we have seen, many RMT therapists encourage this kind of rehearsal. John Bradshaw, the self-described "evangelist of dysfunction," gave this representative advice to women who have no clear recollection of abuse: "Accept the theory that you were sexually abused, live consciously with that idea for six months in context with an awareness of the traits you acknowledge, and see whether any memories come to you."[45] RMT therapists work intensively with clients to recover the dimmest of memory fragments, and in the course of therapy they typically expose their patients to other stories of childhood abuse. Many clients then proceed to expose themselves to yet more stories outside of therapy, through RMT literature such as *The Courage to Heal,* stories on TV talk shows and news shows, and participation in incest survivor groups. This is precisely the sort of context in which we might expect false memories to arise.

Patients are encouraged to search for memories and expected to find them. The authors of *The Courage to Heal* say, "So far no one we have talked to thought she might have been abused, and then later discovered that she hadn't been. The progression always goes the other way, from suspicion to confirmation. If you think you were abused and your life shows the symptoms, then you were."[46] With assurances of this sort from trusted therapists, is it any wonder that suggestible patients manage to find what they have been told to look for?

Therapists can exert influence without being aware that they are doing so. Some clients are so suggestible that they recover memories of childhood abuse with scarcely any prompting. The therapist may simply mention that the client's presenting symptoms are the same as those of another client who turned out to be a victim of child abuse, and the new client may begin confabulating a history of abuse. Some clients enter therapy already fully "suggested" through exposure to media reports of childhood abuse, RMT literature, or friends involved in recovery groups. Preexisting beliefs are critical in the case of both the therapist and the client. RMT therapists characteristically presuppose the existence of repressed memories of sexual

45. Bradshaw, "Incest: When You Wonder If It Happened to You," *Lear's Magazine,* August 1992, p. 43.
46. Bass and Davis, *The Courage to Heal,* p. 26.

abuse in their clients, and, as Richard Ofshe notes, "since patients want to please therapists, that interest reinforces anything the client comes up with in that direction. Then the therapist gets the patient to actively imagine an image of abuse, saying, 'Try to picture this happening to you,' and encourages the patient to elaborate on that fantasy. Then the patient becomes convinced that it was not merely imagination, but a repressed memory of abuse." And once the client begins to report memories of past trauma, regardless of what techniques may have been used to facilitate their recovery, the therapist will be inclined to accept them all as factual: it is an article of faith among RMT therapists that clients do not dream such memories up, and they feel ethically bound to believe and support them. But as Michael Yapko puts it, "The capacity to be therapeutic — to encourage, to soothe, to help shift world views, to change perceptions — is equally the capacity to be anti-therapeutic — to inculcate a mindset and a point of view, to project a vision of reality to the client that may not only be false, but ultimately damaging."[47]

Why do some people, after only a few sessions with a therapist, and having no memories of abuse in their past, believe therapists who tell them that they are victims of child sexual abuse? First of all, people go to therapists because they are suffering some sort of emotional distress. The RMT therapist gains their confidence and tells them explicitly or implicitly, "I am the expert in this area, and your symptoms tell me that something traumatic happened to you in your past." It is a powerful suggestion to a vulnerable person. Further, RMT therapists offer authoritative assurances that specific symptoms reliably point to a specific set of events in the client's past and that "together we will recover them." Responsible members of the psychotherapeutic community maintain that one cannot reliably read the past on the basis of present distress.

Beyond the therapists who make *suggestions* of abuse to their clients are those who believe in repressed memories and the pervasiveness of child abuse so zealously that they cajole or even browbeat clients into accepting the assertion that their parents sexually abused them. As part of a story on RMT, CNN sent an investigative reporter to visit an Ohio therapist. Posing as a new patient, the reporter complained of feeling depressed and having had recent relationship problems with her husband. During that first session, the therapist diagnosed the reporter as an incest survivor, telling her that she was a "classic case." When the reporter returned for a second session, expressing puzzlement that she had no

47. Yapko, "The Seduction of Memory," p. 33.

memories of her abuse, the therapist told her that her reaction was typical and that she had repressed the memory because her trauma had been so awful. Many women who have subsequently retracted accusations elicited on the basis of RMT report similar heavy-handed tactics on the part of their therapists.

Given the vulnerability and suggestibility of many people who seek out the help of a therapist, it is not hard to see how they might forfeit their own perceptions of their lives and family histories in favor of the views of someone they have come to trust, even revere. Every generation produces examples of what can happen when people give their trust over to the wrong sort of individual. In recent years we have seen the likes of Charles Manson, Jim Jones, David Koresh, and others use suggestion, seduction, mind control, peer and authority pressure, and even threats to get and hold their converts. On a much more prosaic level, we see a host of mass media gurus, prophets, and healers spreading a variety of twelve-step gospels to the victims of dysfunctional families, urging the wounded to get in touch with their inner child. Psychotherapists have even greater powers of suggestion than do cult leaders or television counselors to reshape a client's worldview or personal history.

Some individuals need no outside voice to suggest them into recollections of a devastating past. Michael Yapko tells the following true story:

> He told his wife that he simply couldn't deal with the memories of his horrible experiences in Vietnam. In the twenty years of their marriage, she had seen enough strange behavior from him to believe it. One night, he went berserk in an apparent reaction to the sneakers she happened to be wearing. After he calmed down, he told her that his Vietcong captors wore similar sneakers when they regularly dragged him out of his bamboo cage to beat and urinate on him. He told her he had been a prisoner for fifteen days after a carrier-based F-4 jet fighter on which he was the navigator was shot down. He said he escaped after strangling a guard, who was also wearing the same kind of sneakers.
>
> He went to see a therapist, who diagnosed him as suffering from post–traumatic stress disorder and treated him for severe depression and explosive anger. He spent an inordinate amount of time obsessing about his experiences in Vietnam and was unable to make sense of what happened to him there. The therapist succeeded in getting him to talk more openly about the connections between his memories and his present mood swings, nightmares and irrational rages with his wife. Unfortunately, despite lengthy treatment, one day he committed suicide by inhaling carbon monoxide.

After his death, his wife attempted to get his name placed on the state Vietnam War Memorial, declaring him as much a casualty of that war as anyone who had actually died there. To support her effort, his therapist also wrote a letter on his behalf. . . . In response to their requests, his military background was extensively checked, but countless hours spent searching through Armed Forces files failed to turn up any record of the man's service in Vietnam. Much to the shock and dismay of both his wife and his therapist, it became inescapably clear that he had never been in Vietnam at all. The events that were so convincingly at the root of this disturbed man's deep unhappiness were entirely fictitious.[48]

Beyond the fact that people coming into therapy are vulnerable, that their need for approval is often intensified in the one-to-one interchange of the therapeutic setting, that they are offered a generic and elastic list of symptoms — beyond these factors is the magnetic attraction of a root cause for all of one's feelings of inadequacy, low self-esteem, depression, loneliness, and thorny relationships. "Knowing that I was abused explained all my problems so neatly," one woman said. "I didn't have to search for reasons anymore." To someone in deep distress, establishing the cause of the pain, hearing that it is possible to work through it, and receiving the promise of a cure at the end is very appealing indeed. A diagnosis of repressed memories of childhood sexual abuse both gives the client a specific cause for ill-defined feelings of anxiety and supplies the therapist with a justification for what typically turns out to be a very long and costly course of treatment.

Postscript

Mark Pendergrast, who has studied the problem of the recovery of repressed memories for years and has interviewed scores of people on all sides of the question, has written the best and most comprehensive book on this subject, *Victims of Memory*.[49] One of Pendergrast's key conclusions is that *not one* case of massive repression has ever been corroborated or documented. Having already interviewed a large number of self-reported repressed memory subjects for his book, Pendergrast corresponded with RMT expert

48. Yapko, "The Seduction of Memory," pp. 31-32.
49. *Victims of Memory* is the single most comprehensive, widest-ranging volume dealing with repressed memory therapy and its resulting societal problems in America published to date. I am indebted to this book and to Pendergrast personally for many insights into the problem.

Judith Herman in hopes that she would allow him to interview some of her clients as well. Herman sent him a curt note suggesting that he contact the veterans' hospital in his state of New Hampshire. He did contact that hospital, and the state therapist said to him, "It's extraordinarily rare."

Pendergrast himself has been unable to find one documented case. All the evidence he has encountered indicates that people who are traumatized over long periods of time do not forget it: "Real victims always remember their abuse." He did find cases in which individuals had remembered isolated incidents that they had forgotten — or "repressed," if one wishes to use the term — years before (e.g., one woman remembered her father's having fondled her breast while he was teaching her to drive). But he found no cases in which years of abuse were forgotten and then recalled. There have been documented cases of memory loss due to organic brain damage, head injuries, and surgery, but this sort of loss is always permanent. There have also been documented cases of traumatic amnesia, which is a temporary but complete forgetting of a traumatic event, but the memories of such events usually return within a few days. There are simply no medical studies or documented case histories demonstrating that it is possible for anyone to repress years of abuse.

On the other hand, it has been clearly established by numerous studies and confirmed by case after anecdotal case that people can and do remember with clarity and certainty all manner of things that never happened. The one lesson we should take from a century of research on memory distortion, say Garry and Loftus, is that we do not now have any means for reliably distinguishing true memories about the past from false ones. "This is not being unfair to the truly victimized," they say, because they are not questioning the validity of long-held memories. They are talking about only that class of "memories" that emerge in adulthood after extensive "memory work." And they note that "uncritical acceptance of every claim of sexual abuse, no matter how dubious, is bound to have another chilling consequence: it will make trivial the true and ruthless cases of abuse and increase the suffering of genuine victims."[50]

50. Garry and Loftus, "Pseudomemories without Hypnosis," p. 375.

CHAPTER 3

Emily

Katie: When Emily was born, her older brother, Larry, was just starting school, so I was able to devote just as much time to her as I had been able to with him, which was very nice. As a little girl, she always liked to know who was the boss, so that the right person was telling her what to do. And then she would do whatever the boss told her to do. She was in Girl Scouts, and when she was ten, she acted with the Milwaukee Repertory Theater in two different productions. She was a good little actress who had a lot of self-confidence.

Leo: Emily was an absolute joy to our lives, a delight to raise. In her teenage years she had a sense of humor and a twinkle in her eye . . . just a real pep in her step, I used to say. And she was a very logical person with a sharp wit. Just a joy.

Katie: She seemed to go through the high school years very well. I never had to tell her to do her homework; she always did what was expected of her. She was an honors student. She was on the varsity swimming team and lettered all four years of high school, was captain of the team her senior year, and was vice president of her graduating class. She was also in the band for two years. She was a high achiever who could not wait to get to the University of Wisconsin; she didn't want to go to any other, smaller school. She was going to set the world on fire. She was a feminine girl: she dated in high school and had a couple of steady guys. But she was also raised in a feminist home. I was a member of National Organization for Women and supported all the *early* feminist goals. When Emily went off to Madison to start university, she was in very good shape.

52

And the first year went pretty smoothly. The first semester she seemed very much involved in the affairs of her residence hall floor and so forth; toward the end of the year, though, she had lost some interest in that. She had made friends with a girl from the east side of Milwaukee who came from a very splintered family. Perhaps this was a kind of first indication that Emily had become somewhat disaffected from the middle-class group of students she had gone to high school with. That summer she came home and did her usual job, which was a swimming instructor at the recreation department (where she worked for years). By the fall she seemed very anxious to start school again. It was in her sophomore year that I began to notice a big difference in her.

Leo and I have always tried to respect what our children had to say. That doesn't mean that we did not have rules and regulations, simply that we respected their input. We always gave them an option to give their opinion. So Emily and I never really had had fights; we got along very well. But at Thanksgiving time of that sophomore year, Emily came home for the break, and she and I had an altercation that sticks with me because it was something of a milestone. At the time it was fashionable for some teenagers to wear jeans with big holes in the knees. I had made it clear to Emily that I didn't care for that attire out in public with me. I said, "If you want to wear that by yourself, it's fine. Just don't wear it when you're out with me." I thought that was a reasonable way to handle it. Well, I was going to get my hair cut, and she wanted a haircut too, and I was able to get her an appointment on very short notice. She came down to go out with me with those awful-looking jeans on. I said, "Honey, will you please go change — you know how I feel about those."

She went into a rage, an absolute rage. I had never seen her like that. My eighty-five-year-old mother was here for the holiday, and Emily just stood there and screamed at me: all about what a hypocrite I was and all sorts of incredible things. She had never done anything like that in her life. And then she started crying. It was just crazy. All because I didn't want her to wear those jeans. She was nineteen years old at the time.

Finally — I guess because my mother was here — I relented. She was crying upstairs, so I said, "Okay, honey, you can come with me that way." I put my arms around her when she came down, but she was still sobbing. It was very strange to me: she seemed so unhappy, and I didn't know why. She said, "You love me, don't you?" And I said, "Of course I love you." It was a milestone in our relationship because she had never been that way to me before.

But then it was something I just had to let go. I thought, this is an interesting period in a young woman's life, and she's probably making the natural separation that she feels she has to make from her mother. It disturbed me, but I let it go. That's when I first saw a change in her. Leo did not.

Leo: For my part, you could not have had a better relationship than what I had with my daughter. She had no fear of me. We respected each other. We're a humorous family, and Emily loved my sense of humor — and vice versa. For example, she'd point out, like any teenager, how my plaid shorts didn't match my striped shirt: "Nice outfit, Dad." I have a terrible tin ear for music, so when she was little, she'd have me sing Happy Birthday in front of her friends — because it was so off-key. And she'd laugh and laugh. She had a lot of sleepovers. I would be the one up on Saturday mornings making them pancakes and eggs and cracking jokes. You could not have written a better script for a relationship between a father and his daughter. My daughter never said a cross word to me . . . until about six months after she got into the militant feminist stuff.

Katie: That sophomore year, she was just beginning courses in women's studies. Also, although she had never taken any drugs in high school (she might have drunk a little beer), we found out later that she started smoking marijuana during that sophomore year of college.

Leo: Emily had always been so logical and mature. A couple of months after she first went off to college, I asked her if she was going to parties and so forth. She said, "Well, you know, Dad, going out and getting plastered and coming home and throwing up is not my idea of a good time." That response really pleased me . . . and that's the way she was.

Katie: But things really started happening for her that second year of college. You could even call it a disastrous year for her. And our relationship — the mother-daughter bond — seemed to deteriorate greatly. At the same time a strain began to develop in my relationship with my husband, because he did not know, and couldn't really understand, what was going wrong between Emily and me. Around Christmas that year, she started saying to Leo, "Dad, I'm thinking about going to Alaska next summer to work." We were disappointed. We wanted her home during the summer because she was away the whole school year. Privately she said to him, "I have to leave because I can't stand to be around Mom all summer. She's too controlling." Leo was getting mad at me, and I was starting to feel that he was taking her side. It was getting pretty disturbing to me.

54

Leo: I didn't understand the "controlling" part. It didn't make sense to me. We never controlled anything. And Emily's behavior of blowing up at her mother was so unlike her. Ordinarily, if there had been some disagreement about what to wear, for example, Emily would have said, "Oh, lighten up . . . chill out. . . ." She would have changed into a decent pair of slacks, and that would have been that.

During her sophomore year, Emily was living in a room alone in the dorm, and we met some of her friends from down the hall. One of them, Amy, was really into astrology. Now, to my mind, all that business of being a Gemini or a Pisces is just something people make up, like Tarot cards or whatever. But this astrology person was incredibly influential over Emily; one of her old friends told us that she would follow Amy around like a puppy. She brought Amy home in February of that year, and we took the two of them out to dinner. That's when Amy started telling us all about the "third eye."

Katie: Also, at dinner, for the very first time in our presence, Emily lit up a cigarette. We almost fell over. Of course, she was looking for us to raise hell, but we were pretty cool about it. Actually, Leo did give her a small lecture about smoking — but in a very nice way. He told her how bad he felt about ever starting the habit, and that he hoped she would never get addicted like he was. Anyway, this Amy was a latter-day hippie, a flower child. When I said I was happy to meet her, she said, "Oh, I know you quite well already . . . through Emily." At that point, of course, I had to be wondering what Emily might be saying about me.

Leo: Later, when I asked Emily, "Where's Amy from?" her response was: "Oh, you know, she's from one of those typical American patriarchal families where the father goes to a mindless job all day, and the brainless breeder, the mother, stays home and cooks his meals, washes his clothes, and raises his children." She was obviously heavily into women's studies and feminist rhetoric by that time. Her other friend at the time was Tina, a very pretty blond girl who was majoring in physical therapy. Emily had told us how she came from a home where her alcoholic father beat up his wife and also the children. Amy and Tina became important figures in Emily's life.

Also at that time, Emily was "hanging around," as she put it, in a New Age, feminist bookstore in Madison. (We found out later that many places like these, along with serving their coffee and tofu or whatever, try to recruit people into the belief systems of those who run the bookstore.) Emily was saying things like, "Patriarchy is awful, capitalism is terrible, civilization stinks. . . ." She told her cousin, as they looked out a Madison restaurant window, "When I look at cities, all I see is death and decay."

Katie: Now, approaching the end of her sophomore year, her grades were no longer good — by her standards. She had been a high school honors student, and during her freshman year of college she was getting B's and better (a 3-point grade average). Now she was getting C's and was not happy. She had moved from one dorm to another; she insisted that she have a room alone for her sophomore year. Also, during her freshman year she had to have *Time* magazine sent to her at school. During her sophomore year it was no longer *Time;* she asked for *Rolling Stone.* So we were seeing a big shift there.

Leo: And I thought the shift would have been going the other way . . .

Katie: So the next summer she did, in fact, take a job with the Holland-American cruise line working out of Skagway, Alaska. She was staying in a dorm kind of facility in Skagway, which was part of the hotel employment situation. She never called us, but we called her often. Both of us were getting more and more lonesome for her and tense with each other. I was hurt because Leo had as much as said it was my fault she was gone because I was too controlling.

When she came back from Alaska at the end of the summer, she forfeited a bonus by leaving early so she wouldn't miss registration at the university. She flew into Chicago, took the bus home, and we all went down to pick her up. When I saw her, I immediately thought that she was trying to look more manly: she was not shaving her armpits or legs, which was obvious because she was wearing shorts and a sleeveless top. Leo was so happy to see her and so blinded by his love for her that he was unaware of this change. Emily stayed home for only one night and then was on her way to Madison the next day. Maybe Leo blamed me for the brevity of her stay, because things were tense between us.

Leo: A couple of times, on the phone, she said to me, "You see me at my worst, when I'm at home — around Mom." I said, "Emily, I don't see that." I really didn't have a clue about the tension between mother and daughter. But for her it was a repeated refrain.

Katie: I think Emily was trying very hard to get me to tell her to drop dead . . . because her behavior toward me had become outrageous. But I wouldn't

56

do that. Because I loved her, I was having trouble figuring out what was going on. My relationship with her was falling apart, but I was at a loss as to why.

Leo: So she went back to Madison, and we helped her move into this new place, which she shared with three other college girls, one of whom was Tina. A couple of months after we had moved a bed and dresser and other stuff over there with a U-Haul, she called to tell us she no longer had any use for a dresser. So I rented a U-Haul again to carry the dresser back home. And she didn't want her bed either. She wanted a mattress on the floor.

Katie: Sometime during that fall we were in Madison and wanted to take Emily out to dinner. But she said she wanted us to come to her "home" and she would cook dinner for us. She had been healthy her whole life, but she would never touch vegetables. Now, she declared to us, she was a vegetarian. She even had a sense of humor about it: she said that we must just be howling to see her as a vegetarian. We agreed. When we got over to her place for vegetarian spaghetti, it turned out that she had no ingredients. All she had was a head of lettuce. So in the end we did go out to a nutritionally incorrect but good restaurant.

Emily came home for Thanksgiving, and we of course had a turkey dinner. But she said she was "eating lower on the food chain." She said that we all should be eating lower on the food chain. We also found out that Emily was now *working* at the feminist bookstore. She had gotten a job there and she absolutely loved it; it was "the most wonderful place in the world." She was now working with Anita, who had been "incested" by her father. The more we heard, it seemed like everybody who worked at the bookstore had been sexually abused as a child. And they were all on the same track.

At that time she also told us that she was dropping out of college after this first semester (of her junior year) was over. She was not going to go back to school in January because she needed to "zero in more on myself." So as of January she was still in Madison but not in school. The bookstore was able to give her more hours, so she was keeping busy. We all knew that something was wrong, but nobody knew what it was.

At that time, Leo's mother broke her hip and was beginning to require full care, which was being temporarily assumed by Leo's sister; but it was difficult for her because of her own job. Well, Emily called us out of the blue to tell us that she was going to go care for her grandmother, with whom she had never been very close. We thought it was a very nice gesture but at the same time quite peculiar for her at that time in her life. It turned out that she stayed there for about two months, and she and her grandmother got along fine. But every single weekend she would be going back to Madison from River Forest, Illinois, where her grandma lived. Somebody would appear and pick her up and then drop her off again. In the meantime, she was asking her grandmother a host of questions about her father's youth. She was also asking Grandma what she believed and why she believed it. Grandma is a very devout Catholic.

Leo: It was a very good relationship between grandmother and granddaughter, and I was very proud of Emily. She didn't know what she was going to do with her life, but she was down there caring for my mother. (We also figured out later that Emily was seeking the "wise old woman" — the crone — who is such a big deal in the New Age, radical feminist concepts. The figure shows up over and over in feminist and earth worship literature.)

Katie: On Easter Sunday, when we prayed before the meal — as is our custom — I noticed that Emily refused to pray. After dinner I said I needed to discuss something with her: there was some talk of Grandma going back to live with Grandpa. I told her what a great job she was doing caring for Grandma, and she started to cry: "Oh, it's so important that you say that to me . . . that you think I'm doing a good job." It was simply bizarre for Emily to be behaving in this overcharged emotional way; I felt like I was dealing with a whole different person. It was like walking on eggs for me. I was at a complete loss as to whether she was going to scream at me or hug me.

Leo: And I was thinking that maybe this is a woman thing that I'm just not going to get.

Katie: By this time I was just hoping she could be close to *one* of us. But then she left her grandmother abruptly, giving her aunt one day's notice. (We also found out later that at one point she tried to get her two younger cousins to smoke pot, and she told them that LSD was fabulous and that she'd be happy to get some for them. The cousins didn't tell anybody about it then — not until later. But we felt that our daughter's going into her aunt's home and trying to corrupt her cousins was just outrageous behavior.)

That next summer Emily went to work for the recreation department in Madison, and she hardly came home at all. I began to realize that the only time we heard from her was when *we* called, which was every week or ten days. When Thanksgiving came that year, Emily came home, but that was the time she got into a spat with her dad and brother about feminism, rape, and surrounding issues.

Leo: I was driving with her one day and she said, "Dad, what d'you think about rape?" I said, "Emily, I don't know anything about rape, but I've heard throughout my life that it has nothing to do with sex." Whenever we were alone in the car, she would be talking to me about how oppressed women are in society. But she also said, "I'll bet you think I'm getting a little strange, don't you, Dad?"

Katie: After one argument with Leo and Larry about women's oppression (during which I kept quiet because I was a little gun-shy at that point), she said to me in the kitchen, "You know, I really would have appreciated a little help out there, Mom." So I felt like I was between a rock and a hard place.

She had gone back to school briefly that third year, but by that time she was so politicized that when she took the exams, she simply wrote about why the course was no good. She waltzed out of there thinking she was incredibly intelligent and revolutionary — and she couldn't care less about what the report card said. When it did come, she just said, "I hope I flunked badly enough so that I never have to go back. The whole thing is just regurgitating patriarchal crap you've been taught." Contemptuous of everything — of education, of tradition, of the media, you name it. She wouldn't read a paper or watch a TV program. Nobody except her and the bookstore women knew anything.

She came home that Christmas, and there was really kind of an ugly scene. We had a nice Christmas Eve, and Emily was almost like her old self. But Christmas Day she was like Dr. Jekyll and Mr. Hyde, flipping in and out all day. She was rigid, militaristic, combative; she'd look at you with what Leo calls shark eyes, those dead eyes looking right through you. She refused to say "Merry Christmas"; it had to be "Happy Solstice." And she dressed all in black for the holidays.

Leo: We both had to be a little amused at all the astrology and New Age stuff. She talked about using a "Netty Pot" for her sinuses, except she had never had any problems with her nose. Then she was embracing crystals — the whole ball of wax. And her sense of humor was gone. All of our former jokes about my ethnic heritage, my baldness, my height, weight — generally stuff at my expense — all of that had become distinctly unfunny to Emily. Before, she'd always had the ability to laugh at herself. Now everything had to be politically correct. I said to my wife later, "As much as I miss Emily, I also miss myself. I'm gone. Things aren't funny anymore."

Katie: After Christmas dinner, I had forgotten to take my hormone pills for menopause, and I said to Emily, "Would you please bring my pills from the kitchen?" She came back, slammed the pills on the table in front of me, and harangued about how I was addicted to those pills. I told her that I wasn't addicted to Premarin; it's simply a hormone for menopause. "That's the same thing as taking cocaine," she said. "The only difference is that you're rich and you can afford it."

Leo: What she was saying there about us being rich and materialistic and addictive was her *rewriting* of who we are. That was the opposite of what our life was all about. I've always been able to make a good living, but "rich" we were not and are not. We were always able to take very nice family vacations to New York, Florida, the north woods — a lot of tent camping, some wilderness camping. We always had a swimming pool up in the summer, and for about ten years in a row I put up an ice-skating rink in the back yard. We have always lived very active and enjoyable lives. We almost always had dinner together as a family. You don't have to be "rich" to do these things. My point is: she rewrote what we were, our history, in every possible way. Doing and having the things I just mentioned had to be rewritten as undesirable, patriarchal, capitalist activities that "rich" people engage in. This is where the whole business of the *belief creating the memory* comes in: she needed to rewrite our history as a family in order to find the "oppression" she was looking for.

There is a therapist in Milwaukee who claims that the more affluent your parents are, the more likely they will be to "incest" you. She even has a name for this terrible disease of being raised by a wealthy family: "affluenza."

Katie: After Emily railed at me about my "drugs," she stormed out of the house into the snow, madder than hell, and was gone for about ten minutes. When she came into the house, she was standing at the door in her coat, crying. Part of me wanted to slap her silly. But instead I went over and put my arms around her and told her that I loved her. She hugged me and said, "I love you too, Mom."

But every single thing she said was an antipatriarchal and feminist ideological tirade. We had always been football fans, and there was a big game on that night. Of course, Emily told us that she would no longer watch football because it was part of the patriarchal oppression of women. So she just disappeared to her room without saying good night to any of us that Christmas night.

One time, early in college, when she was first taking psychology courses, she had come home and asked us at dinner, very seriously, "Did something traumatic happen to me in my childhood — because I can't seem to remember any of it." Her brother laughed and said that was a classic reaction to Psych 101. Leo treated it rather casually himself, telling her that there were forty picture albums in the family room that she could refresh her memory with.

But by her junior year, she was saying to me that she really thought she might have been sexually abused as a child. I said, "Emily, if you were, I certainly knew nothing about it. I was not unaware of the dangers the world holds for children, especially girls, and I was very careful with you. But that doesn't mean something couldn't have happened." But she was on this track somehow — and I had seen some of this business on talk shows — and it was reinforced by her feminist bookstore. Then sometime during her junior year she told me she had gone to an "incest survivors" meeting. I said, "What in the world . . . ?" But by that point my relationship with her was so odd that I couldn't get through to her much. She also told me that she was working at a battered and abused women's center on a volunteer basis. One evening we were in the den watching a TV show about teen pregnancy.

Leo: I remember I said, "You know, Emily, none of your friends ever got pregnant. I don't get it." She looked at us with tears in her eyes. "I'm glad you brought sex up," she said, "because I have to see a therapist. There's something terribly wrong with me. I have a problem with sexual dysfunction . . ."

Katie: Leo didn't have a clue. But I knew, from some of the shows I'd watched and books I'd read, that she was talking about orgasm. Leo said to her, "Well, honey, if you need some therapy, fine . . ." But I said, "Now wait a minute . . ." That's when she shot up and screamed, "I have to have therapy! You don't know how confused I am. . . ." She used a lot of four-letter words — which she had never done in this home — and she bolted from the room. I was merely thinking, "Before we rush to a therapist, let's check your insurance policy. This is expensive."

So Leo checked his company's coverage, and I got the names of three psychologists in Madison from a friend of mine who is a psychologist. "Be careful," she said to me, "there are a lot of wackos out there, especially in Madison." Emily called from Madison and told Leo she couldn't talk to *me* about money (meaning my concerns about insurance) but that she needed to see a therapist right away. Leo, of course, said, "Honey, go right ahead. We'll pay for everything." And he gave her the three names we had. Later she told us that she had gone to see them: one was too far away; one was a man (and therefore disqualified because she felt uncomfortable); and I don't remember about the third one. "But I did go to a hypnotherapist," she said, "and I really liked her."

Leo: Now I have been around the block a few times in my life, but I found I didn't know diddly squat about this whole world of psychotherapists out there. I know why I'm thirty pounds overweight: it's because I eat too much and don't burn off the calories. You don't have to go to a shrink and be told you have an "eating disorder." Anyway, when Emily mentioned the hypnotherapist and said she was helping her, she wanted to know if we'd pay. Of course we'll pay, I said.

Katie: I didn't like this at all. To me, this hypnotherapy was funny business. But I decided to keep my mouth shut because Leo was willing to pay for it, and I didn't want this to come between him and me. I was just hoping she would come out of it.

Twice a week she went to this hypnotherapist, a person with just a college degree and no psychological credentials — in other words, a self-proclaimed therapist who was advertised in the feminist bookstore and was referred by their network. And that's when Emily came to *know* she had been sexually abused as a child — she just didn't know who it was. Emily said she knew she would eventually be able to put a face on her abuser . . . she just had to work a little harder. Nancy, the hypnotist, taught her how to self-hypnotize. By now she was into dream therapy and body massage as well. I would occasionally ask her how she was doing with an identification of her "incesters" — because she was obviously so unhappy. (We now know that in questioning her grandmother about Leo's past she was trying to discover some history of abuse. And Leo's sisters have always had weight problems, so that showed they were sexually abused . . . and so forth.)

At Christmas she didn't know who had abused her, and in January she still didn't know. She was supposed to come home in February but didn't. I wasn't phoning Emily much anymore. I would call up and she would say something like, "Oh I can't talk, I've got somebody in my room." It was rude. Even our son, Larry, was worried. He said, "She's so weird now, I don't like the person she is now." But I said, "Don't say anything to Dad," because Leo still just did not see her behavior as outrageous.

Then, on the fifteenth of March, I was playing cards with a group of women friends, as I've done for twenty years. Well, Leo called her that night, and she came to the phone and said, "Is Mom there?" He said no, and she hung up the phone. Leo could not believe it. He called back and got her again. She again asked if I was there, he said no, and she said, "Please have Mom call me." And she hung up again. So he called me at my card game. By this time I was getting pretty fed up with the whole thing: mad at him, mad at her, the whole business. I called her, and her voice was like ice; it was like I was talking to a robot: "Listen very carefully because I'm not going to repeat this. Either you stop your pattern of denial and divorce your husband, or I'll never see you or talk to you or write to you again." Then she hung up.

You can imagine how I felt. Our hostess that night was a clinical psychologist. In the hallway I told her about the phone call, and she said, "Oh my God, Katie, the phrases Emily is using are right out of a book — *The Courage to Heal.*" Although I had heard "incest survivors" use that kind of language on talk shows, I did not know about the book. I told my psychologist friend Donna that I had to go to Madison to see what was going on with Emily, and she said, "Look around for books, Katie. See what she's reading, if you can." I remember saying to her, "She's Leo's heart. This will kill him."

As soon as I got home, I asked Leo, "Did you ever touch Emily inappropriately?" He said, "No, what do you mean? That's crazy." I said, "Well, this is what she's saying." He said, "No, you must be misinterpreting what she said. You've got it all wrong." So we got into the car and headed to Madison. We were halfway to Madison, and I said, "Stop, I have to call Larry." I called and said, "I have to ask you this, I'm sorry." I told him what happened, and he told me that he had never touched Emily inappropriately either.

It was midnight by the time we got to Madison. As we got out of our car in front of her place, Emily's roommate Tina was just getting home. It was the only reason we got into the apartment. Because even though Emily said, "You can't come in" when we got to the door, we just walked in with Tina.

It's all still like a nightmare in my memory. There was weird lighting in the apartment, and Emily's hair was so strange, almost like a crewcut.

"What on earth is going on?" we asked.

"You know what's going on," she said. Her stance was incredibly rigid and combative.

"No, we don't know what's going on," we said. So then it was "yes you do" and "no we don't" for a little while. Emily was not going to say anything. Tina asked whether she should leave, and Emily said, "No, Tina, I want you to stay here and see this." But we were getting nowhere, and Leo said it was ridiculous and we might as well leave.

But I sat down on the couch and said, "I'm not going anywhere until I find out what is going on here." I said to her, "From what you said to me on the phone, it sounds like you think your father sexually abused you, and I supposedly knew about it and didn't do anything."

"Yesss," she hissed.

Leo: Her mother had to make the statement, and then Emily could assent to it. We think now that she was preparing for a confrontation, and we just blew her whole routine out of the water by preempting her. So her whole agenda did not flow the way *The Courage to Heal*, which sets up scenarios for this kind of thing, said it would. (In that book they also tell "incest survivors" to go to the father's place of work and force some kind of confrontation, possibly violent. Surround him, they say. If there's a wedding, you go to the wedding and hand out letters in envelopes detailing what the accused father has supposedly done to you. Same thing for funerals.)

Then I said, "Emily, you're crazy!" And Tina looked me right in the eye and said, "My roommate is not insane." Emily said, "I am not crazy — now get out of here! I'm calling the police." The whole scene was a nightmare.

Katie: As I recall things, I said, "Honey, this isn't right." She was standing across the room from me. She had actually called the police, and she handed me the phone. Someone on the line said, "This is 911 and you're going to have to leave there. There's something wrong there."

"Oh, there's nothing wrong here," I said. "I mean, there's no violence or anything." Emily started coming across the room screaming at me: "Get out! Get out!" I thought she was going to hit me — honest to God. I went to touch her cheek, and I said, "Honey, I love you." But she recoiled from me as if I were a snake. "I know something's wrong," I said. "I don't know what it is, but please get some help. We love you."

Then we did leave, but my legs gave out on me when we were on the front porch. Leo thought I had decided to wait for the police, but I said I just couldn't move. I finally did get up, and we got in the car and drove home.

Leo: What a drive that was! We didn't know what to do. When we got home, the phone was ringing and we thought, Oh God, she's committed suicide.

Katie: It was Larry, and we told him what happened. He went to Madison the next morning and was with Emily for about an hour. He said that she appeared hysterical, that she was crying the whole time. But there was no doubt in her mind that it was true: she told him she had had a tremendous flashback when she was reading *The Courage to Heal*, but she didn't go into any detail. Larry did not believe her accusations, but he said he was sure that she believed it. He was terribly torn: this was the sister he loved who was in such obvious distress and was saying such terrible things. And he knew that it couldn't possibly have happened.

The first call I made was to Donna, my clinical psychologist friend. She said, "Oh my God, you've got to talk to someone, Katie. I'll get you in to see somebody." So then we started a new nightmare of trying to figure out what had really happened. All we did was cry. We were in shock.

That Saturday or Sunday — two days later — we talked with both our families. My niece called me back the next day and said, "Aunt Kate, I think that Emily must be involved in a New Age cult." So she and her mother, my sister, gave us the name of a cult expert in Madison. And Donna (who said she did not want to get involved with it professionally because she wanted to remain a friend to me) got us an appointment with a psychologist here in Milwaukee.

Leo: So the week after we were accused, the three of us were in the office of a psychologist who was an expert on child sexual abuse. He particularly worked with people who had been through a trial and were convicted. I said to him on that first visit, "We're sure our daughter believes this happened to her. What advice do you have for us?"

"First off," he said, "Don't try to get in touch with her. Just leave her alone. She's going to misconstrue anything you try to say or do. If you must send her a card for her birthday, make it very brief: just say that the door is always open and we love you."

So we did just that. Larry said later that Emily told him she had received the card, and her reaction was, "Yeah, the door to his bedroom is always open." But we did continue to send her cards and little notes saying that our love for her was unconditional, realizing all along that whatever we sent, she would take in a hostile vein.

At the psychologist's office, I noticed *The Courage to Heal* on his file cabinet. I said, "I know our daughter's reading that book you have up there.

What do you think of it?" He said that it wasn't written by professionals but that at the end of each chapter they recommended that women go to a therapist. I had been reading the book myself, and I asked him whether I should quote it to Emily to show I was reading it and taking her seriously.

"No," he said, "let this be her discovery — her thing. Let her be in control on this." He also said to Larry (the only one Emily would talk to), "Tell her you believe that she believes. That way you will be able to keep a dialogue going with her."

I asked him whether he knew anything about "New Age," and he said he thought it had something to do with music. Somebody had shown me a copy of *Time* magazine with Shirley MacLaine on the cover and a feature article on New Age stuff, with a stack of books on the inside. That's the kind of article I wouldn't have read in a million years before this happened. But now I was devouring stuff like that to try to get a clue to Emily's behavior.

We did go back to see that psychologist with the three of us one other time, but he was not much help. So we went to Madison to see the cult person, who, it turned out, was a couple who were supposedly experts on cults and thought reform. They charged 100 bucks an hour and saw us for two hours at a time. (Incidentally, we've spent $25,000, minimum, on stuff our insurance didn't cover over the four and a half years since Emily made her accusation.) He put his hand on my shoulder and said, "I'm very sorry, your daughter has been conned." I'll never forget that.

Katie: The cult experts told us that there were some very militant feminist cult groups in Madison. One was noted for its violence; it was made up mainly of women who were actually running guns and even assassinating people. So we had an enormous amount of anxiety that our daughter had taken up with people engaged in horrible activities like the things we had read about and heard from these cult experts in Madison.

Leo: I kept saying, "*Some*thing must have happened. *Some*one must have done this to her and she's just put the wrong face on him."

Katie: And I would go crazy. I wasn't yelling at him, but I would say, "What do you mean? Would you believe it if she said it was your father's or someone else's face? This *didn't* happen!"

Leo: If I thought that she was lying about this to get at me for some reason, I would tell her not to come near me until she got her head on straight. That's not the case. Emily believes this. And what is so interesting about her rewriting her past: she is not only rewriting what and who we were as the rest of her family; she is rewriting who *she* was. She was a strong young woman; you didn't push Emily around. She would demand to know what was going on. Her uncles, aunts, and cousins, her friends — none of them could believe that *she* had succumbed to the mind games. She was a logical thinker. Of course, they emphasize again and again in this "mind warfare," it's not the airheads or spaced-out kids who get caught in this. It's the ones who supposedly were thinking for themselves.

Katie: Of course, one can't forget that "the rational" is allied with "the patriarchal," and she was getting rid of all vestiges of that. She had talked a lot about left brain/right brain stuff, about the "third eye."

Leo: Well, we devoured everything written in this subject area that we could get our hands on. Over the first year and a half to two, I averaged ten hours a day, seven days a week on basic research. And I was working full-time at the same time. Weekends were 16-hour-a-day marathons for at least a year — reading, phoning, searching all over the place. Because once you start to learn about something, you find out how much you don't know.

Katie: We were really blessed for a couple reasons. First, we were accused together; we had each other to lean on, and love, and hold up. Every night we hugged each other. I think we would have died without that. And our family stood behind us 100 percent. We were very fortunate in that. We've talked to many families where good marriages split up when the husband was accused, because the wife said, "Why would my daughter lie?" Even if your marriage was okay until your wife believed something like that, how would you put things together after that? Trust has been destroyed.

Similarly, if our daughter were to come through that door today — and we would welcome her with open arms, of course — there are simply things that would never be the same. How could her father be in the same room or the same house with her alone again?

Leo: And if we were to have a grandchild, I would never be alone with the child. I wouldn't risk it. There are certain things that are just plain changed for all time.

Katie: So we pursued the mind control direction and talked to many people, although at that point we had not found anybody else who was in the same situation we were in. We thought, maybe this is just a small cult in Madison. We felt that it was connected to the New Age bookstore where Emily worked — that and the two girls she had been hanging around with. Everything seemed to fit a New Age picture. Of course, we had no idea what would motivate somebody to send Emily in these directions. So we spent the next year or so studying all the time and trying to contact people who could give us information. We even thought about getting a deprogrammer. We almost always knew where Emily was. I became a regular detective. I would call everywhere. I had asked somebody from the Cult Awareness Network (somebody who may have worked for the CIA at one point) about hiring a detective, and he said, "Well, you can do a lot of that yourself." He told me about getting information through the phone company and other fairly simple stuff, all of which I did. Another thing he told me: keep track, document everything, because you'll find that you'll forget things.

Leo: I said, "We've got to get a different perspective on this." Poor Katie had to listen to all this — night after night. Then I'd get angry — and that could be overwhelming — angry at the fact that this could be happening in this day and age. The way we look at the witch trials at the end of the seventeenth century, that's the way people two centuries from now are going to be laughing at what is going on here . . . this witch hunt.

Katie: We'd wake up in the middle of the night — this was about three months after the accusation — and we'd talk almost all night, hardly sleep at all. Leo would be in bed for a little while; then he'd get up and sit in a chair for over an hour. He would get up four or five times a night (after a year, maybe it was down to twice a night).

I'm a heavy sleeper, and I remember waking up to see Leo in the chair just sobbing. He was crying a lot. I even got him on some medication for a while which helped him, thank God. He was on it for a few months, and he has not cried much since then. He still does, but not anything like that first few months.

Leo: Funny thing, up until a few years ago, I seldom even took an aspirin for anything. Well, I used Prozac for about three or four months and I never cried while I was on it. It was dry-up medicine.

Katie: For me, it just made it so I could get through the day, which was a blessing. Prozac is still saving my life. Sometimes I can feel my blood pressure shooting up, and I'm in a terrible way for a day or two. This has really been costing me, emotionally and physically. Leo's therapy was to sit at this dining room table for months, and when he wasn't reading, he was writing. That's how he got through it.

Leo: *The Courage to Heal* tells women to write and write, and so I figured, if it's supposed to work for trauma, I'll try it.

We ended up concluding that Emily had been seduced by a new kind of hybrid cult that would be militant feminist, lesbian, and into earth worship. That's about all we knew. The cult and thought-reform experts we talked to would say, "There are all types — they're all different, and they're popping up all over the place." Larry has kept in contact with Emily (about four times a year on average over the last four years), and all the things she has said to him led us to the conclusion that it was a militant feminist cult.

Cult experts also told us that sometimes a cult can be made up of just two or three people, that the person is sold her own cell, mentally. Many cults are very, very loose; and there are a lot of hybrids. Often there is what is called "cult-jumping": people going from one group to another to find one that suits them. Especially in a place like Madison, where there is so much oddball stuff, much of it connected with feminism. (The largest coven of witches in America is in Mount Horeb, a half hour away from Madison. But those people are really pretty benign.)

We've never been able to identify the exact group that our daughter may be in. There was one group — OWL (Oregon Women's Land) — a militant feminist, lesbian group that had us worried. We talked with a woman whose daughter was involved with that group. They had her living in a chicken coop. They were feeding their cats (which they refer to as "power animals") before her, and she almost died before they got her out. We thought this might be connected to what Emily was into — the nature thing, earth worship, etc.

Of course, every expert on thought reform and totalist belief systems would say, "Find out who they're seeing, where they live, and so forth, but most importantly, *what are they reading?* What was she reading? *The Courage to Heal,* naturally, which I firmly believe would have put Emily where she is today by itself. Add to that Sonia Johnson's *Going Out of Our Minds: The Metaphysics of Liberation.* Johnson started out heterosexual — she has two sons — but now she feels sorry for her sons because they are men. It turns out she's a lesbian and proud to be: it's the "only way you can really know love." And much of the literature that Emily was reading was all about "forming circles, going to the menstrual hut as they did in the old days of matriarchy," and so forth. So that's why we thought it was that kind of cult, though everyone we talked to said it didn't fit into any particular niche.

We also found out later that Emily had met a woman on her first trip to Alaska who had made quite an impression on her. One of Emily's friends told us later that she came back from Alaska and all she talked about was this woman she had met there. Still later, she told her brother in a phone call that she is now a lesbian. Being a lesbian would simply be a non-issue in this family. You are what you are. But I want to tell you, Emily is no more a lesbian than I am.

Katie: I feel that what happened to her was a confluence of women's studies, the environment at the feminist bookstore and the people she hung around with there, the hypnotherapist, the incest survivors' group she was going to — and mainly *The Courage to Heal.*

Emily stayed in Madison for about a year and a half after the accusation, and then she moved up to Alaska, and that's where she's been ever since. We lost her at one point, but then we found her again and now know where she is.

Our son has been able to stay in touch with her. He's done a wonderful job. He went to dinner with her within the first six months of this accusation, and said to her, "Tell me just exactly what you think it is that Dad did or Mom did." She said, "You want me to be lying on the floor screaming?" Larry would come over at times and see us sobbing (because we were so involved in our own forms of "therapy"), and he wouldn't know what to do. Poor guy. He has stood in front of one of our support groups and given a little talk about what it's like being a sibling; he took questions and did a wonderful job. We were very proud of him. We understand very well that Larry has very different feelings from ours because he had a totally different relationship with Emily. And the fact that he loves us enough to continue to try to communicate with her is very touching. If my sister had done this to my father, I don't think I'd ever forgive her.

If Emily walked back into our lives today, our friends would be kind to her for our sakes, but everything would be changed, everything different, forever now. You know that you love your child and will always love that child, but a whole level of trust has been eroded. For my part, I have been going back through Emily's life and retelling her story, the one I know to be true, as opposed to her re-creation of it.

Leo: What I'm proudest of in my life is my parenting. I was damned good at it. I don't know whether I was good at it because I liked it, or I liked it because I was good at it — but both are true. I was a scout leader, and am very good with kids. I will not go near a kid now — unless there is an adult right there. That's how my life has changed.

That's what hurts the most. I'm still a good parent: it came easy to me, and still does. Some people would say it's so difficult to be a good parent. It wasn't for me, and I still want to be. Our kids were good kids, so you could say there was luck involved. But in terms of the happiness and pride I had about how my kids turned out as adults — up to when they were eighteen and twenty-three years old, respectively — I wouldn't have written the script of their lives any differently if I could have written it myself.

Katie: That's one of the great tragedies of this. And to think that some people who are supposed to know what they're doing are still out there practicing this repressed-memory mumbo jumbo — that's almost unbearable. I really thought in the beginning that most of them were well-meaning. And I'd still like to think that the better trained people are well-meaning. It's just that when they're exposed to our side of the story and still reject us so blatantly as though we were a group of pedophiles, as several individuals and whole groups have done, I find that unconscionable. I don't know how they're able to live with themselves.

Leo: One therapist trained in hypnosis told me she stopped handing out *The Courage to Heal* to her patients when her own thirty-eight-year-old daughter accused her of molesting her as a child. Her daughter made the accusation after reading that book. This therapist told me she was doing a profound rethinking of feminism, body therapies, and hypnosis. She said she was embarrassed!

If the repressed-memory therapists who encourage their clients to produce false memories study how men who were never in Vietnam come to believe that they were, and then compare that process with the process they are using, they will understand the damage they have done and the lives they have destroyed. Some of those therapists have had the backbone to apologize and stop. The others belong in jail.

Postscript

Leo: On May first, 1995, I saw my daughter for the first time in over five years. Katie and I, Larry and his wife, and a friend of Emily got together for dinner at a local restaurant. We all made polite small talk for forty-five minutes, when Emily stood up, said "That's it," and ran out the door. We have not seen her since. I handed this letter to Emily's friend, who followed her out. A few days later, her friend told me that Emily did read the letter. I hope she saved it. I fear it is our last communication.

5/1/95

Dear Emily:

If and when you read this, we will already have had our 7 p.m. visit. Here are some of the things I hope I had a chance to say.

If you ever examine how you came to believe whatever it is you believe about your childhood and are uncomfortable and/or questioning about the process you went through, *please* do not despair or think you are alone. Mom and I will always be here for you. (Unless, of course, we croak before you call.)

I promise you I will not write, visit, phone, or fax unless you ask. Just pick up the phone and ask Larry, Bonnie, Bob, Mom or me, or any of us in your family, and we/they will wire a plane ticket, bus fare, or whatever to you. You can take a six-week, six-month, twelve-month, or however long a sabbatical you want. We or they can help you get started with a place to live, a job, education, insurance, and so forth.

I am writing a book on thought reform and could use your help. I already have a publisher, and most of the research has been done. There are so many new books, articles, and professional papers coming out every day that it makes it tough to keep up. It will be a few years before we go to press. There will be a chapter that for now I am simply calling "Emily's Chapter"; it will contain whatever you write. If you choose not to, there will simply be blank pages that you may want to fill in some other time in your life.

At one in the morning of March 16th, 1990, as your mother and I drove home from your Madison apartment, I said, "Katie, what we have just been through is life-altering, and I will use every fiber of my being for as long as I live to understand and expose whatever or whoever has taken our child from us." I will not have it! You were never abused by me or anyone in our family.

Emily, I do not like the process that has been used on you to rewrite the lives of my wife, my son, my daughter, my mother, my father, my sisters, or myself.

I miss you, I love you — and this will not change. Be well, stay in touch, and lighten up!

Dad

CHAPTER 4

The Radical Feminist Influence

Everything begins in feeling and ends in politics.

— *Charles Péguy*

Feminist consciousness is a consciousness of *victimization* . . . to come to see oneself as a victim.

— *Sandra Bartky*

In her book *Revolution from Within,* Gloria Steinem states that in the United States alone, "about 150,000 females die of anorexia each year."[1] In her best-selling book *The Beauty Myth,* Naomi Wolf cites the same figure and states that this huge number of young women is being "starved not by nature but by men." Likening the death toll from eating disorders to the Holocaust, Wolf says that "women must claim anorexia as political damage done to us by a social order that considers our destruction insignificant . . . as Jews identify the death camps."[2] Wolf and Steinem got the death toll figure from *Fasting Girls,* a book in which the author, Joan Jacobs Brumberg,

1. Steinem, *Revolution from Within: A Book of Self-Esteem* (Boston: Little, Brown, 1992), p. 222.
2. Wolf, *The Beauty Myth: How Images of Beauty Are Used against Women* (Garden City, NY: Doubleday, 1992), pp. 207-8.

says that she and other women studying eating disorders are seeking "to demonstrate that these disorders are an inevitable consequence of a misogynist society that demeans women . . . by objectifying their bodies."[3]

Some feminist publications have claimed that as many as 75 to 90 percent of young women suffering from anorexia and bulimia were sexually abused as children. One is left to infer that childhood sexual abuse indirectly causes vast numbers of deaths — more than three times the number of fatalities from car accidents for the total population per annum — by producing lethal eating disorders.

As it turns out, however, these figures are completely unsubstantiated. Actual documented evidence indicates that in America the average annual death rate from anorexia during the past decade was less than one hundred, and it has been declining rather than increasing through the period.[4] On August 11, 1994, Connie Chung's TV news magazine program *Eye to Eye* reported on this and other bits of misinformation that have appeared in radical feminist literature and subsequently have been picked up and repeated by the popular media to the point that they are now being widely cited without question. Chung's guest, Christina Hoff Sommers, exploded three specific myths.

1. The figure of 150,000 annual anorexia deaths cited by Brumberg, Steinem, and Wolf and subsequently repeated in an Ann Landers column and many other places (including in textbooks currently used in college classrooms) is off by a factor of more than a thousand. The National Center of Health recorded 101 such deaths in 1983, 67 deaths in 1988, and 54 deaths in 1991. There is nothing like the epidemic being claimed by the radical feminists. Steinem and Wolf have promised to remove this statistic from future editions of their books, but they have not yet publicly acknowledged that the figure is in fact wrong. What they have done is to denounce Sommers as a traitor to the feminist cause. They charge that, by setting the record straight, Sommers effectively reduced the public's concern about the seriousness of eating disorders. The implication seems to be that the public would be better served by the dissemination of falsehoods that support a more appropriate point of view on the issue.

2. On February 23, 1993, Patricia Ireland, president of the National Organization for Women, told a national audience on PBS's Charlie Rose

---

3. Brumberg, *Fasting Girls: The Emergence of Anorexia Nervosa as a Modern Disease* (Cambridge: Harvard University Press, 1988), pp. 19-20.

4. See Christina Hoff Sommers, *Who Stole Feminism? How Women Have Betrayed Women* (New York: Simon & Schuster, 1994), p. 12.

show that physical abuse of pregnant women was the primary cause of birth defects in the United States. Ireland was repeating a statistic that she apparently got from the Women's Studies Electronic Bulletin Board. On November 4, 1992, Deborah Louis, president of the National Women's Studies Association, had posted the following message on the bulletin board: "According to the last March of Dimes report, domestic violence (vs. pregnant women) is now responsible for more birth defects than all other causes combined." Having received Ireland's endorsement, the statistic was subsequently cited in many major publications, including *Time* magazine, the *Boston Globe,* the *Chicago Tribune,* and the *Dallas Morning News.* When Sommers called the March of Dimes to check the accuracy of the statistic, she was told that the organization had never seen such research before. Later a March of Dimes spokesperson characterized it as a rumor "spinning out of control," noting that governors' offices, state health departments, and Washington politicians were flooding her office with calls. The March of Dimes asked *Time* to set the record straight, but a retraction did not appear until December 6, 1993, almost a full year after the original story had run.

The false statistic was later traced back to a domestic abuse advocate at Harvard Law School who said she had misinterpreted a report from a March of Dimes representative. The original report had actually contained nothing at all linking domestic abuse with birth defects. Nevertheless, the statistic was soon circulating through feminist channels — and far beyond — as fact. "Why was everybody so credulous?" asks Sommers. "Battery responsible for more birth defects than *all* other causes combined? More than genetic disorders such as spina bifida, Down syndrome, Tay-Sachs, sickle-cell anemia? More than congenital heart disorders? More than alcohol, crack, or AIDS — more than all these things *combined?* Where were the fact-checkers, the editors, the skeptical journalists?"[5]

3. In January 1993, newspapers and television networks reported that the incidence of men battering women rose by 40 percent on Super Bowl Sunday. Pundits were quick to highlight the link between the national testosterone fest and violence against women. Nancy Isaac, a Harvard School of Public Health research associate, told the *Boston Globe,* "It's a day for men to revel in their maleness and unfortunately, for a lot of men that includes being violent toward women if they want to be."[6]

But Ken Ringle, a reporter for the *Washington Post,* discovered that

5. Sommers, *Who Stole Feminism?* pp. 14-15.
6. Isaac, quoted in *Boston Globe,* 29 January 1993, p. 16.

this statistic was unfounded, too. A little research into police records indicated that on average no more domestic violence was reported on Super Bowl Sunday than on any other day of the year.[7] Once again, an unsubstantiated assertion was given credibility through repetition in the popular media and entered the culture as fact. Sommers contends that these false statistics are "typical of the quality of information we are getting on many women's issues from feminist researchers, women's advocates, and journalists." Time and again, a search for corroborating evidence raises "grave questions about credibility, not to speak of objectivity."[8]

Setting aside the issue of how these false statistics first come to be reported, it is understandable that, once established, they would be embraced by proponents of RMT. They obviously affirm the ideological presuppositions of such individuals, and we are all inclined to embrace evidence that supports our view of the world. Recall how, in the preceding chapter, Emily criticized her family for loving football. This was one more bit of evidence affirming her view of things over against theirs. Many radical feminists believe that Western culture is essentially and exhaustively misogynist, and so they expect to hear statistics like those cited above and are not inclined to question them.

We get into another area altogether, though, when partisans go beyond endorsing their own point of view and undertake efforts to subvert other points of view. At the end of her *Eye to Eye* broadcast, Connie Chung felt duty-bound to report that Gloria Steinem, Patricia Ireland, and Naomi Wolf, having caught wind of the subject of the program before it was shown, all tried to convince her not to air the material. Chung was clearly uncomfortable, even distressed, reporting these attempts to call off the broadcast. Steinem, Ireland, and Wolf had argued that it "would do women no good" to refute the false statistics, implying that it would set the women's movement back. People who are willing to ignore the truth and overlook lies in order to promote a message are by definition nothing more than propagandists.

A significant group of radical feminists promotes the view that Western culture is endemically patriarchal and not only condones but encourages violence by men against women as a means of exercising and maintaining their position of superiority. These feminist ideologues insist that acts of brutality against women such as rape and domestic assault are part of the fabric and legacy of Western culture — indeed, the logical ex-

---

7. *Washington Post*, 31 January 1993, p. A1.
8. Sommers, *Who Stole Feminism?* p. 15.

tension of the Judaeo-Christian tradition — rather than the aberrant behavior of individual criminals and misfits. They dismiss as irrelevant or
disingenuous the tradition's explicit condemnations of the mistreatment of
women and children and its explicit calls for their protection. In support
of their belief, some feminists have asserted that men are generically and
innately evil and that women are generically and innately good, the innocent victims of men's will to power. They reject the thesis that both genders
harbor hostility and engage in violence. Some go so far as to insist that all
heterosexual relationships are pathological and demeaning if not dangerous
to women. Catharine MacKinnon, for example, has stated that "what in the
liberal view looks like love and romance looks a lot like hatred, a torture
to the feminist. Pleasure and eroticism become violation . . . admiration of
natural physical beauty becomes objectification."[9] They deny the validity
of crime statistics indicating that only 3 percent of households report
domestic violence, and they ignore statistics indicating that violence occurs
in lesbian and gay male relationships at the same rate as or at a greater rate
than it does in heterosexual relationships.

Can lies advance the cause of women? Does it serve a valid purpose
to compare the death toll from anorexia to that of the Holocaust? Wolf,
Steinem, Ireland, and Brumberg apparently feel justified in using such
strategies to bolster their assertions that "men, not nature," are starving
young women to death, that we live in a "misogynist society that demeans
women." Sommers has characterized their mind-set this way:

> American feminism is currently dominated by a group of women who
> seek to persuade the public that American women are not the free crea-
> tures we think we are. The leaders and theorists of the women's move-
> ment believe that our society is best described as a patriarchy, a "male
> hegemony," a "sex/gender system" in which the dominant gender works
> to keep women cowering and submissive. The feminists who hold this
> divisive view of our social and political reality believe we are in a gender
> war, and they are eager to disseminate stories of atrocity that are designed
> to alert women to their plight. The "gender feminists" (as I shall call
> them) believe that all our institutions, from the state to the family to the
> grade schools, perpetuate male dominance. . . . To confound the skeptics
> and persuade the undecided, the gender feminists are constantly on the
> lookout for proof, for the smoking gun, the telling fact that will drive
> home to the public how profoundly the system is rigged against women.

9. MacKinnon, *Toward a Feminist Theory of the State* (Cambridge: Harvard University
Press, 1989), p. 198.

To rally women to their cause, it is not enough to remind us that many brutal and selfish men harm women. They must persuade us that the system itself sanctions male brutality. They must convince us that the oppression of women, sustained from generation to generation, is a structural feature of our society.[10]

Not surprisingly, gender feminists have found a cause célèbre in the issue of childhood sexual abuse. Many view such abuse as the quintessential expression of the sort of brutal mistreatment that women routinely receive in an oppressively patriarchal culture. Moreover, the issue provides an effective bridge to the sympathies of the larger culture. Mainstream America may not be prepared to endorse much of the radical feminist program, but virtually everyone agrees that the sexual abuse of children is abhorrent. To the extent that feminists combat such abuse, their efforts are more broadly endorsed. Unfortunately, there is evidence that some authors have made inflated claims about the frequency of the molestation of young girls on the order of the inflated figures for eating disorders. Furthermore, the altogether appropriate condemnation of child abuse has been politicized in many ways and in some cases made hostage to larger agendas. For example, Harvard psychiatrist Judith Herman, one of the most visible and vocal proponents of repressed-memory therapy, has argued that "the study of trauma in sexual and domestic life becomes legitimate only in a context that challenges the subordination of women and children. Advances in the field occur only when they are supported by a political movement powerful enough to legitimate an alliance between investigators and patients and to counteract the ordinary social processes of silencing and denial." She goes on to define this "political movement" as "a collective feminist project of reinventing the basic concepts of normal development and abnormal psychology."[11] In effect, she is saying that we cannot lay claim to being genuinely concerned about child abuse unless we are willing to accept her ideology.

Given this politicization of the issue, it is becoming increasingly difficult to conduct any sort of practical discussion of child abuse. Many radical feminists staunchly endorse the dictum that children never lie and that allegations of sex abuse must never be questioned. Many cite questionable statistics in support of the view that *all* men constitute a serious threat to children and women. It must be acknowledged that some women adopt

10. Sommers, *Who Stole Feminism?* p. 16.
11. Herman, *Trauma and Recovery* (New York: Basic Books, 1992), pp. 9, ix.

views of this sort on the basis of personal experience, having themselves been subjected to cruel abuse in childhood at the hands of their fathers and/or other men. But while this explains the phenomenon, it does not validate it. Charges that half the human race is in fact subhuman and that child abuse is epidemic serve only to divide people unnecessarily and create an atmosphere in which false and mistaken accusations will proliferate.

The Rise of the New Radical Feminism

In every great movement for social change, the pioneers are perceived by the status quo as radical. Early feminists were pilloried for seeking the right to vote. During the 1960s and early 1970s, prominent feminists were considered radical for leading the drive for equal opportunity and compensation in the workplace and a greater degree of self-determination in reproductive decisions. Always diverse, the women's movement has broadened yet further during the past few decades to include a considerable variety of emphases and ideological points of view. There are significant differences of opinion among feminists about what the goals of the movement should be and what strategies should be used to attain them. Disagreements among various factions have made it more difficult than ever to achieve any consensus on who the leaders of the movement actually are. An argument could be made, however, that the most visible leadership roles have fallen to a comparatively small group of radical feminists including the likes of Andrea Dworkin, Catharine MacKinnon, and Susan Faludi, who are now denouncing such longtime feminist luminaries as Betty Friedan, Joan Didion, and Germaine Greer for failing to endorse a new, more astringent feminist orthodoxy. This new radical fringe (it must be fringe if it is drumming out the likes of Friedan and Greer) seems to have developed an influence far out of proportion to its numbers, largely because it has chosen to focus its attention on the realms of academia and public policy (the latter typically by way of the former). And it is largely by way of the academic realm that this new radical feminism has also established significant connections with RMT.

One of the key defining characteristics of the new radical feminists I have in mind here is an essential divisiveness in their view of the sexes: they characterize *all* males in our culture as oppressors and *all* females as victims of male oppression. Some go so far as to postulate a genetic predisposition on the part of men to evil and a genetic predisposition on the part of women to virtue. Robin Morgan has attributed "sexism, racism, hunger, war, and ecological disaster" to "the Man's competitiveness and greed."[12] Susan Brownmiller has defined rape as "a conscious process of fear and intimidation by which all men keep all women in a state of fear."[13] Some maintain that the reality of collective male guilt renders the issue of individual guilt irrelevant. Marilyn French, for example, has asserted that

> as long as some men use physical force to subjugate females, *all* men need not. The knowledge that some men do suffices to threaten all women. Beyond that, it is not necessary to beat up a woman to beat her down. A man can simply refuse to hire women in well-paid jobs, extract as much or more work from women than men but pay them less, or treat women disrespectfully at home. He can fail to support a child he has engendered, demand the woman he lives with wait on him like a servant. He can beat or kill the woman he claims to love; he can rape women, whether mate, acquaintance, or stranger; he can rape or sexually molest his daughters, nieces, stepchildren, or the children of a woman he claims to love. *The vast majority of men in the world do one or more of the above.*[14]

One begins to detect here some echoes of RMT rhetoric: childhood molestation is a lot more common than you have been led to believe; the vast majority of men in the world are up to something along these lines, so you have every reason to suspect that you may have been abused, whatever the initial clarity of your recollections. In her book *Going Out of Our Minds,* a staple in feminist bookstores and gender courses, Sonia Johnson more pointedly insists that in our male-dominated culture, "incest is not only encouraged, it is insisted upon; not just condoned but blessed. . . . It is an institution of patriarchy — like the church, like the law: absolutely necessary to maintaining male privilege and power."[15] In another book influential in gender studies circles, *The Great Cosmic Mother,* Monica Sjoo and Barbara Mor similarly assert that rape is a "culturally mandated" form of punishment for women who will not accept the taboos of a patriarchal culture.[16] And Catharine MacKinnon essentially classifies every female sexual experience in every context as abusive:

---

12. Morgan, *Going Too Far* (New York: Random House, 1978), p. 93.

13. Brownmiller, *Against Our Will* (New York: Simon & Schuster, 1975), p. 16.

14. French, *The War against Women* (New York: Summit Books, 1992), p. 182.

15. Johnson, *Going Out of Our Minds: The Metaphysics of Liberation* (Freedom, CA: Crossing Press, 1987).

16. Sjoo and Mor, *The Great Cosmic Mother: Rediscovering the Religion of the Earth* (San Francisco: Harper & Row, 1987), p. 151.

If one believes women's accounts of sexual use and abuse by men; if the pervasiveness of male sexual violence against women substantiated in these studies is not denied, minimized, or excepted as deviant or episodic; if the fact that only 7.8 percent of women in the U.S. are not sexually assaulted or harassed in their lifetimes is considered not ignorable or inconsequential; if the women to whom it happens are not considered expendable; if violation of women is understood as sexualized on some level — then sexuality itself can no longer be regarded as unimplicated. . . . The male sexual role, this information and analysis taken together suggests, centers on aggressive intrusion on those with less power. Such acts of dominance are experienced as sexually arousing, as sex itself. They therefore are. . . .

To be clear: what is sexual is what gives a man an erection. . . . Whatever else does this, fear does, hostility does, hatred does, the helplessness of a child or a student or an infantilized or restrained or vulnerable woman does, revulsion does, death does. . . . All this suggests that what is called sexuality is the dynamic of control by which male dominance — in forms that range from intimate to institutional, from a look to a rape — eroticizes and thus defines man and woman, gender identity and sexual pleasure. It is also that which maintains and defines male supremacy as a political system.[17]

In fact, MacKinnon believes the male influence to be so invasive in our culture that it leaves its mark even on sexual relationships in which men are not physically involved. "Some have argued," she writes, "that lesbian sexuality — meaning here simply women having sex with women, not with men — solves the problem of gender by eliminating men from women's voluntary sexual encounters. Yet women's sexuality remains constructed under conditions of male supremacy: women remain socially defined as women in relation to men; the definition of women as men's inferiors remains sexual even if not heterosexual, whether men are present at the time or not."[18]

Andrea Dworkin, one of the most prominent and aggressive of the radical feminists, has a similarly bleak view of male-female relationships in a patriarchal culture, as we see in this representative passage from her book *Intercourse:*

Violation is a synonym for intercourse. . . . Intercourse occurs in a context of a power relation that is pervasive and incontrovertible. . . . Be-

---

17. MacKinnon, *Toward a Feminist Theory of the State*, pp. 127, 137.
18. MacKinnon, *Toward a Feminist Theory of the State*, pp. 141-42.

cause of their power over us, [men] are able to strike our hearts dead with contempt or condescension. We need their money; intercourse is frequently how we get it. We need their approval to be able to survive inside our own skins; intercourse is frequently how we get it. They force us to be compliant, turn us into parasites, then hate us for not letting go.[19]

Throughout her writings, Dworkin preaches an essential antagonism between the sexes and a relentlessly dark view of men. "Men are rapists, batterers, plunderers, killers," she says.[20] Moreover, "Becoming a man requires that the boy learn to be indifferent to the fate of women. Indifference requires that the boy learn to experience women as objects."[21] And, she writes, "Men hate intelligence in women. . . . Girls are taught in order to make them compliant: intellectual adventurousness is drained, punished, ridiculed out of girls. . . . To the orthodox of male culture, [woman] is animal, the antithesis of soul. . . . The price of exercising creative intelligence for those born female is unspeakable suffering."[22]

Dworkin's bombast is typical of much of the new radical feminist literature. It is drawn almost exclusively in shades of black and white. There is no spectrum, no gradation, no qualification of the absolutes. All men are indifferent to the fate of women. All men hate intelligence in women. All men are rapists, batterers, plunderers, killers. Rhetoric of this sort effectively puts an end to any further communication between the sexes on the issue. What response can a man make when he is literally asked, "When did you stop beating your wife?" In the spring of 1993, female students at the University of Maryland put up posters all over campus with pictures of male students and this message: "Notice: These men are potential rapists." The male students pictured on the wanted posters had no history of date rape or abuse or of being especially objectionable in *any* sense; the female students had simply selected their names at random from the university directory. Presumably they did this with a clear conscience, out of a sincere conviction that all men are at the very least *potential* rapists. That's the party line.

---

19. Dworkin, *Intercourse* (New York: Free Press, 1987), pp. 122-27.

20. Dworkin, *Pornography: Men Possessing Women* (New York: E. P. Dutton, 1989), p. 49.

21. Dworkin, *Pornography*, p. 48.

22. Dworkin, "The Politics of Intelligence," in *Ethics: A Feminist Reader*, ed. Elizabeth Frazer, Jennifer Hornsby, and Sabina Lovibond (Cambridge: Blackwell, 1992), pp. 102, 106, 108, 113.

Revisioning the Family

Given the degree to which the new radical feminists have demonized men, it is quite understandable that they tend to take a dim view of marriage and the traditional family. What could one conceivably find to bless in the union of evil and innocence, after all? "Marriage is an institution developed from rape as a practice," says Dworkin. "No honest woman can live in marriage: no woman honest in her will to be free. Marriage delivers her body to another to use; and there is no basis for self-respect in this carnal arrangement, however sanctified it may be by church and state."[23]

Historically, the family has been inextricably bound up with a host of other social institutions and with traditional sexual roles, and as a result it has been a target of criticism for feminists since the beginnings of the movement. Betty Friedan once asked Simone de Beauvoir if she didn't think that women should have the option to stay home and raise children if that's what they wanted to do. "No," de Beauvoir responded, "we don't believe that women should have this choice. No woman should be authorized to stay at home to raise her children. Society should be totally different. Women should not have that choice, precisely because if there is such a choice, too many women will make that one."[24] Generally speaking, however, the movement has gone beyond this sort of doctrinaire thinking to embrace the idea that women should indeed have the freedom to build whatever kinds of lives they want.

But while American society in general has been singing the praises of the traditional two-parent family a lot in recent years — as witness the attempts on the part of both of the two major political parties to capitalize on "family values" issues during the past few major elections — many feminists have remained critical. At the height of public interest in the O. J. Simpson, Lorena Bobbitt, and Lyle and Erik Menendez trials in 1994, Barbara Ehrenreich took a shot at traditional family values in a *Time* magazine essay. Her basic thesis was that Americans were fascinated with these trials because they laid bare in lurid ways a truth we all recognize "at some deep, queasy Freudian level" — namely, that the families we profess to love can turn out to be lethally dysfunctional. "Only with the occasional celebrity crime," she writes, "do we allow ourselves to think the nearly unthinkable: that the family may not be the ideal and perfect living arrangement after

23. Dworkin, *Pornography,* pp. 19, 121.
24. De Beauvoir, quoted by Betty Friedan in *Saturday Review,* 14 June 1975. The quotation is from *The Second Sex.*

all — that it can be a nest of pathology and a cradle of gruesome violence." However inclined we may be to think of home as a stronghold of love and nurture in a cruel world, the fact remains, she insists, that "for a woman, home is, statistically speaking, the most dangerous place to be. Her worst enemies and potential killers are not strangers but lovers, husbands and those who claimed to love her once. Similarly, for every child like Polly Klaas who is killed by a deranged criminal on parole, dozens are abused and murdered by their own relatives. Home is all too often where the small and weak fear to lie down and shut their eyes."[25]

Whatever the validity of Ehrenreich's assessment of the family, it is shared by a significant segment of feminists today — even those who have chosen to promote their agenda under the rubric of "family issues." We can see indications of the spread of this point of view in *The Hite Report on the Family: Growing Up under Patriarchy.* The book, which author Shere Hite describes as an attempt to show "how the family has been a repressive, authoritarian institution for too long," makes little pretense of being a serious scientific study. Its conclusions are based on responses to anonymous surveys solicited from magazine readers, student groups, feminist groups, and the like. These self-selected listener opinion polls — SLOPs in the pollsters' jargon — are commonly understood to have little more than entertainment value; no social scientist of any standing takes them seriously. But even if Hite's findings don't give us any sense of the extent to which the reported opinions have pervaded our society in general, they can at least serve to give us a sense of some of the opinions that are holding sway in the responding groups. In general, the respondents to Hite's questionnaire believed, among other things, that (1) there are benefits for the majority of children living in single-parent families, (2) it is better for children to grow up in an atmosphere that is not "poisoned by gender inequality," (3) many people who flee the nuclear family do so for valid reasons, and (4) nontraditional families may be healthier than traditional families.

These are, of course, all matters of continuing debate. The degree to which we perceive the family to be "a nest of pathology and a cradle of gruesome violence" will depend on what we believe about the nature of men and women, what they are capable of, and what sorts of behavior they are actually engaging in on a regular basis. What statistics do we believe to be valid, and how do we interpret them? Citing established government-reported crimes figures, Stephen Chapman has questioned radical feminist claims that domestic abuse is epidemic in America. "About 3 percent of

25. Ehrenreich, "Oh, Those Family Values," *Time,* 18 July 1994, p. 62.

women living with men in America suffer a violent domestic incident during any given year," Chapman reported, "which means that 97 percent don't. Seeing violence as endemic to family life is like seeing airplane crashes as the essence of commercial aviation. It is very much the exception."[26] But radical feminists don't trust government statistics, and they have statistics of their own to cite.

This matter of perception is very important when it comes to evaluating the claims that arise out of RMT, because sooner or later in that therapeutic process, everyone has to face a difficult question: Is it credible that the accused individual was actually capable of committing such abuse? Is it credible that these "recovered memories" are actually genuine? The authors of contemporary radical feminist literature have no difficulty answering such questions. Of course it's credible. All men are rapists (or at the very least potential rapists). All families are pathological associations. Abuse is common, even culturally mandated. It's happening everywhere, and there's every likelihood that it happened to you. The National Organization of Women has gone on record endorsing the idea that "incest within the family is a direct outgrowth of the traditional patriarchal view that women and children are a man's property and that it is a male prerogative to abuse family members."

As we can see in this book's narratives, many of the lost daughters have embraced the works of Dworkin, MacKinnon, Bartky, and the like. Many college-age women are being introduced to RMT through women's study groups, feminist literature classes, rape survival groups, and similar contexts in which these books are read as gospel. Indeed, radical feminist literature has so dominated the reading lists of certain disciplines in American universities for the past twenty to twenty-five years that a whole generation of educated young women has come to view it as *the* literature of feminism. Even though on average the views of these young women tend to be more moderate than those of the authors they are reading, many have come to view the radical feminists as true pioneers, trailblazers in a movement to which they are personally indebted. They feel an implicit obligation to give credence to these views. At a minimum they are inclined to accept as fact the host of statistics presented in these books — statistics that, as we have seen, often show up in the mainstream media as well, even when they are acknowledged by the authors to be false and misleading. In a number of

26. Chapman, "Concern for Family Provokes Backlash from Some Feminists," *Chicago Tribune*, 24 July 1994, sect. 4, p. 3.

ways, then, this literature exerts a force on many women's perceptions of self, society, and relationships between the sexes.

The views of radical feminists have entered mainstream culture in other ways as well, such as the widely publicized views of the comedienne Roseanne. The *New Yorker* recently validated Roseanne's status as a popular feminist icon not only by doing a feature on her but also by making her a celebrity consultant for a special issue on women. "Can this be?" asked *New York Times* columnist Maureen Dowd.

> The magazine of Dorothy Parker and Hannah Arendt joining forces with the boorish TV star who urges women to kill bad husbands and children to kill bad parents? . . .
>
> There is something disagreeable about turning this Rabelaisian back-lot brat into a feminist ideal.
>
> Roseanne stands for things that self-respecting women should disdain: Tyrannical behavior, lording it over the help, disguising a love of power as a love of equality.
>
> She equates all criticism with misogyny. She takes on the guise of victimhood when it suits her. She promotes herself as a tribune of blue-collar women, while she lives the profligate, plastic-surgeried life of a spoiled star.
>
> Even her humor is a religion of grudges.[27]

A good part of Roseanne's credentials as a feminist are based on her assertion that she was sexually abused by her parents. She claims to recall details of abuse dating back to when she was just six months old (an age from which memory experts agree no genuine memories survive in any-one). Her parents and siblings both deny that anything of the kind ever happened, and there is no sort of evidence apart from her accusations that it ever did.

Given her fondness for over-the-top rhetoric (e.g., "I think women should be more violent, kill more of their husbands"), few would probably accord Roseanne the status of mainstream model for American women or of a spokeswoman for feminist ideals. Still, the popularity of her television series and her appearances on the talk-show circuit have made her influen-tial way out of proportion to the merit or cogency of her sentiments. And, perhaps in hopes of attracting more public interest in their own views and concerns, some public feminists have been quick to canonize her. *New*

---

27. Dowd, "Please, Don't Hold up Boorish Roseanne as the Feminist Ideal," *Chicago Tribune*, 4 September 1995, sect. 1, p. 11.

Yorker editor Tina Brown does not belong to the ranks of radical feminists, but she professed to be inspired by Roseanne's "embodiment of the gargantuan woman's experience," and she ratified and promoted the celebrity's radical eruptions by showcasing them in the pages of her magazine.

Radical feminists pointedly set out to change women's perceptions of men and the family, but it may well be that they have effected changes of a more lasting and significant nature by influencing the ways in which women view themselves. By arguing that women in a patriarchal society are relentlessly bombarded on all sides by threats to their well-being, radical feminists have fostered a growing sense of victimhood in many women, a kind of siege mentality that some feminists have suggested is as crippling as the sexism that underlies it.

The Emergence of a Sense of Victimhood

In an essay entitled "Sexual Terrorism," Carole Sheffield describes an "ordinary" event that she experienced early one evening in a laundromat. She was alone in the brightly lit building, and her car was the only one in the lot. "Anyone passing by could readily see that I was alone and isolated. Knowing that rape is a crime of opportunity, I became terrified." She left her clothes in the machine and ran back to the security of her car, where she sat with the doors locked and the windows up.

> When the wash was completed, I dashed in, threw the clothes into the dryer, and ran back out to my car. When the clothes were dry, I tossed them recklessly into the basket and hurriedly drove away to fold them in the security of my home. Although I was not victimized in a direct, physical way or by objective or measurable standards, I felt victimized. It was, for me, a terrifying experience. . . . Mostly I was angry at being unfree: a hostage of a culture that, for the most part, encourages violence against females, instructs men in the methodology of sexual violence, and provides them with ready justification for their violence. . . . Following my experience at the Laundromat, I talked with my students about terrorization.[28]

We have here a good example of the power of perception. Most of us, men and women alike, would probably experience some degree of

---

28. Sheffield, "Sexual Terrorism," in *Women: A Feminist Perspective*, ed. Jo Freeman (Mountain View, CA: Mayfield, 1989), p. 4.

anxiety if we were the sole occupant of a laundromat in a tough neighbor-hood at night. Depending on our assessment of the threat, we might feel anything from edginess to terror, as Sheffield did. Most of us would at the very least feel vulnerable, and to that extent victimized: the criminals have robbed us of our freedom even to wash our clothes in peace when and where we wish. Moreover, I think most of us would acknowledge that a woman would rightly feel herself to be at greater risk than a man in such a context, properly apprehensive about the possibility of sexual assault, among other things. But when Sheffield asserts that the real danger she faced in the laundromat came from "a culture that, for the most part, encourages violence against females, instructs men in the methodology of sexual violence, and provides them with ready justification for their vi-olence," she is clearly no longer giving voice to concerns that most people would feel in this context. This is ideological rhetoric; some might call it paranoia. And it feeds on itself. I think we can safely assume that Sheffield already felt like a hostage of a patriarchal culture when she entered the laundromat, but it seems clear that the terror she experienced there served to heighten her convictions in that regard, to confirm in her own mind the validity of her beliefs about the culture. And then she proceeded to pass her fear and anger along to her students and others. Sheffield's essay is the first selection in an anthology entitled *Women: A Feminist Perspective,* which is said to be the best-selling women's studies textbook of all time. Persuading women that they are oppressed and victimized often appears to be the first step in the new radical feminist consciousness-raising.

In recent years, the biggest disagreement between mainstream femi-nists and the new radical feminists involves the degree to which women can be said to have been victimized and rendered powerless in our society. New feminist writers such as Susan Faludi (sometimes calling themselves the "third wave") say that women are victimized and held powerless by a male cabal of "backlashers" with a premeditated design to keep women down. Older feminists such as Betty Friedan and Elizabeth Fox-Genovese see a different picture: they say that North American women have come a long way in a generation. Christina Hoff Sommers has argued that many of today's new feminists, "women who are all free and protected by law, many of them privileged," and many of them either students or teachers in institutions of higher learning that now boast more female than male students, are preoccupied with their sense of vulnerability and hurt. They speak of their privileged lives as a state of siege. "When they speak of their personal plight they use words appropriate to the tragic plight of many American women of a bygone day and of millions of contemporary, truly oppressed women in other countries," says Sommers. "Their resentful rhetoric discredits the American women's movement today and seriously distorts its priorities." Sommers pointed out to one of these new feminists, a young woman still in college, that she and her friends were among the world's most privileged people. The young woman responded, "We still suffer psychological oppression. If you feel like the whole world is on top of you, then it is."[29]

Once again, we see the key role played by perception here: the sentiment seems to be that if I feel that something is true, then it is true. This has important implications for our understanding of the dynamics of RMT, especially given the close relationship between RMT and gender feminism. We will do well to take a closer look at the sense of victimization that many of the new radical feminists are experiencing in the areas of rape, domestic violence, pornography, and sexual harassment.

Rape

The new radical feminists regularly characterize American society and Western culture as a "rape culture." Specific figures for the prevalence of rape are difficult to assemble with any accuracy for a number of reasons, including significant differences of opinion about what sorts of acts constitute rape and the reluctance of many women to report any such incidents. In 1990, the FBI recorded 102,560 rapes or attempted rapes in America, and the Bureau of Justice came up with an estimate of 130,000 — but these included only *reported* crimes. A Harris poll of women for the same period suggested that the actual number of rapes was about three times the reported number — 380,000. Figures supplied by the National Victim Center for 1990 almost doubled that number again, to 683,000. Generally speaking, however, gender feminists tend to set the figures much higher still. For example, whereas the U.S. Justice Department estimates that 8 percent of all American women will be raped in their lifetimes, Catharine MacKinnon contends that, "by conservative definition, [rape] happens to almost half of all women at least once in their lives."[30]

Perhaps because radical feminism is strongest in academic settings, rape activists have evidenced a special concern about sexual violence and "date rape" on college campuses. Some assert that the crimes have reached epidemic

29. Sommers, *Who Stole Feminism?* p. 47.
30. MacKinnon, "Sexuality, Pornography, and Method," *Ethics* 99 (January 1989): 331.

proportions. Responding to stories of an outbreak of rape at Columbia University, Peter Hellman, a reporter for *New York* magazine, went there to do a story on the subject. He found no evidence of a crisis. The Columbia security police had reported only two rapes in all of 1990. National figures for 1990 indicated fewer than a thousand reported rapes on campuses in the entire country — on average, less than one rape for every two campuses that year.[31] Writer Katie Roiphe conducted a study similar to Hellman's at Princeton University and found that campus police reports showed only two rapes during the entire decade between 1982 and 1993. The statistics indicated that male students were more frequently victims of violence than were females.[32] Wendy Kaminer has suggested that the term "date rape," like the term "addiction," no longer has much literal or objective meaning. It tends to be used figuratively, as a metaphor signifying that all heterosexual encounters are inherently abusive of women, a popularized form of the Dworkin-MacKinnon dogma that in a male-dominated culture that has "normalized" rape, yes can never really mean yes.[33]

Whatever the source of the crisis mentality, I believe Sommers is right when she says that the "findings being cited in support of an 'epidemic' of campus rape are the products of advocacy research."[34] Probably the most-cited source for figures in this area is the Ms. Magazine Campus Project on Sexual Assault, a study conducted in 1985 by Mary P. Koss, a professor of psychology at the University of Arizona. Working with a broad definition of rape, Koss concluded that 15.4 percent of college-age respondents had been raped and 12.1 percent had been victims of attempted rape, making a total of 27.5 percent who had been victimized by sexual assault. But many researchers have questioned Koss's methodology and conclusions in the study. For one thing, Koss admits that the majority of the women who were classified as having been raped did not themselves believe that they had been raped. In fact, only 27 percent of the women so classified characterized themselves as rape victims. (Of the remaining 73 percent, half said that the incident Koss had classified as rape was actually a matter of "miscommunication," 14 percent said it was a "crime but not rape," and 11 percent said they didn't "feel victimized.") Thus, by Koss's own admission, only 27 percent of the original 27.5 percent — about 7.4 percent of all the respon-

31. Hellman, "Crying Rape: The Politics of Date Rape on Campus," *New York*, 8 March 1993, pp. 32-37.
32. Roiphe, *The Morning After: Sex, Fear, and Feminism* (Boston: Little, Brown, 1993), p. 45.
33. Kaminer, "Feminism's Identity Crisis," *Atlantic Monthly*, October 1993, p. 67.
34. Sommers, *Who Stole Feminism?* p. 222.

dents in the study — actually believed they were victims of rape or at-tempted rape. And, beyond that, we must bear in mind that the study was based on self-reporting respondents (answering ten questions on a survey) — that is, it was based on how these women *felt* about what happened to them rather than on objective evidence. And, for what it's worth, Koss also found in follow-up interviews that 42 percent of the women she counted as rape victims subsequently had consensual sex with the men who they originally said had raped them.[35]

Despite all these caveats to the Koss study, which have repeatedly been pointed out by other rape researchers and by Koss herself, the initial figure of 27.5 percent reported in *Ms.* — "one in four," as the battle cry goes — has been accepted as the official statistic almost everywhere. It commonly appears in date-rape brochures handed out to first-year students at colleges and universities, for instance, and has been cited regularly by politicians from Democrat Senator Joseph Biden to Republican Congressman Jim Ramstad in support of legislation such as the Violence against Women Act of 1993, which allocated $20 million in federal funds to combat rape on college campuses.

There is a huge disparity between public funds designated for rape crisis centers on campuses and for centers in the nation's inner cities, where statistics indicate that most rapes actually occur. "There were three rapes at the University of Minnesota in 1992; in New York City there were almost 3,000," notes Sommers. "The University of Minnesota has a rape crisis hot line, but New York City does not." She attributes the disparity not to insensitive politicians but to shortsighted activists: "The dispropor-tionate and ever-growing share of the scarce public resources allocated for rape prevention underscores how disproportionately powerful and self-preoccupied the campus feminists are despite all their vaunted concern for 'women' writ large."[36]

Many studies of rape victimization have been conducted in the wake of the Koss study, but those finding lower figures have tended to receive a good deal less notice in the press. A 1993 Harris poll found that only 2 percent of the respondents indicated that they had "been a victim of rape or sexual assault" during the previous five years. Margaret Gordon of the University of Washington produced similar findings in a separate study:

35. The Koss study is summarized by Robin Warshaw in *I Never Called It Rape* (New York: HarperPerennial, 1988), published by the Ms. Foundation. For more on the study, see Sommers, *Who Stole Feminism?* pp. 210-15.

36. Sommers, *Who Stole Feminism?* p. 221.

about 2 percent of respondents reported having been raped. In addition to garnering little interest in these findings among the popular media, Gordon encountered criticism from rape activists for reporting them at all. "There was some pressure — at least I felt pressure — to have rape be as prevalent as possible. . . . I'm a pretty strong feminist, but one of the things I was fighting was that the really avid feminists were trying to get me to say that things were worse than they really are."[37]

Given the convictions of gender feminists that Western culture is endemically misogynist, a "rape culture," it is understandable that they would be inclined to accept and defend the highest estimates of the incidence of rape in our nation. And, given differences of opinion about the definition of rape and the percentage of sexual assaults that go unreported, it is not likely that we will ever achieve a consensus on the extent to which their numbers are exaggerated. There is one area, however, in which an objective assessment clearly shows that their ideology has led them to some false conclusions. Susan Faludi, for example, has asserted that the "highest rate of rapes appears in cultures that have the highest degree of gender inequality, where sexes are segregated at work, that have patriarchal religions, that celebrate all-male sporting and hunting rituals, i.e., a society such as us." The evidence suggests otherwise. The incidence of rape actually tends to be far lower in cultures that are far more patriarchal than North America. As Sommers points out,

> American society is exceptionally violent, and the violence is not specifi- cally patriarchal or misogynist. According to *International Crime Rates,* a report from the U.S. Department of Justice, "Crimes of violence (hom- icide, rape, and robbery) are four to nine times more frequent in the United States than they are in Europe. The U.S. crime rate for rape was . . . roughly seven times higher than the average for Europe." The inci- dence of rape is many times lower in such countries as Greece, Portugal, or Japan — countries far more overtly patriarchal than ours. . . . The international studies on violence suggest that patriarchy is not the pri- mary cause of rape but that rape, along with other crimes against the person, is caused by whatever it is that makes our society among the most violent of the so-called advanced nations.[38]

Those who are invested in exaggerated statistics of sexual abuse are increasingly vicious in denouncing researchers who produce contradictory findings. Katie Roiphe has been called a "traitor who has sold out to the

---

37. Gordon, "The Making of an Epidemic," *Blade,* October 1992, p. 3.
38. Sommers, *Who Stole Feminism?* p. 223.

white male patriarchy." Neil Gilbert, a long-time rape researcher who had the temerity to question the "one in four" dictum in a critical analysis, has been targeted for demonstrations and denunciations. Students on the Berkeley campus where he teaches chanted "Cut it out or cut it off" and carried signs reading KILL NEIL GILBERT! A date-rape "clearinghouse" in San Francisco has been set up with the sole purpose of refuting and attacking Gilbert. On most college campuses today, victims of date rape are joining "survivor groups" along with women who believe themselves to be incest survivors. Thus many additional women are being motivated to explore the possibility that they, too, were abused in childhood. In this highly politicized atmosphere, people inevitably develop strong feelings, and they are being encouraged to believe that if they feel something is true, then it *is* true, regardless of any evidence to the contrary. It is just the sort of context in which we would expect RMT to thrive.

Domestic Violence

Feminists have long been concerned about forms of abuse in addition to rape to which women are disproportionately subject as well. Gender feminists tend to argue that domestic battery is the most common variety of such abuse. Their basic argument is that men use physical violence in the home, as they use rape outside the home, to terrorize women and keep them in a constant state of fear. "Patriarchy *requires* violence or the subliminal threat of violence in order to maintain itself," says Gloria Steinem. "The most dangerous situation for a woman is not an unknown man in the street, or even the enemy in wartime, but a husband or lover in the isolation of their own home."[39]

Because domestic violence tends to be underreported, and because determinations of what constitutes this sort of abuse vary widely, there is a fair amount of disagreement about just how prevalent such violence actually is. Here is a cross section of estimates:

- 626,000 women are assaulted by intimates in the United States annually — U.S. Department of Justice
- 1.8 million women are physically assaulted by their husbands or boyfriends each year — *Behind Closed Doors: Violence in the American Family*

39. Steinem, *Revolution from Within*, pp. 259-61.

- 3 million women are battered annually — Sen. Joseph Biden, 1991
- 4 million women are affected by domestic violence, reported and unreported, each year — Senator Biden's staff report, 1992
- 3 to 4 million women are brutally beaten each year in the U.S. — *Feminist Dictionary*
- 6 million wives are abused by their husbands annually — *Time*, 5 September 1993
- 8 to 12 million women a year are assaulted by their partners — Clarence Page, *Chicago Tribune*, 2 June 1996
- More than 50 percent of all women will experience some form of violence from their spouses during marriage, and more than one third are battered repeatedly every year — National Coalition Against Domestic Violence.

Excluding the Justice Department figure, since it does not include any estimate of *unreported* domestic assaults, we still have a vast range of numbers here, the differences scaling by more than a factor of ten. Part of the disparity can be attributed to the different sorts of abuse being described: abuse, physical assault, battery, brutal beating, repeated assaults. But there are genuine differences about the extent of the overall problem in these numbers. The last figure — the NCADV's assertion that more than one-third of all married women in America, a total of more than eighteen million women, are repeatedly battered every year — is the most dramatic. By any standards, that would indeed constitute an epidemic of domestic violence. Are all these numbers valid?

Richard J. Gelles and Murray A. Straus have been studying domestic violence for more than twenty-five years, and within the scientific community their research is among the most respected in the country. Their work was also highly regarded by feminist activists for many years, although more recently it has come under increasing criticism from radical feminists who contend that it does not accurately indicate the severity of the problem. Part of the reason that Gelles and Straus have reported figures that are lower than other sources is that they have tended to make more distinctions concerning levels of violence. As Christina Hoff Sommers notes in an extended discussion of their work,

They distinguish between minor violence, such as throwing objects, pushing, shoving, and slapping (no injuries, no serious intimidation), and severe violence, such as kicking, hitting or trying to hit with an object, hitting with fist, beating up, and threatening with a gun or knife —

94

actions that have a high probability of leading to injury or are accompanied by the serious threat of injury. The vast majority of family disputes involve minor violence rather than severe violence. In the 1985 Second National Family Violence Survey, sponsored by the National Institute of Mental Health, they found that 16 percent of couples were violent — the "Saturday Night Brawlers" (with the wife just as likely as the husband to slap, grab, shove, or throw things). In 3 to 4 percent of couples, there was at least one act of severe violence by the husband against the wife. But in their surveys they also found that "women assault their partners at about the same rate as men assault their partners. This applies to both minor and severe assaults."

Gelles and Straus are careful to say that women are far more likely to be injured and to need medical care. But overall, the percentage of women who are injured seriously enough to need medical care is still relatively small compared to the inflated claims of the gender feminists and politicians — *fewer than 1 percent*. Murray Straus estimates that approximately 100,000 women per year are victims of the severe kinds of violence shown in the TV film *The Burning Bed*. That is a shockingly high number of victims, but it is far short of Senator Biden's claim, derived from feminist advocacy studies, that more than three or four million women are victims of "horrifying violence."[40]

Using the same questions that Gelles and Straus had used in their national survey in 1975 and 1985, the Commonwealth Fund and Louis Harris conducted a phone survey of 2,500 women in 1993. They got basically the same results as Gelles and Straus did, but they interpreted the results in a way that made them sound a good deal more like the higher numbers reported elsewhere. The pollsters got a 34 percent positive response to the first two questions on their survey (Did your partner in the last 12 months [1] insult you or swear at you; or [2] stomp out of the room or house or yard), and the report classified all these respondents, representing 20.7 million American women (34 percent of the approximately 55 million women married or living with someone as a couple) as victims of "emotional and verbal abuse." (Since Gelles and Straus have always found that women are just as likely to engage in those activities as are men, we

---

40. Sommers, *Who Stole Feminism?* pp. 194-95. The Gelles and Straus conclusions can be found in *Physical Violence in American Families* (New Brunswick, NJ: Transaction Publishers, 1990) and *Intimate Violence: The Causes and Consequences of Abuse in the American Family* (New York: Touchstone, 1989).

should presumably conclude that an equal number of men suffered abuse at this level during the same period.)

Having received a 5 percent positive response to a question about whether their partner "pushed, grabbed, shoved, or slapped you" (which Gelles and Straus did not classify as severe abuse), the Commonwealth Fund concluded that 3.9 million women are "physically assaulted" every year. This figure, interpreted as such, was widely reported in newspapers around the country, including the *Wall Street Journal*, the *Washington Post*, the *Detroit News*, and the *San Francisco Chronicle*. The Gelles-Straus research found this level of violence in approximately 15 percent of all relationships — and, once again, it found that men are as likely to be recipients of this sort of assault as women.

Perhaps the most interesting responses to the poll involved the level of violence that Gelles and Straus classified as severe. The questions were, "Has your partner (8) beat you up? (9) choked you? (10) threatened you with a knife or gun? (11) used a knife or gun?" Of the 2,500 respondents to the Harris/Commonwealth survey sample, not one person acknowledged experiencing this level of assault. The Gelles-Straus research indicated that violence of this sort occurs in less than 1 percent of domestic relationships. "This finding does not, of course, mean that no one was brutally attacked," says Sommers. "But it does suggest that severe violence is relatively rare. . . . Clearly the interpreters of the Harris/Commonwealth poll data were operating with a much wider conception of 'abuse' than Gelles and Straus."[41]

Many people appear to be interpreting the basic data broadly. A number of different sources, including government agencies, the American Medical Association, and the popular media seem to have settled on the estimate of 4 million physical assaults on women by intimates annually in America. But many of these sources are implying if not directly asserting that these are 4 million *severe* physical assaults, whereas the results of the Harris/Commonwealth survey and the Gelles-Straus studies both indicate that the severe category of assaults accounts for only 2.5 percent of the total 4 million.

In pointing all this out, I am by no means attempting to downplay the gravity of domestic abuse. It is a scandal that 100,000 women are being severely beaten every year in an ostensibly civilized nation. The point I want to get at, though, is that different groups are interpreting the data on domestic violence in different ways on the basis of their perceptions of what the world is really like. It is quite understandable that a gender feminist, convinced that she lives in a patriarchal culture that mandates violence by

41. Sommers, *Who Stole Feminism?* p. 197.

96

men against women, will be inclined to accept and endorse higher estimates of the prevalence of such violence. But when groups such as the National Coalition Against Domestic Violence promote the idea that America is in the grip of an epidemic of spousal abuse in which one third of all married women are repeatedly battered each year, they are helping to instill in the minds of many women a level of fear, suspicion, and rancor that is not warranted. Those who are convinced that huge numbers of women fall victim to violence at the hands of men who ostensibly love them and that we as a nation are deeply in denial about the problem will naturally find it easier to accept the idea that significant numbers of women were abused as children and that they may have repressed all memories of such abuse.

I should also note in passing one reason to question the assumption of many radical feminists that violence against women and children can be attributed to a patriarchal mind-set, that men use violence as a tool to subjugate women and children both inside and outside the home. If that were the case, one would expect to see lower levels of domestic abuse in gay and lesbian relationships. But in the past few years evidence to the contrary has appeared in mainstream publications including *U.S. News & World Report* and *Time* and books such as Claire Renzetti's *Violent Betrayal: Partner Abuse in Lesbian Relationships*. These sources have reported that the frequency of violence is at least as high in intimate lesbian and gay male relationships as in heterosexual relationships — and this includes the whole range of abuse from verbal threats and insults to stabbings, shootings, and sexual violence, including rape. Two large centers for domestic violence victims in San Francisco, Communities United Against Violence and the Women's Domestic Abuse Shelter, have reported a huge caseload of homosexual domestic violence cases, and the gay directors of these centers admit that the phenomenon is very much underreported. Already feeling itself under siege by the AIDS epidemic and the activities of conservative politicians, the gay community apparently doesn't want to expose itself to attack on another flank. Nevertheless, the lesbian director of the Women's Domestic Abuse Center said that the large reported incidence of domestic abuse in the lesbian community has caused her to rethink the whole issue of domestic violence.[42] There is increasing reason to believe that in many cases battery has very little to do with patriarchy or gender bias. As Sommers has put it, "Where noncriminals are involved, battery seems to be a pathology of intimacy, as frequent among gays as among straight people."[43]

42. Interview on Minnesota Public Radio broadcast 15 April 1996.
43. Sommers, *Who Stole Feminism?* p. 200.

Pornography

Although they probably have little else in common, Andrea Dworkin and Ed Meese share the distinction of having gotten involved in well-publicized campaigns against pornography. The partnership between radical feminists and political and religious conservatives in the battle against pornography is more striking from a distance than close up, however: these confederates are approaching the issue from decidedly different angles and promoting decidedly different agendas. Meese's 1986 Commission on Pornography was a part of the Reagan administration's vaunted attempts to stem the tide of moral decay in America. Dworkin's efforts are aimed at halting the degradation of women and putting an end to what she believes is one of the chief causes of sexual assault on women.

Catharine MacKinnon, who has worked closely with Dworkin in a number of national and local efforts to draft legislation outlawing pornography, offers a representative argument on this issue when she says that "men treat women as who they see women as being [and] pornography constructs who that is. Men's power over women means that the way men see women defines who women can be. Pornography is that way. . . . It is not a distortion, reflection, projection, expression, fantasy, representation or symbol, either. It is a sexual reality."[44] The essential problem, according to Dworkin and MacKinnon, is that men exercise comprehensive and ruthless control over women as objects; the specific problem with pornography, they say, is that it is the chief means by which men develop their understanding of the nature and role of men and women in their world. Dworkin and MacKinnon are convinced that pornography teaches men to disregard the essential humanity of women and encourages them to be abusive in their relationships to the point of sexual assault and murder. Because of the importance and pervasiveness that MacKinnon assigns to pornography, she characterizes the world as an essentially "pornographic place."

> Pornographers' consumers make decisions every day over women's employment and educational opportunities. They decide how women will be hired, advanced, what we are worth being paid, what our grades are, whether to give us credit, whether to publish our work. . . . They raise and teach our children and man our police forces and speak from our

44. MacKinnon, quoted by Pete Hamill in "Woman on the Verge of a Legal Breakdown," *Playboy*, January 1993, p. 140.

pulpits and write our news and our songs and our laws, telling us what women are and what girls can be. Pornography is their Dr. Spock, their Bible, their Constitution.[45]

One observer has suggested that assertions of this sort belie "an almost clinically paranoid view of reality (try substituting 'communists' or 'Jews' for 'pornographers' consumers')."[46] These assertions have alarmed many within the women's movement as well. In 1984, several prominent feminists, including Betty Friedan, Rita Mae Brown, and Adrienne Rich, formed an organization called the Feminists Against Censorship Taskforce (FACT) to oppose the point of view being promoted by Dworkin and MacKinnon on this specific issue. And when FACT went to court to challenge an Indianapolis antipornography ordinance that Dworkin and MacKinnon had helped to write, the organization was joined by the Women's Legal Defense Fund, law professor Susan Estridge, battered women's advocate Susan Schechter, and other well-known feminists. The FACT coalition maintained that the threat to freedom of speech implicit in the legislation far outweighed the threat to women posed by the sorts of pornography it sought to restrict. MacKinnon denounced them all: "The labor movement had its scabs, the slavery movement had its Uncle Toms, and we have FACT." Elsewhere she described women who had differed with her on this issue as "house niggers who sided with their masters."[47]

It will not serve our purposes here to rehearse the arguments over pornography any further. Suffice it to say that many aspects of the issue remain a matter of hot debate — including the degree to which pornography pervades our society and the degree to which it affects male behavior, including specific links between exposure to pornography and sexual assaults on women. My interest once again is in the way in which radical feminist thought on this issue feeds into an overarching sense of the victimhood of women in our culture. Dworkin and MacKinnon paint the picture of a world in which all men construct their understanding of sexual relationships and gender roles from pornography, in which all women are oppressed by a male conspiracy to render them powerless and submissive. Women who accept the thesis that all men are sexual monsters will naturally be more receptive to the tenets of RMT.

---

45. MacKinnon, quoted in "Woman on the Verge of a Legal Breakdown," p. 185.
46. Hamill, "Woman on the Verge of a Legal Breakdown," p. 185.
47. MacKinnon, quoted in "Woman on the Verge of a Legal Breakdown," p. 186.

Sexual Harassment

The Clarence Thomas Supreme Court hearings helped sensitize many Americans to the realities of sexual harassment. It was the first time that many people found out what sorts of behavior count as sexual harassment. Any person who has power over another in the workplace (or comparable settings, such as the classroom) and uses that power to get dates, procure sex, press unwanted intimacies, or the like is guilty of sexual harassment. I think most Americans would agree that behavior of this sort is simply wrong and that it should be punished. On the other hand, I think most would agree that it is possible that people of good conscience might disagree about whether sexual harassment has occurred in a given situation, particularly if the only evidence available is the testimony of the involved parties. But beyond this, there are also some significant differences of opinion about what sorts of behavior should be considered unacceptable. There is a growing number of cases in which radical feminists are contending that men should be punished for behavior that most other people would consider benign. I will cite just two cases.

At Chicago Theological Seminary, Graydon Snyder, a professor of New Testament and former dean, told a story from the Talmud, the Jewish book of laws, a story he has used as an illustration for thirty-four years of teaching. In the story, a man falls from a roof into the arms of a woman, and they accidentally have sexual intercourse. The Talmud uses the story to illustrate the idea of intentional acts, and Snyder used it to illustrate the difference between Talmudic wisdom and what Jesus advocated in the Sermon on the Mount. But the last time Snyder told the story in class, one of his female students accused him of sexual harassment for having done so. The seminary put Snyder on probation for "engaging in verbal conduct of a sexual nature" and warned him that he could be fired; he was also told that he had to undergo psychotherapy and take sexual harassment workshops, and he was advised not to meet alone with any student or staff member.[48]

The distinguished poet and novelist Stephen Dobyns was sued for sexual harassment after he was alleged to have used "salty language" outside the classroom. His friend and colleague Francine Prose described the hearing:

48. Adrienne Drell, "Bible Scholar Sues to Fight Taint of Sex Harrassment," *Chicago Sun-Times,* 25 March 1994, p. 5.

There was much talk of protecting women from blunt mentions of sex. And the young women who testified were in obvious need of protection. They gulped, trembled and wept. . . . Victorian damsels in distress, they used 19th-century language: They had been "shattered" by his rude, "brutish" behavior. . . .

Are these the modern women feminists had in mind? Victorian girls, Puritan girls, crusading against dirty thoughts and loose speech? I thought of all the salty words I have used in class — words that could apparently cost me my job. . . .

Soon after the hearing, [Dobyns] was informed that he had been found guilty of making five sexually harassing remarks. The committee recommended that he be suspended from his job without pay for two years, banned from campus except to use the library, required to perform 200 hours of community service and to pay one of his accusers $600 to compensate for the wages she lost because of the mental suffering he caused her.[49]

I will grant that it is almost always possible to find some anecdotal evidence to discredit a position, but that is not my intent here. The point I want to make is that the mind-set behind the charges of sexual harassment in these two cases and others like them is consistent with the radical feminist perspective I have been describing throughout this chapter. Implicit in these accusations is the belief that whatever makes a woman *feel* bad is wrong — in these cases, criminally wrong. And, since different things make different people feel bad, there is no way of clearly defining what constitutes harassment. Not only is the category of genuine crimes diminished by trivial charges, but everyone's freedoms are diminished when we stand under threat of reprisals for unintended offenses. It is understandable that gender feminists would pursue charges of this sort first of all in academic settings, since that is their stronghold — but it is nonetheless regrettable that they are starting there, because their success in that arena can be especially destructive to essential freedoms. As Prose puts it, "Feminists, academics, intellectuals — those who stand to lose the most from restrictions of free expression — are ignoring the possible consequences of the precedent they are setting."[50]

49. Prose, "Bad Behavior," *New York Times Magazine,* 26 November 1995, p. 36.
50. Prose, "Bad Behavior," p. 36.

Postscript

In a telling essay in the *Atlantic Monthly*, Wendy Kaminer offers a thorough-going analysis of the movement of the new feminism in the direction of victimhood:

> Vying for power [in the feminist world] today are poststructuralists (dominant in academia in recent years), political feminists (office-holders and lobbyists), different-voice feminists, separatist feminists, pacifist feminists, lesbian feminists, careerist feminists, liberal feminists (who tend also to be political feminists), anti-porn feminists, eco-feminists, and womanists. . . . New Age feminists and goddess worshipers widen the array of alternative truths. And the newest category of feminism, personal-development feminism, led nominally by Gloria Steinem, puts a popular feminist spin on deadeningly familiar messages about recovering from addiction and abuse, liberating one's inner child, and restoring one's self-esteem.
>
> The marriage of feminism and the phenomenally popular recovery movement is arguably the most disturbing (and potentially influential) development in the feminist movement today. It's based partly on a shared concern about child abuse, nominally a left-wing analogue to right-wing anxiety about the family. There's an emerging alliance of anti-pornography and anti-violence feminists with therapists who diagnose and treat child abuse. . . . Gloria Steinem has blithely praised the important work of therapists in this field without even a nod to the potential for, well, abuse when unhappy, suggestible people who are angry at their parents are exposed to suggestive hypnotic techniques designed to uncover their histories of victimization.
>
> But the involvement of some feminists in the memory-retrieval industry is only one manifestation of a broader ideological threat posed to feminism by the recovery movement. Recovery, with its absurdly broad definitions of addiction and abuse, encourages people to feel fragile and helpless. Parental insensitivity is classed as child abuse, along with parental violence, because all suffering is said to be equal (meaning entirely subjective); but that's appropriate only if all people are so terribly weak that a cross word inevitably has the destructive force of a blow. Put very simply, women need a feminist movement that makes them feel strong. . . . [But] victimism is likely to become an important organizing tool for feminism in the 1990s.[51]

51. Kaminer, "Feminism's Identity Crisis," p. 66.

102

Are the radical new feminists oblivious to ways in which they are helping to make women feel vulnerable instead of strong, the ways in which they are encouraging young women like Kristin and Emily of the preceding narratives — women who are among the most privileged people in the world — to feel oppressed and at risk? Certainly they are making it difficult to discuss this issue. As Kaminer notes,

> in some feminist circles it is heresy to suggest that there are degrees of suffering and oppression, which need to be kept in perspective. It is heresy to suggest that being raped by your date may not be as traumatic or terrifying as being raped by a stranger who breaks into your bedroom in the middle of the night. It is heresy to suggest that a woman who has to listen to her colleagues tell stupid sexist jokes has a lesser grievance than a woman who is physically accosted by her superior. It is heresy, in general, to question the testimony of self-proclaimed victims of date rape or harassment, as it is heresy in a twelve-step program to question claims of abuse.[52]

Among those who are convinced that oppression and suffering of women are woven into the fabric of all human relationships, the conviction of an all-encompassing victimization of women begins to look very much like religion, a controlling belief system. People who question that belief system — regardless of their credentials as feminists in other contexts — are typically vilified as everything from "right-wing conservatives" to "clandestine perpetrators." The classic response of the true believer to those who question their assertions regarding rape, domestic abuse, sexual harassment, and so forth is that they are "in denial," a charge against which there is no effective defense. Some go further and contend that anyone who questions an article of their faith must be guilty of oppressing women in some specific way; a man who questions the ultimate reliability of RMT, for example, is often charged on that evidence with being the sort of person who wants to molest young girls. This kind of reaction is nothing new. It goes back to the witch hunts in the sixteenth and seventeenth centuries, when the greatest heresy was to question the existence of witches and to say that innocent people were being executed solely because they were *thought* to be witches. The charge in itself was enough to get one branded as a witch. As it was then, questioning a true believer's claims today can amount to a self-indictment.

I have tried to point out some of the ways in which the emerging sense of victimhood among radical feminists has helped to create an en-

52. Kaminer, "Feminism's Identity Crisis," p. 67.

vironment in which RMT could take root and attain credibility. Sadly for many of those involved, RMT also serves to reinforce this sense of victim-hood. RMT therapists typically warn their clients that recovering their repressed memories will be an unpleasant process but that, for their own good, they will just have to ride out the storm. But, as Frederick Crews notes, "For too many women the storm doesn't end, or else it ends all too abruptly in suicide. And even in the best cases, a 'survivor' is coached to reject the happiest actual memories of her childhood as being inconsistent with the stark truth of molestation. The result is a lasting sacrifice of resilience, security of identity, humor, capacity to show affection, and con-nection to the *people who have cared most steadily about this woman's hap-piness.*"[53] RMT is supposed to lead to healing, but it almost inevitably destroys the lives of the clients *and* those who love them most.

---

53. Crews, *The Memory Wars: Freud's Legacy in Dispute* (New York: New York Review of Books, 1995), p. 198; italics in original.

CHAPTER 5

Susan

We had arrived in Anycity on the previous afternoon after a six-hour flight from our home. This was our seventh holiday visit to Susan and Steve's home, a pattern begun before they had their first child. As in past years, the weeks before our flight had been bustling with happy conspiratorial coast-to-coast phone calls about secrets for presents and plans for our two grandsons.

An unusual winter storm had disrupted the ordinarily mild Anycity winter with bitter cold and dangerous icy roads, but it was warm and wonderful to hug and kiss everyone. Susan seemed thinner than when I had seen her in October and she seemed tense, but this was a very busy time for her. Emotions run high in most families at holiday times. I was soon alternating between the playroom, where five-year-old Bobby was watching Sesame Street, and the living room, where I could be generally grandmother-foolish with two-year-old Paul and at the same time try to converse a little with Susan as she cooked dinner.

There was the normal dinner talk that brought us up to date on news and gossip not important enough for phone calls. After dinner, Alex helped Bobby put together a potato clock we had brought, and I pretended to be a dog, a cat, and a sheep until little Paul turned red with laughter. But Alex and I were tired and soon left to get ready for sleep. As she usually did, our daughter had left presents for us from the boys on our bed — drawings that they had made. We were a close family in so many ways.

Still on our usual Eastern time zone sleep hours, I awoke early in the morning, in time to see Susan stumbling out of the house carrying two-year-old Paul. "He was sick during the night," she said. "I'm taking him to the doctor." The phone call from our son-in-law, Steve, came to the house a few hours later.

"We lied," Steve said. "We're not at the doctor's office. We're at a friend's home. We want you to leave our house and fly home. We've made reservations on the 3:30 flight. The taxi will arrive in an hour and a half. Susan now remembers that she was seriously abused as a child by Alex."

Steve delivered that terrible message unemotionally over the telephone at 9:30 a.m. on Friday, December 21, 1990. No explanation, no justification, no details, no offer of joint counseling — just our exit visas. Neither our daughter nor her husband has looked at me or spoken to me since those stinging words accusing Alex of serious abuse and ordering us to leave their house. That has been as painful as the expulsion from their home and the accusation, because Susan and I shared so much of our ordinary day-to-day lives. For a few months we continued to communicate using e-mail, the communication mode of academics in the nineties, but our letters all focused on abuse — her belief and my lack of belief in her revelation. She has cut off any contact I might have with my grandsons Bobby and Paul.

My husband Alex and I have only just begun to overcome the heartache, the anxiety, the shame, and the confusion enough to be able to share our story with a few people. "How do you cope?" we are inevitably asked. Every day has been hard and nothing has been resolved. Perhaps the most haunting question has been, "How could this have happened?" I have read and reread my letters to and from Susan, trying to understand something, anything, about how this could have happened.

What Were We Supposed to Have Done?

Nothing else in my life has ever had so many "worst parts." So much that has happened seems so unnecessary. I don't suppose there is really any nice way to accuse your father of incest, but the cruel, dramatic, gestapo-like techniques that included our trip across the continent, the surprise accusation, the ostracism, and the lack of details set in motion reactions that have made dealing with the revelation more difficult.

"My therapist suggested that I ask you and Dad not to come visit," our daughter wrote later, "but I couldn't bring myself to do that." What kind of professional advice had she been getting? I thought that therapists were supposed to help patients work to determine their own minds, not put them in conflict by suggesting that they do something contrary. Could a conflict between what she wanted and what her therapist expected have caused Susan to act in such an unnatural and cruel way?

Alex and I clung to each other to keep our hearts from breaking, too shocked to cry. We had arrived without a clue as to what was about to happen. We packed our bags and again negotiated the perils of the icy Anycity roads, of holiday crowds and airline overbookings, to get to the safety of our home. In retrospect, the chill and storm were a fitting backdrop for our own chilling experience.

Should we have left Anycity? But who would want to stay where they were not wanted? What should we do next? After such humiliating treatment, how could we ever speak to Susan and Steve again?

Reason and love dictated that something was obviously deeply wrong with Susan and her husband. We had had thirty-three years of love and affection from Susan, too much love to let pride shut us off after a single incident. We had too much concern for her well-being at a time when a complete and sudden switch in her behavior seemed to reflect some kind of nervous breakdown, a fact recognized by Steve in a letter weeks later. We didn't even know what we were supposed to have done. "Serious abuse" must certainly mean sexual abuse.

Susan had been really stressed by the earthquake of 1989 while they were living in San Francisco. She was also struggling between the pressures of career and motherhood, and I knew she had had some fundamental problems in her marriage because she had confided in me a year earlier. Steve was very unhappy in his job and resented Susan's impulsive decision to make the move to Anycity in order to get her early tenure. Perhaps Steve was so quick to accept something as horrible as this story of childhood abuse because for him it could explain his dislocation from the job he loved and the town where he had family. Surely this confusion would be corrected quickly. I sent Susan an e-mail message and she responded.

December 22

Dear Susan,
　　I love you. I hope that we can keep some communication going.

December 23

Dear Susan,
　　I'm glad that we can write. I love you. I cannot deal with your memories — because I don't know what they are. We have been accused of

something, but I could hardly go to a therapist, as you ask, without knowing what the details are. What is supposed to have happened? You asked me to tell you about your teachers in elementary school. . . .

December 24

Susan, you have made serious charges against us. I don't have the slightest idea what you are upset about enough to have initiated this crisis. I don't know where to begin to do what you ask and see a therapist like yours, who is a young clinical psychologist, a female, and a specialist in sex abuse. I don't know if your memories are from the time of nursery school or later. You are going to have to tell us specifically what you remember. We are devastated by the accusations and by being thrown out of your house.

We went through Christmas in a surreal holding pattern. There seemed nowhere to turn. The library was closed. Doctors were away on vacation. A wonderful friend came when we called, and we survived. Could there be anything worse than having a child you have loved and cared for accuse you of abusing her? Her death perhaps. Her suicide certainly. Our daughter wasn't dead. There was hope. I still felt in my heart that this had to be some kind of horrible mistake.

December 27

Dear Susan,

I do not doubt that you have painful memories, but I do not remember you ever being abused by Alex. What do you remember? I have no desire to deny any truth as you claim. You asked me to write about my own childhood. . . .

December 28

I thought that you should know that we finally have heard some specifics of the charges. Your grandmother told me. You think you were sexually abused by Alex. Why could you tell her and not us? Perhaps, by analogy, you can understand where I am. It is as inconceivable to me that this could be true as it would be to you that Steve would do such a thing to Bobby and Paul.

We do love you deeply. Please understand that. We understand that you are hurting terribly. The depth of your pain can be judged by the fact that you were willing to throw away our relationship on the basis of a vague memory that occurred after a suggestive probe by your therapist, rather than act in any way that would leave doors open.

Susan

Our hearts are heavy because we feel that there is nothing we can do or say that is going to make a difference. . . .

Doubt finds fertile soil in confusion and ignorance, and so doubts sprouted in my mind. Maybe something did happen to Susan and she had transferred that memory to Alex. Susan had done lots of experimenting with drugs when she was a teenager. Could that have caused memory confusion? Could Alex have a side to him that I didn't know about? No, that wasn't possible. I have known this person since he was nine years old. But why would anyone make up such a horrible accusation? How could I have been unaware of sexual abuse? What had really happened? What was Alex supposed to have done?

December 29

Dear Susan,

We are struggling to understand. As you asked us to do, we are reading *The Courage to Heal*. We have been searching our souls and our pasts. We have an appointment with a therapist next week. But we don't know what we have done.

You may be right, perhaps my last message sounded as though I were closing doors. I don't want to do that. But I could not bear to see my grandchildren as I last saw them with their mother secreting them out so that there could be no good-bye.

You asked about what I remember of the years when you were in nursery school and we lived in New York City. . . .

December 30

Dear Susan,

All we have wanted to do is help. We have felt so cut off and in the dark and hurt. Alex said on the plane coming home, "If I take sodium pent, will that get at the truth, will that help?" We haven't had a clue of where to begin. You have given us some information in your last letter. Maybe something happened in our family that we have repressed. I hope not, but we will certainly try to find out.

I don't happen to agree with you that the past is an enormous tragedy. I have found joy in most of my life and am proud of overcoming the problems. I count myself unbelievably fortunate that I have had Alex and you to accept my love. I count myself fortunate that you have been an intelligent, kind, and beautiful person. I hardly know anyone who has not been thrown some curve balls.

109

You don't have a history of inflicting pain. You have been wonderfully supportive of us. We love you. That is why what has been happening has been such a confusing mystery to us. From my perspective there are so many things that do not add up. There are some things that seem so very inconsistent to me. When you share with us what you know, perhaps we will be better able to help you.

Susan, you asked why Alex has not contacted you after you evicted him and accused him of abuse. Why do you think that Alex should be the one to initiate contact with you?

Susan did initiate contact with Alex, and they wrote many letters to each other. She reported that she felt confused by the contrast of her memories and her feelings of love for Alex. She complained that she didn't think he was proud of her. As she had with me, she delved into details of his childhood. Why this fascination with our childhoods? It was months before I understood that "the notion of intergenerational transmission of violence has become the premier development hypothesis in the field of abuse and neglect," even though longitudinal research has shown that the vast majority of children who are abused do not go on to repeat the offenses. Our daughter decided that Alex and I had been abused and that therefore her abuse must have happened.

New Year's Eve brought with it our wedding anniversary. We kept our long-planned dinner engagement. We did not tell our younger dinner companions what had happened. They would hate us, I thought. We could not tell them. Exercising the human spirit to endure, we put aside the madness and chatted about other things. It was a joy to be distracted for a few hours. Clearly, it was going to be important to maintain some part of life that didn't involve this insanity.

Who Would Believe Us?

The problem, of course, with accusations of sexual abuse is that the accused person is assumed to be guilty. It's like the old joking rhetorical question, "When did you stop beating your wife?" How do you prove a negative? We live in a country in which people are supposed to be assumed innocent until proven guilty, but that is not the case with sexual abuse. Even the legal system has changed on this highly charged subject — changed but at the same time neglecting to provide any mechanisms for the change. Many people find these changes dangerous and alarming. That's why groups like

Victims of Child Abuse Laws (VOCAL) have formed. I was lucky, I thought, that I had a previous relationship with a wise and respected psychiatrist who already knew much about me. It wouldn't seem so shameful to talk to him. I was lucky, I thought, that we had the financial and educational resources to find qualified support.

As I have since learned, however, revelations of sexual abuse made many years after the fact are considered by some sex abuse therapists to be common in just such successful families. "He or she [the adult victim of child abuse] is likely to have pursued a higher education and to be successful in the professional or business world, often holding a very responsible job. Frequently, the person will be married and have children who may also appear to be well adjusted and asymptomatic." Isn't there something inherently puzzling in this? Doesn't sex abuse cut across class, economic, and professional distinctions? If abuse is more frequent in successful families, why do the data show increased abuse in times of economic downtrends? Perhaps only people from successful families have "revelations." Are revelations of past sexual abuse only for the privileged and the educated? That seems hard to believe.

Alex and I had had our share of problems in the past. Alex's drinking had increased over the years, but at my pressure he had stopped a decade ago. That history didn't lessen the anxiety before we went to our early morning appointment. We were well aware of the connections between alcoholism and abuse. "Will the therapist believe me?" Alex asked. "When I met with him ten years ago, I assured him that there was no abuse of any kind," I replied. But what did our story look like? We couldn't give any details. All we could say was that we had been expelled from Anycity and that Alex had been accused of some sort of sexual abuse, but we didn't know what. The fact that such an accusation was actually made, even if false, must be evidence of some terrible family trouble.

January 3

Dear Susan,

As a child you were one of the most adventurous and exploratory and energetic human beings I have ever met. You were also one of the most trusting. Our guiding philosophy, if you can call it that, was to try to provide environments in which those qualities could be nurtured, but environments in which you would be safe. Raising a child who was a teenager in the culture of the sixties was not the easiest of tasks. I worried more than you can ever understand, and I had so many conflicts between my own conservative beliefs and the ambient culture or counterculture pressures about what probably led to future happiness. You know how I disapproved of your taking drugs, and you told me how old-fashioned I was when you embarked upon your sexual explorations with a variety of partners. Yet, all in all, we felt we had an easier time than most of our peers. Valedictorian of your class in addition to completing high school in three years — your explorations seemed within the bounds of the time and did not seem to hurt you.

The therapist listened. He probed. He empathized. He was obviously distressed by our situation. He was supportive. We should come back in a week. He would do some checking, and he encouraged us to continue writing to Susan. He seemed surprised that we had not asked Susan to tell us who her therapist was since it was our understanding that the therapist had brought up the subject of incest, recommended that she read *The Courage to Heal,* and was the one who had made the diagnosis. We were still in emotional limbo as we received more painful details from Susan.

January 4

Dear Susan,

The letter you wrote to Ralph when you were living with him as a freshman in college is terribly painful. It is heart-wrenching to feel the depths of your despair because of your hunger and extreme desire to be thin — your anorexia. Is that the evidence of abuse? You told me at the time that Ralph wanted you thin. Why isn't your relationship with him a partial explanation for your anorexia? What about your headstrong decision to marry him when you were a senior, only to get divorced nine months later?

You asked me to respond to a story you wrote in the fifth grade. Is this your evidence of sexual abuse? I must ask, What was the assignment? What books had you been reading at the time? Your story does not seem unusual to me, given the lifetime I have spent reading children's stories.

Is the evidence for sexual abuse, which you think I missed, your anorexia as a freshman in college? Your stories from fifth grade? Your teenage journal entries?

January 6

Dear Susan,

Thank you for the information about calling a social service agency to find a therapist who is female, young, a clinical psychologist, and an expert with issues of sexual abuse — a therapist like yours. Thank you also for the reference from *The Courage to Heal* about what the "mother"

112

is supposed to do and feel. I cannot lay all the blame on your father. I cannot blame anyone but myself for failing to see your pain and for being unaware of the terrible circumstances, the hell, you must have been living through. And the hell you are living through now. I am so sorry. I love you.

I have had the feeling that ever since this sad business began, my daughter has been trying to fit me into the paradigm of the wife of a child abuser, and I have found it insulting. Financial independence, academic and professional achievement, political activism are mine. What does Susan really know about the challenges to achieving those things for women who came of age during the 1950s? How much of the changed cultural expectation for women has she mapped on to me personally? Has she mistaken the fact that I viewed my professional options less broadly than she did hers as evidence that I am subjugated? So much does she try to put me in her image of the mother of an abused child that she even makes the suggestion that I did not write my own letters.

The pain of her degradation of me has been profound. The insults in her letters, the accusations of my incompetence not only as a mother but also as a woman have created wounds that will be difficult to heal. But I have also understood that from her perspective it was necessary to dismiss me. Then it would be just her word against Alex's word. By thinking of Susan as temporarily deranged, I have been able to keep feelings of love alive; but I have not been able to find the same excuse for Steve.

On January 6, seventeen days after our expulsion from their house, we finally received a letter containing Susan's alleged details of her abuse. It was horrible. I responded.

Dear Susan,

My poor dear Susan. No one should have to have such secrets locked away. How horrible! My poor child. You have memories of being abused starting at age 3, of being forced into sexual intercourse between ages 14 and 16, of being raped at age 16, a few days before you left for college. I struggle for understanding. My heart weeps for you. I am so sorry for you. Alex has no memories of all this. I have no memories of all this. In our small house, for so many years, how could all this have happened without my awareness? Finally you have given us the details that you remember.

I write my own letters. I'll tell you what I remember about our early years. . . .

I love you. I am struggling.

It was crazy. None of this made any sense to me. Where was I when all this was supposed to have taken place? How could someone blot out thirteen years of incest going on in a little house where every sound can be heard? How could two people blot out the same thirteen years? No, this was bizarre. This just didn't make any sense.

We had more to deal with at our next visit with the therapist. We had the details of the accusation. In the interim our therapist had spoken to an expert on memory who believed that it was highly unlikely that a 16-year-old would repress memories such as Susan claimed. That expert said that he had recently been getting many other such calls about accusations of sexual abuse from families with a child claiming repressed memories and dissociation. There is some comfort in learning that you are not the only one to suffer the same situation, I guess. It occurred to me that if this could happen to us, then our problem could represent just the tip of an iceberg.

"How many people who are accused of sex abuse have either the resources or the resolve to get even as far as a therapist?" I asked Alex. The shame that comes with being accused of sexual abuse is so intense that every inclination is to keep quiet about it. Even if you know that it didn't happen, the pain and the shame that your very own child is making such a claim is so great that most parents we have heard about in similar situations quickly disown and disinherit. It becomes a way to survive.

At this point our therapist and the expert had no more than our word against Susan's word. "Would you be willing to take a lie detector test?" the therapist asked. "The expert could arrange it." Would Alex do it? You bet. Alex is a kind and loving person. Whatever his faults, lack of courage to face the truth was not one. It was six very long weeks, however, before the test actually was administered. Alex's memories — or lack of the critical memories — were confirmed. But what is the value of a lie detector test? We were still discussing that months later. Our daughter felt it was irrelevant.

Dear Susan,

I know that such tests are not admitted into court as evidence and that they can be unreliable. I know that their reliability depends greatly on the administrator of the test and that they are more an art than a science. That is why we went to the effort and expense of paying for someone to come from Washington to do the test. The administrator has about as high a reputation for reliability in this field as anyone could have. The results of his tests are taken seriously by people in the field and by psychiatrists and lawyers.

If you were to take a lie detector test on these issues, I would fully expect you to pass. You believe what you say about abuse. Whether your memories are accurate or delusions, you would pass a lie detector test. A lie detector test for you would give us no information. We agree that you believe what you say about your memories of abuse. It is, however, effective to administer such a lie detector test to the father in these cases. A lie detector test can give some determination as to what a person believes. Alex was being tested against what he said he believed. Alex said that he did not sexually abuse you. The lie detector test showed that he believes what he said and is not lying. Thus, for him to have abused you means that he would have had to repress all the memories. He has no history of blackouts, memory loss, or physical aggression.

We are left, then, with the following: the situation that Alex is lying (less probable given the lie detector test) or that two people repressed exactly the same memories that extend over a period of thirteen years. What do you think is the probability that that has taken place — memories that would have been highly charged for both. What is that probability when coupled with the fact that no one else seems to have had a clue that all this was going on?

Up until the lie detector test, we had remained in limbo. We were relieved when Susan's twenty-seven-year-old sister, Sandra, whose bedroom had been next to Susan's, told us that she personally had no memories of Susan's sexual abuse. She certainly had told none of her friends at the time. But we were heartbroken to hear her say, "In my experience, people don't make up stories like that. Susan must be telling the truth." Sandra's "experience" was from hearing the stories of other women in the twelve-step self-help groups in which she participated and from reading *The Courage to Heal*, which someone in one of her groups had recommended to her. Until the lie detector test, we had only our story, though our friends believed us. Alex had a reputation for telling the truth. In fact, colleagues frequently complained that Alex told the truth even when others did not want to hear it. Imagine, just a few months earlier, I would probably have assumed that if someone were accused of such a crime, that person would in all likelihood be guilty.

We were not especially happy to learn that, under the law of our state, Susan had two years after her midlife revelation in which she could bring legal charges against us. Legal charges! Had Susan's therapist made a formal report of her diagnosis because of mandatory reporting laws on sexual abuse? We still do not know the answer to that question. Do we have any rights at all in all of this?

To the Library

I needed to know more, and I desperately wanted to keep contact with Susan. I found security in the familiar stacks of the library. Article by article, book by book, shelf by shelf I went, trying to grasp some larger picture.

January 10

Dear Susan,

    I am curious about your therapist for a number of reasons. I love you and want you to have the very best care. My concern was first raised by being informed that (a) the therapist had raised the subject of incest rather than taking it from you, and (b) that you have been using hypnosis. There is much debate about the reliability of memories recalled under those circumstances. Also, I am aware that there is a Clinical Incest Group in Anycity whose members enter the therapeutic situation with the bias that 50 percent of their patients will not remember sexual abuse and incest and so the therapist has to draw it out. This type of therapy is outlined in a book by Maltz and Holman. Don't you think that there might be some dangers in such preconceived assumptions?

    I am puzzled by your desire to keep the identity of your therapist from us. What are you trying to hide? I do hear you. I love you. I can feel your pain and hurt.

In the library I awakened to the social and political dangers of the current crusade to wipe out sexual abuse. Belief that the "rightness" of one's cause justifies any means is an eternal danger. It goes without saying that human beings should not abuse each other, sexually or in any other way. But zealots who lead crusades based on their belief of their own moral virtue and superiority have a history of bringing much oppression to the world.

    I found an overabundance of articles and books in which the authors lack respect for the boundaries between therapy and politics and in which they pander to emotions. *The Courage to Heal,* which Susan had referred to as a bible, tells the reader, "If you think you were abused and your life shows the symptoms, then you were" (p. 22). This is a political statement, not a scientific one. No empirical evidence exists to support such an assumption. In fact, there is actually much dispute in the literature on just what signs actually are related to sexual abuse. These signs were so broadly defined in most of the sex-abuse articles, however, that some of them could certainly be found at various times in most people. Wendy Maltz asserts that, due to memory loss, only about half of female incest survivors in your practice may be able to identify themselves as victims during your initial inquiry. . . . If you suspect the possibility of childhood sexual abuse based on physical symptoms and other clues, even when the patient has no conscious memory of sexual violation, share this information with your patient . . . set the stage for hidden memories of incest to surface. . . . [The signs include] physical problems: chronic pelvic pain, spastic colon, stomach pain, headache, dizziness, fainting, chronic gynecologic complaints, sleep disturbances, depression, asthma, heart palpitations.

Belief in these signs of sexual abuse represents very muddled thinking on the part of therapists. I learned that the signs referred to are based on symptoms described in "post-traumatic stress disorders" of people who have suffered known attacks or other disasters in life. Writers like the authors of *The Courage to Heal* have taken these signs and reinterpreted them to predict that sexual abuse has actually occurred if any of the signs are evident in a patient. Just because known victims of sexual abuse may suffer from anorexia, obesity, or sexual problems, it does not follow that having anorexia, obesity, or sexual problems implies that a person was sexually abused, as they seem to assume. There are too many other circumstances in life in which people display these symptoms.

Fortunately, I also found some literature that I could respect, literature that did not seem to pander and that attempted to document arguments and recommendations with research. It was a great relief to find *Accusations of Child Sexual Abuse* by Wakefield and Underwager and *Witness for the Defense* by Loftus and Ketcham, for example. The problem, however, was that this body of work pertained only to accusations made by young children. There was a void when it came to current research articles about women claiming to have had revelations of long-past sexual abuse even though the *manuals* for treatment of this condition have proliferated. Even so, if the evidence of recent research showed that neither adult eye-witness testimony nor children's memories are always reliable, how could therapists, trained and certified, be so sure that women who had gone for years without remembering could suddenly have memories that were always accurate?

Gaining some sense of perspective and security from the reading, Alex and I finally broke our silence and began to tell a few of our friends, our older friends. One couple in particular provided the love and emotional support that we needed to keep up our fight to love our daughter and not take shelter by disowning or disinheriting her. The wife, an outspoken feminist, was deeply concerned about the effects on the women's movement if many false accusations such as ours began to take place. She gave me a recommendation of a young therapist, a social worker, who specialized in sexual abuse matters. The social worker was described as a very fair person and sounded like the kind of person Susan had been asking me to see. Perhaps if I spoke with this woman, Susan would know that I was trying to understand.

I was excited and hopeful on the drab February afternoon before the appointment. I certainly did not expect this young therapist's absolute belief that Susan's story must be true. "Children don't lie about these things," she said. But Susan was not a child. She was a thirty-three-year-old woman entering midlife. Is a thirty-three-year-old woman incapable of delusions?

"It is so painful for a person to remember these things that she would never invent them. It is just too painful," she said.

"What is the research evidence for all this?" I asked.

"It's all so new," she replied. "We're just getting to the point where women are not afraid to talk about these secrets."

She was anti-Freud but seemed not to know Freud's work, and she gave me a publication from *Women Organized Against Rape* from 1980 that stated the feminist position that family-oriented therapy in incest put the responsibility on a faulty family rather than on the offender. The feminist position is that only the adult male offender is at fault. Then I began to wonder if one side effect of Masson's critique of Freud (*The Assault on Truth: Freud's Suppression of the Seduction Theory,* New York: Farrar, Straus & Giroux, 1984) was to give feminists the additional idea that anyone making a claim of long-repressed memories of childhood sexual abuse is to be believed.

Hey! I'm against rape and incest too, I screamed silently. Didn't this young woman see the irony in her argument that if some memories are too painful for people to invent and thus must be true, then it had to follow that these very same actions would surely be too horrible for someone to actually do and thus are to be disbelieved. Unless, that is, she actually believed that men were capable of thinking and doing these things but that women were not. Both points are unsupportable.

I was crushed. It was difficult to get out of that office fast enough to get away from this woman whose melodious voice was overflowing with patronizing sympathy for my plight. She was pitying *me* because I was a victim! I was so crushed by this woman's total disbelief in my recollections that for the first time I thought that life was not going to be worth living if this was the kind of reaction I was going to get. I lost all hope. I cried. I thought about suicide. I felt profoundly insulted. *I can deal with rape or incest*, I thought, *but I cannot deal with being a nonperson*. Neither my daughter nor this therapist seemed to feel that I was a conscious conspirator in all that was supposed to have happened. Instead, there was the assumption that I was "out of it," was somehow absent as a sentient human being and was pitiful and of no account. Young women seeking therapy claiming — after explicit probing and perhaps even hypnosis — to have long repressed memories of sex abuse were to be believed, while older women whose lives have attained some balance and a semblance of order were not to be trusted to have reliable memories or judgment. Is this what the feminist movement had come to?

My despair turned to anger and the anger to action. I set as a goal to change this one young woman's view of the situation. I returned after the lie detector test. She spent a long time reading every word of the copy that I brought with me. Like me, she had never seen the results of a lie detector test before. She admitted doubt. Surely, I thought, our daughter and her husband would now come to their senses too. But that was not to be.

April 12

Dear Steve,

You feel that the e-mail interaction is driving Susan and me apart. I would support alternative interaction that would help resolve this. I would have stayed and had joint counseling at Christmas. I would talk on the phone. Once Susan, as she herself wrote, finally got "bored" with keeping the name of her therapist from us, we tried to get her therapist to talk to ours. You and Susan have set the limits on the conditions of communication, not me.

I have tried to make the point that the general climate around the issue of sexual abuse is highly charged and politicized. For a number of years, for example, therapists have insisted that children don't lie about these things. Yet there have been many false accusations of sexual abuse. In fact, in the March 4 issue of *Time* on page 76 there is a short rehash of the subject with the information that the "controversy is sure to escalate this spring, when the American Psychological Association publishes a book called *The Suggestibility of Children's Recollections*." There is even more controversy about the validity of repressed memories and dissociation.

Steve, it seems that there is nothing we can do. You are convinced by the "gestalt of symptoms." I simply am not impressed by your list of symptoms:

• Anorexia: That could have many different underlying causes.
• Susan uses a fan at night to sleep: Some people take sleeping pills.

- She has difficulty dealing with "your family": Until this, she got along just fine with us. I can't follow your logic here.
- Childhood stories: These were reinterpreted by people looking for evidence, not given blind evaluation.
- Susan chose to leave your former town when she was not given tenure. That is the usual response to not getting tenure. Frankly, I think you are having difficulty accepting the fact that she chose her career over your stated preferences.

Are We the Only Ones?

As I have asked and asked myself how this could have happened to us, a family that was loving for so many years, a family that shared so much of life even after the children had grown up and the responsibilities had shifted, I have made lots of lists of possible reasons. Of course, the truth will be somewhere in the shuffle of a whole context of interacting factors. Nevertheless, my explanations seem to fall into four general categories: our faults as parents, some physical problem, stresses my daughter and her husband have been under, cultural context.

Have Alex and I failed as parents? I can't help but ask this question. I can think of a million things that I would do better a second time around if life let me sign on again. But in spite of this terrible mess, I really don't think that Alex or I did fail. We can all do only our best as we muddle through life. We did our best with what we knew at the time, and until the "revelation," that was better than okay. Agonizing over whether I should have interfered more or interfered less, or done this or done that, is not going to get anywhere now. We simply don't know what the result of other decisions might have been. Agonizing after the fact in a situation not to be replayed is a waste of effort. Who could it help?

We have learned a tremendous amount in recent decades about the biological bases of many behaviors. The chemistry of a host of behaviors such as depression is beginning to be laid bare. Our culture approaches so many problems from this perspective: "Take a pill. Feel better." I can't assume that Susan's problem is chemical any more than I can assume it is emotional. I would feel better, though, if I knew that she had had a complete physical examination.

I know that Susan has been under tremendous stress on many fronts. She has cried out in her letters her feelings of having been violated and her feelings of inadequacy. She begged for our belief and approval. She accused me of not hearing. But though I have heard and as her mother been privy to so many shared confidences, I happen to see other more immediate reasons for her stress. Some of the thoughts that have gone through my head:

About her feelings of inadequacy:

We did have very high standards and expectations about her achievement, but our love and respect did not depend on grades or honors. Intellectual families tend to be achievement oriented. We have been tremendously proud of her achievements, but our pride is greater because we have seen Susan make the world a little bit better than she has found it. But I do think that some of her stress was because she wanted us to be proud of her work.

Could Susan be exhausted and frustrated from the problems of trying to find adequate day care for the past several years? I know, because she told me, that she sometimes wished that she could just stay home and be with her children. Could she be under stress because she felt torn between her work and her children?

About her feelings of having been violated:

The earthquake severely damaged the house Susan was living in last year. One whole section had to be blocked off. The traumatic effects of the earthquake were obvious to many people who were with Susan. Even before her revelation, I felt that she was especially upset because the bed in which I, while visiting her, had been sleeping less than twenty-four hours before the quake, was virtually destroyed by the hundreds of books and four huge bookcases that fell on it. Earthquakes violate people.

Susan told me that fall that a student who was supposed to have completed work for a joint conference presentation with her had not done so. Did she feel betrayed by this person? Was there a connection between what was going on in Susan's mind and this student's claim that she was late with the project because she had been sexually abused by a professor?

Susan came to visit me for three days with the children in October on her way to a wedding. It was during the week, and it turned out that I had less time to spend with her than I'd anticipated. The obligations that came with recent changes in my work had surprised and overwhelmed me. Susan told me she was hurt because I didn't have more time for her.

Is "violation" a feeling that comes when one does not get tenure? It is well known that issues involving tenure are exacerbated for women.

However we may have shaped it initially, Susan has ultimately created her own adult life and she is responsible for it. I can understand latching onto an explanation that gets both Susan and Steve "off the hook," as it were. One person even suggested to me that Susan felt so close and secure in her relationship to Alex and me that she knew at some level that, even after this horrid accusation, we would still be there for her. It is a thought that had occurred to me, but it seemed too self-serving to maintain. I would feel so much better if I knew that Susan had had a second consultation with a politically neutral, older therapist of either gender. For any other serious medical problem, the profession recommends a second opinion. Why not for therapy if the diagnosis is as serious and devastating to all involved as is incest?

I suspect that the contemporary cultural and social climate has set the scene for what has happened to us. Susan went to a therapist when she was vulnerable. Could she have been especially susceptible to suggestion in those circumstances? Research is full of examples of how people are influenced by the expectations of the people they are with and by the way questions are posed. To be against child sexual abuse is a "politically correct" position, especially for activist women. To be a "victim" of something is almost a social necessity on college campuses. So much support and so much zeal abound for such accusations that more and more unjust ones, such as in our case, are being made. The current climate surrounding child sexual abuse is so politically charged that it has even been referred to as a "witch hunt." I have come to believe that our very sad situation happened because of my daughter's mental stress during this politically charged time in our culture.

June 29

Dear Susan,

We really do seem to have reached a stalemate of your memory versus Alex's and my memory. I am sure that is why you have to keep trying to put me in the position of being a "dodo," a nonsentient, pathetic being who was unaware of all that was happening to you and thus did not save you. If I won't support your belief that you were abused, and if you dismiss me, it is just your word against Alex's; and the climate is such that most people will probably believe you — at least for a while.

But think of what you know about memory. Memory is reconstruction. Memories can be altered. Memories recalled in a time of present

122

personal depression are known to be reinterpreted in a highly negative fashion. Memories recalled in a time of happiness are likewise positively interpreted. This is the way human memories work. Memories are reconstructed in terms of the facts, and they are reinterpreted in terms of their emotional impact.

I love you, Susan.

Getting On with Life

Last November, Susan lovingly sent us boxes of pears from the tree in her yard so we could share. In December, Alex spent days turning those pears into candy for Susan. A few weeks later, a phone call from her husband took all the sweetness from our lives. I really don't know how I have coped, but somehow I have — better than I would have expected. Certainly the love and respect that Alex and I share for each other is the foundation. I have gained a new understanding of the depth of our relationship. My sense of humor affords perspective and most of the time a positive view of life. Our friends, therapists, and the caring people I have met both in person and through the literature in my quest for understanding have made living through the past six months possible.

Turning my anger to action has surely helped. That has translated into writing this piece. I don't really want the world to know what a rotten mess has taken place in my life, but perhaps by sharing my story I can alert others to the fact that false accusations of sexual abuse are being made and that the results of such accusations result in major tragedies for all the people involved, but especially for the person making the charge. I write this because I am disturbed at the lack of critical thinking that seems to abound in the area of sexual abuse in people who are otherwise very rational. I write this because I am concerned about how ready the population is to accuse people of sexual abuse. The media have whipped people into a frenzy on the subject. I write this anonymously only because with all my heart I hope that we will be reunited with Susan, and I don't want to embarrass her.

I don't feel angry at Susan, although sometimes I just want to shake her to get some sense in her head. I am, however, very angry with her young therapist, whom I know only through the few defensive comments Susan has shared. I suppose it is to be expected that I would want to blame the therapist instead of my daughter. Susan may have been vulnerable when she went to this person, but she deliberately chose a therapist who represented a strong feminist political perspective rather than a therapist who was family oriented on issues of sexual abuse. I feel that something is terribly amiss, even so. From my perspective, the therapist seems to lack wisdom, compassion, understanding, and basic scientific knowledge of memory and mind that should be prerequisites for a license to practice psychotherapy. Probably, in fact, she is just young (thirty-two), inexperienced, and full of righteous anger at all the sexual abuse of women in the world.

To me it seems immoral that this woman has been willing to label Alex a sex criminal but unwilling to make a phone call and talk to us. Is that how it is supposed to be in therapy? I have noticed in the magazine and newspaper accounts that many revelations involve women accusing fathers who are dead. Is that why the therapist and Susan will not talk to us? Is it cowardice in a new wrapper? Do young therapists not have the courage to face the people they so hastily accuse and whose lives they are ready to destroy?

To me, it seems cruel that the therapist advised Susan to tell our grandsons that Alex had done terrible things to her and that Alex and I had been keeping terrible secrets about it for many years. Can it possibly be good for a two- or five-year-old to be told that a grandparent he has loved is really a monster? How can a young child digest information like that? Wouldn't it have been better to tell the children that we were dead? We live six hours away by plane and visited the children at most three times a year in their parents' home. Where is the rational thinking in believing there was danger to warrant giving such traumatic information to children — even believing in the alleged events of thirty years past? What was the reason for such advice? It seems so unnecessarily cruel to my grandsons.

To me, it seems slanderous that the therapist advised Susan to tell the children's teachers that we had been abusers. Never even a phone call to us? Never a check about a distraught young woman's dramatic "revelations"? Such arrogance in her own diagnostic ability!

To me, it seems irresponsible to have made such a serious "diagnosis" on the limited information that was available.

To me, it seems unethical to give a patient a book as self-consciously suggestive as *The Courage to Heal* before that patient has had a clear revelation of her own abuse.

To me, it seems incompetent to have made such a "diagnosis" given what is known about the vagaries of human memory. It seems incompetent that a psychologist whose training is supposed to be "scientific" would recommend a book to clients whose premise is without empirical foundation: "If you think you were abused, then you were."

124

To me, this whole episode seems cruel and unnatural and unnecessary. For the last four months material to be used in filing complaints against this therapist has taken space on the right-hand corner of my desk. I have not acted on it only because people I respect warned that it might jeopardize an eventual reconciliation with Susan. . . .

I am angry with the establishment that has been responsible for the training and certification of my daughter's therapist — training that has resulted in Susan's being in the terrible position she is in now, rather than having been guided in a more gentle way through her disturbance. It seems wrong to me that clinical training programs and certifications boards license therapists to deal with issues of the human mind without assuring that they have an understanding of the reasonable limits of what they might legitimately know. That is giving license to incompetence. It seems wrong to me that programs do not ensure that the therapists grasp the ethics involved in imposing their opinions on patients. That is giving license to unethical behavior. I am going to work to change that.

I am going to get on with my life because I think that will be the best for my daughter. I will wait for her. I cannot change what has happened, and I am not going to let it destroy the other good things in my life. If Susan makes a sincere opening, I will accept it.

I am about to put this story in the mail. In the same mail I will post a letter to Susan's therapist inviting her to talk to us and offering to pay for her airfare and time to come to our city, under any conditions with which she feels comfortable, to see for herself the little house in which the alleged abuse was supposed to have taken place, to meet the people who knew Susan as she was growing up, and to see three hours of tapes from the lie detector test. Wouldn't Susan be the beneficiary of the insights we might gain from each other? Isn't it appropriate for us to speak with each other inasmuch as her diagnosis of incest has so totally devastated our lives?

July 12

Dear Susan,

I will come when you want me to.

I have such deep sadness for the lovely, kind, brilliant thirty-three-year-old woman who now has such terrible memories and who sees her parents as people to fear.

Love, Mom

CHAPTER 6

Changing Perceptions
of the Child Abuse Problem

Every society, regardless of how technologically advanced or culturally sophisticated, is susceptible to mass hysteria.

— *John Taylor*

If the sexual abuse of children went underreported, underexposed, and underpunished for three-quarters of a century after Freud abandoned his seduction theory — and women suppressed their suffering of real, well-remembered abuse in the face of male therapists' skepticism — that situation changed dramatically in the early 1970s. In response to growing public concerns about child abuse, Congress passed the Child Abuse Prevention and Treatment Act (CAPTA) in 1974. The new legislation provided federal funding to combat child abuse for all states that met two basic conditions: they had to grant legal immunity to anyone reporting child abuse, and they had to require educators, health care workers, law enforcement officers, psychiatric care providers, and other professionals to report abuse to appropriate child protection authorities or be subject to fines or imprisonment. Minnesota Senator Walter Mondale, who was then seeking the Democratic party's nomination for president, pushed hard through congressional hearings for the passage of CAPTA, which became popularly known as the Mondale Act.

One of the experts called to testify before the congressional hearings that preceded the passage of CAPTA was sociologist David Gil, who had

126

conducted a groundbreaking survey of child abuse in the 1960s and concluded that the problem was "intimately tied to poverty." Gil suggested that the government could most effectively combat child abuse by working to "correct social and economic inequality." Senator Mondale knew that President Nixon and other conservatives would never support the passage of CAPTA if they believed its emphasis would be on poverty and inequality. He interrupted Gil in the middle of his testimony and said, "This is not a poverty problem; it is a national problem."[1]

At the time, many were inclined to characterize the problem in the same way Mondale did. The increase in concern about child abuse can in large measure be traced back to the growth in influence of the women's movement and of the therapeutic community in America. Activists in the women's movement tended to view child abuse — and particularly sexual abuse of children — principally as a crime committed by men against girls. Viewed in these terms, it had a natural place on the feminist agenda that increasing numbers of Americans adopted during the seventies. At the same time, Americans were becoming more accepting of and interested in a large range of post-Freudian psychotherapies, among them RMT. Both the feminist and the therapeutic communities were sensitive to the problem of child abuse, and, as their influence grew, their concern about this issue was publicized and taken seriously. People were quick to acknowledge that abuse was often hushed up and that the problem was bigger than society had been willing to admit in the past. Many people were willing to give a sympathetic hearing to charges that the problem was widespread or even epidemic. Well-known RMT proponent Judith Herman could get people to listen when she asserted that "any serious investigation of the emotional and sexual lives of women eventually leads to the discovery of the incest secret."[2] And, as popular culture embraced psychotherapeutic concepts and terminology, more people understood and were willing to accept assertions like that of Renee Fredrickson that a repressed history of childhood sexual abuse "lurks in the background of millions of ordinary, high functioning Americans."[3]

The passage of CAPTA, in turn, served to vastly extend the public's awareness of the problem of child abuse. Some critics charge that the

1. CAPTA, S. 1191, Hearings before the Subcommittee on Children and Youth of the Committee on Labor and Public Welfare, U.S. Senate, 93rd Congress, 1st session.

2. Herman, quoted by John Taylor in "The Lost Daughter," *Esquire,* March 1994, p. 78.

3. Fredrickson, *Repressed Memories: A Journey to Recovery from Sexual Abuse* (New York: Fireside/Parkside, 1992), p. 71.

legislation has helped turn speculation about a possible epidemic of abuse into a self-fulfilling prophecy. By requiring public servants to report all suspected abuse, CAPTA has led to the reporting of huge numbers of cases on the basis of questionable evidence, as the various groups of professionals affected by the legislation choose to report any and all suspicions rather than risk fines or imprisonment for failing to report. And, by offering immunity from prosecution to all who report suspected abuse, the law has inadvertently encouraged false reporting by a host of troubled, malicious, and ill-informed people. Social workers across the nation have been handed huge caseloads; many offices are months behind on even initiating investigations of the reports stacked up on their desks. To many observers, it certainly has the appearance of an epidemic.

How big is the problem really? No one can say for certain. A 1992 study by the National Committee for the Prevention of Child Abuse (a well-respected child advocacy group) reported nearly three million suspected victims, but the Committee itself subsequently determined that fewer than half of those reports merited further investigation. Still, we know that even in the wake of CAPTA, with more public awareness of the problem and more incentives for everyone to report suspected abuse, many cases continue to go unreported. On the other hand, the number of mistaken reports and false accusations also seems to have increased significantly. A 1992 U.S. Department of Health and Human Services study tallied 1,227,223 *false* reports of child abuse during the previous year — most of them against parents. It is in the nature of the problem that child abuse is often difficult to detect. The sort of clear evidence traditionally needed for criminal prosecution is often hard to come by in domestic cases. Abused children may well be intimidated by the legal process or reluctant to accuse even abusive family members for fear of reprisals or abandonment. Spouses of perpetrators and other family members may be similarly intimidated or may be motivated to cover up the abuse for any number of other reasons. It is only right that we should be making greater efforts than we have in the past to protect children from abuse. But it is also true that in doing so we have a responsibility to see that innocent people are not falsely accused of this ugly crime.

The effects of CAPTA have been far-reaching. It has changed not only the ways in which Americans perceive the problem of child abuse but also the ways in which we are attacking it. In the years following the enactment of the new legislation, as the number of reported cases of child abuse skyrocketed, overworked social service agencies had to hire additional personnel to handle the caseloads. Given the rapid rise in demand for such positions, there was a shortage of qualified individuals to meet the need. As Debbie Nathan and Michael Snedeker have pointed out, "the shortage was especially acute when it came to experts in sexual abuse, which in the early 1970s was child protection's newest subspecialty. The gap was at first filled by a pioneering group of feminist-minded social workers who addressed the problem of incest and molestation in their work to reduce violence against women."[4] Like Senator Mondale, many of the new experts in this expanding field elected not to focus on the link between poverty and child abuse. For a variety of reasons, some growing out of their preexisting ideological convictions, they focused much of their efforts and resources on uncovering abuse in middle- and upper-middle-class settings. This partly helps to explain a string of sensational investigations of daycare facilities that took place during the eighties. One of the best known of these investigations — at the McMartin Preschool in Manhattan Beach, California — is representative of the sort of unfortunate investigative misdirection that took place around the country during this period.

Hysteria in Low Places

In August 1983, a seemingly insignificant preoccupation initiated what was to become the longest and most expensive trial in U.S. history and touched off a social hysteria that is still with us today. Judy Johnson, a woman later diagnosed as a paranoid schizophrenic, became preoccupied with a redness around her two-year-old son Matthew's anus. At the time, Johnson had an older son dying of a brain tumor, she had just recently separated from her husband, and her income was not good. At first, in July, she had thought she'd transmitted her case of vaginitis to her younger son. But one mid-August morning she inspected Matthew's anus and it looked normal to her; when he returned from his day at the McMartin Preschool, she found that it was red again. Judy was suddenly seized with the idea that her son's male teacher at the preschool, Ray Buckey, had sodomized Matthew that day — and had, in fact, been doing so all summer.[5]

---

4. Nathan and Snedeker, *Satan's Silence* (New York: BasicBooks, 1995), p. 15.

5. The McMartin story can be found in many sources. Among others that I have found helpful are Nathan and Snedeker's *Satan's Silence*, pp. 67-92 and 124-28; and Mark Pendergrast's *Victims of Memory: Incest Accusations and Shattered Lives*, 2d ed. (Hinesburg, VT: Upper Access Books, 1996), pp. 362-66. HBO also aired a dramatic motion picture account of the story entitled *Indictment*, produced by Abby Mann.

Although Johnson questioned her son all evening, he would not confirm her suspicions: he insisted that nothing bad had happened at preschool that day. Nevertheless, Johnson called the police the next day and told them of her suspicions. Matthew was not yet three and slow in verbal development, speaking only in single words or fragments of sentences, and so the police had nothing more to go on than his mother's allegations. Apparently they believed her, because they opened an investigation. Johnson proceeded to take Matthew to a hospital for an examination. A doctor listened to Mrs. Johnson's theory about sodomy but did not confirm it. His examination of Matthew turned up none of the sort of physical trauma that occurs when an adult male penetrates the anus of a two-year-old child. One would at the very least expect to find anal tears and severe bruising in such cases; the worst incidents involve maiming and even death. Matthew's anus was merely red and irritated.

But Judy Johnson did not give up her anxiety or her accusations. Within several days she returned to the police with more stories of what she believed had been done to her son at McMartin. The police recommended that she take Matthew for another physical examination, this time to UCLA, where a group of doctors and social workers who specialized in child abuse had recently organized the Suspected Child Abuse and Neglect (SCAN) team. The doctor who oversaw SCAN's evaluation program at UCLA's Neuropsychiatric Institute, Dr. Michael Durfee, had a special interest in "sexually abused infants and toddlers who were too young to describe their experience to anyone, psychiatrists included." His work with the SCAN team had attracted the attention of psychiatrists and graduate students who were researching cults, multiple personality disorders, and the sorts of incest "survivors" who had begun emerging in significant numbers since the publication of the book *Michelle Remembers*. The institute assigned a young, comparatively inexperienced intern to examine Matthew, and she concluded that the redness and scratches on his anus were indeed the result of penile penetration. Johnson now had the confirmation she desired.[6]

The intern never managed to get Matthew to say that he had been molested, and, as investigative reporter Debbie Nathan discovered, "later court reports indicate that Manhattan Beach police detective and sex abuse investigator Jane Hoag was never able to get Matthew to admit anything to her" either.[7] So, it was on the basis of the intern's questionable determina-

6. Nathan and Snedeker, *Satan's Silence*, p. 70.
7. Nathan and Snedeker, *Satan's Silence*, p. 70.

tion alone, and without any corroborating accusations from the child himself, that the Manhattan Beach police pursued its investigation of Ray
Buckey.

On September 2, 1983, the police searched the McMartin Preschool
and Ray Buckey's property for signs of pornography and child molestation.
They found nothing, but they arrested Buckey anyway. When he vigorously
denied the charges, they had to release him for lack of evidence. Then,
without any further investigation, the police sent a letter to the two hundred
families who had or had had children in the McMartin Preschool. The letter
stated that Ray Buckey was under investigation for child molestation, and
it encouraged parents to question their children about being witnesses or
victims of sexual molestation. The letter specified "oral sex, fondling of
genitals, buttock or chest area, and sodomy, possibly under the pretense of
'taking the child's temperature.'"[8]

During the parents' initial questioning of their children, not a single
child said that anything bad had happened at the preschool. But the anxious
parents kept pressing their children, and they also talked among themselves.
By the end of September, after continued questioning and suggestions from
their parents, some of the children started changing their stories. Bizarre
and impossible scenarios began to emerge, such as "poo" coming out of
Ray's penis and behavior that smacked of satanic rituals. A number of the
children said that Buckey had photographed them in the nude, but the
police never found any pictures or any evidence that Ray had ever taken
any. Then parents of the "remembering" children called parents of other
children and urged them to question their children again and more
vigorously. Even though all these interrogations initially met with denials
from the children, police urged the parents who suspected anything to take
their children to UCLA for SCAN team evaluations.

Some parents who had initially been skeptical of and disgusted by the
charges against the McMartin Preschool started to believe the charges when
other parents persuaded them or their own children began to mimic the
stories of the other children. The police appear to have believed all the
juvenile stories from the outset and never to have wavered in their conviction that Ray Buckey was a child molester. The whole community seemed
ready to believe the worst. Less than a month after Buckey was arrested, a
survey of Los Angeles County residents indicated that their chief fear —
surpassing their fear of the effects of drugs or drunk driving — was child
abuse. Almost a decade after the enactment of the Mondale Act, public

8. Nathan and Snedeker, *Satan's Silence,* p. 72.

awareness of child abuse was high. And Los Angeles boasted some of the most media-exposed "experts" in child sexual abuse in the country.

Los Angeles District Attorney Robert Philibosian, who was facing a tough reelection contest, stepped into this charged atmosphere in October 1983. He assigned the McMartin case to Assistant District Attorney Joan Matusinka, a Los Angeles prosecutor who specialized in child abuse cases. A decade earlier, Matusinka, along with Dr. Roland Summit, had helped found Parents Anonymous, an organization designed to promote self-help for abusive parents in a context of professional counseling and support services. Matusinka's Los Angeles chapter of the organization had been concentrating on the sexual abuse of very young children.

Here we see an example of the way in which the interests of the investigator can narrow the focus of an investigation. By concentrating on sexual abuse of very young children, Matusinka's group was setting itself up to overlook most of the abuse that was actually occurring, since, as Nathan and Snedeker point out, abuse is most common among older age groups. "Statistically, the younger a child is, the less likely is the chance that he or she will have sexual contact with an adult. By far the most common period for such experience is adolescence. It is rarer among prepubescent children, and significantly less common for preschoolers, toddlers, and infants. Forcible rape of preschool-aged victims is extremely infrequent."[9] Moreover, this kind of narrowing of the focus can lead an investigator to make an increased number of false accusations. As we have seen in the case of RMT therapists, a passionate belief that a given kind of abuse is common can lead people to detect it wherever they look, even where the evidence is thin or ambiguous.

Matusinka was also a member of the Preschool-Age Molested Children's Professional Group, which had been assembled by Drs. David Corwin and Roland Summit to provide alternative ways for children to provide legal evidence in criminal child-abuse trials. The founders of the group worked from the assumption that putting an abused child through the rigors of the traditional legal process could impose additional trauma. To avoid this, they proposed to videotape the child's testimony outside of the courtroom, out of sight of the suspected molester, and then submit the recorded statements in lieu of actual testimony in the trial. To help elicit testimony, the group designed and used toys, dolls, and "projective techniques" intended to put the child at ease in this context. More controversially, they also introduced another pioneering device, the so-called anatomically correct dolls.

9. Nathan and Snedeker, *Satan's Silence*, p. 75.

These dolls, for those who have not seen them, specifically show genital parts, including pubic hair. Female dolls typically have large breasts with prominent nipples; male dolls typically feature an erect penis. The dolls are designed to help the children describe in a nonthreatening context the sorts of sexual contact they have had with an adult. But many critics charge that the presence of the doll itself profoundly affects any testimony that it helps to elicit. As Richard A. Gardner, head of child psychiatry at Columbia University, points out, the dolls

> are different from just about anything the child has previously seen and are likely to produce strong emotional reactions. This serves to obfuscate and suppress other emotions (having nothing to do with sex abuse) that may be at the forefront of the child's mind. Also, they transmit to the child the message that the examiner is interested in discussing matters related to naked bodies, and this serves to draw the child's thoughts, feelings, and fantasies into that path. . . . Many [of the dolls] have gaping orifices (vagina, anus, and mouth); many cannot be justifiably called "anatomically correct" because of the disproportion between the size of the genitals and the rest of the body. . . . They are a serious contamination to any meaningful psychiatric interview . . . a contamination that already makes it unlikely that the examiner will truly find out whether the child has been genuinely abused. . . . The likelihood of the child's ignoring these unusual genital features is almost at the zero level. Accordingly, the dolls always demand attention and predictably will bring about the child's talking about sexual issues.[10]

The exposure of these children to such dolls also ignores what Freud (in 1905) called their "polymorphous perversity." Before young children have been socialized into appropriate public and private behaviors, they exhibit all imaginable sexual behaviors: heterosexual, homosexual, bisexual, and autosexual. Infants have no problem touching and caressing any part of anyone's body, whether a private or a public part. Says Gardner,

> They will put into their mouths any object that will fit, whether it be their own or anyone else's. They touch all parts of their own bodies, and attempt to touch all parts of other people's bodies. In short, they touch, suck, insert, smell, and feel all the parts of their own as well as other human beings' bodies and make no particular discriminations regarding

10. Gardner, *Sex Abuse Hysteria: Salem Witch Trials Revisited* (Cresskill, NJ: Creative Therapeutics, 1991), p. 50.

the age, sex, or relationship to them of the object of their "sexual" advances. . . . If one gives a child a peg and a hole, the child is going to put the peg in the hole unless the child is retarded or psychotic. Give a child a wooden doughnut, and the child will inevitably put his/her fingers in the hole. Give a child one of these female "anatomically correct" dolls with wide open mouth, anus, and vagina; the child will inevitably place one or more fingers in one of these conspicuous orifices. . . . In the course of playing with these dolls, it is almost inevitable that the child will take the penis (often erect) and place it in one of the orifices of the female doll. . . . For many of these "validators," such an act is "proof" that the child has indeed been sexually abused. The assumption is made that what the child does with these dolls is an exact, point-by-point replication of what has occurred in reality. The argument goes that these dolls "help" the child verbalize what has happened. . . . This is crass rationalization. It justifies the use of these materials to verify what the examiner believes in the first place, namely, that the sex abuse did occur. No competent psychologist or psychiatrist believes that the child's projections on the Rorschach, Thematic Apperception Test, or doll play necessarily reflect reality. What they do reflect is the child's cognitive processes, wishes, aspirations, and distortions.

Gardner concludes that the use of anatomically correct dolls is "such a significant contaminant that I would consider any examiner who utilizes them to be incompetent."[11]

By the time Joan Matusinka was assigned to the McMartin case, fifteen children had said that they were sexually abused by Ray Buckey. She decided that this was the perfect test group for the new techniques of the Preschool-Age Molested Children's Professional Group. To conduct the testing, she called in evaluators from Children's Institute International (CII), a non-profit child-abuse diagnostic and treatment facility in Los Angeles run by Kee MacFarlane, who was also a member of the Preschool-Age Molested Children's Professional Group. A former lobbyist for the National Organization for Women who was hired as a sex abuse specialist by the National Center for Child Abuse and Neglect (NCCAN) while still in her twenties, MacFarlane was on the cutting edge of the child-protection movement in this country. Her credo in all cases of suspected child abuse was "Believe the children."

MacFarlane was the main "facilitator" at CII when the McMartin children came in to be evaluated. Typical sessions involved role-playing and

11. Gardner, *Sex Abuse Hysteria*, p. 51.

the use of anatomically correct dolls. CII videotaped the sessions, and the following passage is a description of a representative taped interview with a little girl named Tanya. MacFarlane begins by introducing Tanya to a group of puppets and dolls representing characters from *Sesame Street* and popular cartoons.

Not until Tanya was deeply absorbed in the world of pretend did Mac-Farlane present her with a collection of "very special dollies in this little bag . . . they look like real people underneath . . . we can take off their clothes." Tanya then identified the dolls' "wee-wees," "chee-chees" (breasts), "butts," "wienie," and the "naugus hole," or vagina. MacFarlane proceeded to ask Tanya if she had ever seen a man's weenie. Her daddy's, Tanya answered. MacFarlane was not satisfied. "How about somebody else? . . . I know who else . . . another man." Still, Tanya insisted she had seen only her father's. "Well, I know some secrets," said MacFarlane, "that I know you know 'em, too. You know what? I know some secrets about your old school." When Tanya still didn't respond, MacFarlane added that she had seen the little girl's friends from McMartin's, and they told her "all the bad secrets." "We can have a good time with the dolls," MacFarlane coaxed, "and, you know, we can talk about some of those bad secrets, if you wanted to. And then they could go away. Wouldn't that be a good idea?" Urging puppets on Tanya, she again asked if she knew bad secrets. "Uh-uh," Tanya shook her head. Then maybe she could figure them out, MacFarlane said. She showed off her "secret machine" [a microphone connected to a video recorder] and assured Tanya that she would feel better if she told it bad things about Ray. "I hate those secrets," Tanya finally said, addressing a bird puppet on MacFarlane's hand. "Ray-Ray did bad things, and I don't even like it."

Now MacFarlane took a doll with genitals, named it Ray, and told Tanya to use Mr. Animal to explain what Ray did to her. Tanya began manipulating the doll and simulating a voice for it, while MacFarlane pretended that a female doll was Tanya. "Oh, Mr. Ray — Ray-Ray, you're touching me, huh? Where are you touching me?" MacFarlane squealed. "On the wee-wee," Tanya answered, and it was not clear who she thought was making this reply. Herself? A doll? A puppet?

The session became a scene of naked dolls with genitals touching, poking and threatening each other. Cloth penises were being inserted into mouths. "Did that happen? Ooh, that must have been yucky," Mac-Farlane said. "It didn't happen," corrected Tanya, "I'm just playing." . . .

Toward the end of the interview . . . MacFarlane . . . asked Tanya, "Do you know the difference between the truth and a lie? What's a lie?" "Umm,

135

it has big teeth, and it — and it's kind of brownish," answered the little girl. At that, MacFarlane asked whether Tanya had "told the truth to the secret machine." The little girl was mute. She only nodded, with her mouth wide open.

Following the session, MacFarlane led the child out to her mother, and verified that Tanya had been molested. She urged [the mother] to tell her daughter how proud she was that she had told the secrets and how much she loved her. Then CII notified the DA's office that Tanya . . . had been a victim of Ray Buckey. The process was repeated with dozens of other children. In every case, MacFarlane and her colleagues found sexual abuse.[12]

Even apart from this sort of leading, young children are dubious witnesses to specific events. A recent study of children's suggestibility by Stephen J. Ceci and Maggie Bruck involved forty three-year-olds who had visited their pediatrician for an annual checkup. Half the children had an exam that included the physician touching their buttocks or genitals, and half did not. Immediately after the exam, an interviewer pointed to the genitals of an anatomically correct doll and asked whether the doctor touched them there: of those who had not been touched, half incorrectly said that they had been touched; when they were given the dolls to handle themselves, even more reported that they had been touched. At the same time, fewer than half of the children who *had* been touched said that they had been. And when those from this group who reported that they had been touched were asked to show on the dolls where they had been touched, their identifications were in many cases incorrect; for example, several of the girls stuck their fingers into the dolls' anuses and vaginas.[13]

This, then, was the sort of evidence that was being marshaled to convict not only Ray Buckey but everyone else associated with running the McMartin Preschool as well. Eventually, the McMartin allegations grew to include Ray's sister, Peggy Ann; his mother, Peggy McMartin Buckey; his seventy-seven-year-old grandmother and founder of the school, Virginia McMartin; and three other staff members. And the charges against them escalated beyond simple abuse as the children went on to tell MacFarlane that they had been forced to kill animals, drink blood and urine, and take part in a variety of satanic rituals. In the spring of 1984, District Attorney Philibosian announced to the press that "the primary purpose of the

12. Nathan and Snedeker, *Satan's Silence*, pp. 79-80.
13. Ceci and Bruck, "Children's Recollections: Translating Research into Policy," *Society for Research in Child Development Social Policy Report* 7 (Fall 1993): 1-30.

McMartin Preschool was to solicit young children to commit lewd conduct with the proprietors of the school and also to procure young children for pornographic purposes." Unaccountably, one of Philibosian's assistants added that there were "millions of child pornography photographs and films" of the victims.[14]

The McMartin case became a feeding frenzy for the media, but there is no indication that any of the reporters covering the story ever asked to see the millions of photographs. The fact is that not one single photo has ever turned up, despite substantial reward offers and international searches by the FBI and Interpol. There was no physical evidence of any sort in the case — nothing beyond the testimony of the children. Perhaps the media failed to investigate in any real depth because they didn't want to look as though they were in any way doubting the testimony of the ostensible victims. Perhaps they simply couldn't imagine that charges of this magnitude would be brought without compelling evidence. In any event, almost no members of the media asked the prosecution any tough questions — or even asked to see any evidence. On the other hand, they didn't fail to exploit the story. *People* magazine called McMartin "California's Nightmare Nursery"; *Time* headlined its story with the word "Brutalized"; on ABC's *20/20,* Tom Jarriel characterized the preschool as a "sexual house of horrors," and when co-host Hugh Downs asked, "How deeply marred are these children, Tom, and will they ever recover from it?" Jarriel replied, "Psychologically, perhaps never, Hugh."[15]

In March 1984, Ray Buckey, his sister Peggy Ann, their mother, Peggy McMartin Buckey, their grandmother Virginia McMartin, and three other teachers at the preschool were arrested. By that time, members of their community had already tried to burn the school down and had sprayed graffiti such as "Ray Must Die" on it. Ray's middle-aged mother, Peggy, had been stabbed in the crotch by a stranger on the street. Some parents had formed vigilante squads and were searching for other accomplices, driving their children around town looking for "molestation sites," and taking down addresses and license plate numbers of possible suspects. Parents began accusing each other. There were rumors that the mayor's wife was driving around town with dead bodies in the back of her station wagon. One community parent patrolled nearby commuter airports and took down airplane registration numbers, reporting such suspicious characters as a "female pilot who may be a lesbian."[16]

14. Nathan and Snedeker, *Satan's Silence*, p. 88.
15. Nathan and Snedeker, *Satan's Silence*, p. 88.
16. Nathan and Snedeker, *Satan's Silence*, p. 89.

One of the actors in the drama was Dr. Bruce Woodling, who had testified as an expert medical witness in two significant California child-abuse cases preceding McMartin. Woodling believed in the moral significance of his work and told coworkers never to make a diagnosis of "no child abuse," because, he said, the case would never go forward if they did. Woodling had learned in medical school that the "anal wink," or dilated rectum, constituted proof of sodomous activity in gay males. He proceeded to use this as a test to determine whether abuse had taken place in child-care facilities: he would rub the anuses of young boys and girls with cotton swabs, and if the tissue dilated, he interpreted it as proof that they had been sodomized. One of the children who was examined by Woodling in connection with one of the earlier cases, Tricia McCuan, remembers the examination. Woodling informed her that she had been molested, and when she denied it he told her, "This examination will tell who's right and who's wrong." The eight-year-old girl became distraught and did not want the exam; she was embarrassed, frightened, and tearful, but Woodling insisted on going ahead with it. When he was finished, Woodling told the little girl that he had proof she had been molested. Years later, Tricia remembered this encounter as a violation, "the worst thing that ever happened to me." Some condemned Woodling's methods as unscientific, but they were afraid to testify for the defense for fear of being labeled child-abuse sympathizers.[17]

While in prison awaiting trial, the McMartin child-care workers lived in constant fear for their lives. Riding in a bus to a hearing, Peggy and Peggy Ann had their hair set on fire by other convicts while guards sat by, paying no attention. Ray had worse experiences in the men's prison, including intimidation by body-building cellmates who had been paid by the prosecutor's office to get the goods on him.

Meanwhile, Judy Johnson's reports of what had happened to her son Matthew had grown continually more elaborate and bizarre. She was now asserting that female members of the staff had stapled the boy's ears, nipples, and tongue, had jabbed scissors into his eyes, and had killed a baby and forced him to drink the blood. There were, of course, no physical signs that Matthew had suffered any of this kind of abuse. Little more than half a year after Judy's first accusations against Ray Buckey, and with the witch hunt she had initiated in full fever, Judy's life took another bad turn when her estranged husband divorced her. After Matthew spent a weekend with his father, Judy accused her ex-husband of having sodomized the child.

17. Nathan and Snedeker, *Satan's Silence*, p. 188.

This time the police filed no charges. Judy continued to make wild accusations: now male models and AWOL servicemen were following her around, she said, and someone had broken into her house and buggered the family dog.

Toward the end, Judy barricaded herself and her sons in their small house, insisting that it stood on sacred ground. When her brother showed up to try to ease the situation, she aimed a shotgun at him. Police and hostage negotiators eventually managed to subdue her. A subsequent psychiatric evaluation produced the diagnosis of paranoid schizophrenia. Within two years Johnson was dead of liver disease brought on by alcohol abuse.

From our perspective today, it seems clear that Judy Johnson was delusional from the very beginning. Her initial charges against Ray Buckey were groundless — unsupported by any physical evidence and unsubstantiated even by the boy who was supposed to have been molested. Why, then, were so many people drawn into the delusion — police, medical practitioners, the district attorney's office, the media? We could attribute political motives to some of the players. Philibosian might have viewed the prosecution as a ticket to publicity and support for his reelection bid. Matusinka might have been seeking to make a name for herself with a popular, high-profile case. It's possible that some of those involved may simply have been taking the easiest course. Police and medical care providers may have been hesitant to question Johnson's accusations out of a fear of prosecution under CAPTA guidelines. Some, such as Kee MacFarlane and Bruce Woodling, may have been driven by their prior beliefs to suppose that accusations of any sort are bound to be true, that children never lie about such things. But it is also possible that everyone involved had nothing more in mind than seeking the best interests of Matthew Johnson. Had they all simply pursued that end *without regard to any other considerations,* it would have been enough to produce the same result: they rendered themselves captives to a delusion. Six months after the McMartin staff had been arrested, and with the trial under way, Kee MacFarlane helped to spread the paranoia yet further by testifying at a U.S. Congressional hearing that the country was in the throes of organized child-molestation conspiracies. The McMartin Preschool, she said, had become "a ruse for larger unthinkable networks of crimes against children." Her views were broadcast the next day by the national media as the perspective of an expert in the field.[18]

Some of those involved in the McMartin incident managed to resist the

18. Nathan and Snedeker, *Satan's Silence,* p. 91.

hysteria, however. Glenn E. Stevens, one of the prosecutors in the McMartin case, eventually quit in disgust. Denouncing the prosecution as a massive hoax, he was one of the first to testify about the coercive nature of the child interviews: "If a child said no, nothing ever happened to them, the interviewer would then say, 'You're not being a very bright boy. Your friends have come in and told us they were touched. Don't you want to be as smart as them?'"[19] After viewing videotapes of interviews with forty-six McMartin children, psychiatrist Lee Coleman said, "I can state categorically that the children were *in every single session* outrageously manipulated by their interviewers."[20]

Despite the publicity surrounding the McMartin trial, Robert Philibosian was unsuccessful in his bid to be reelected as district attorney for Los Angeles. He was replaced by Ira Reiner, who quickly dropped all charges against five of the female defendants, calling the evidence against them "incredibly weak." Peggy Buckey was finally acquitted after more than twenty-eight months of trial. The charges against Ray Buckey were dismissed after a combination of hung juries and not-guilty verdicts. He was released after having spent five years in prison, universally despised as a vicious child molester. After he was released, many people remained convinced that he was guilty as sin. No one can say what damage was done to the children in the case; we have to assume that many of them still carry "memories" of abuse confabulated under duress by court-appointed facilitators.

In some ways the McMartin Preschool trial was unique. It was, as I have mentioned, the longest-running and costliest trial in the history of the American legal system. But it was certainly not the only one of its kind. In its wake came nearly a hundred similar abuse trials of individuals in child-care facilities around the nation, most of them based on equally flimsy evidence and all of them marked by the same sort of hysterical suspicion and accusations. The fears generated by publicity surrounding the initial trials spread, creating a sense of anxiety in other communities and setting the stage for yet more investigations and more trials. This anxiety was further deepened by the pronouncements of ostensible experts such as Kee MacFarlane that the whole country was in the grip of an organized conspiracy of child molesters. It provides us with an object lesson in what can happen when people accept the key initial belief that abuse is epidemic in our culture: in cases like this, as in the area of RMT, we will almost always find what we expect to find.

19. Stevens, quoted by Lawrence Wright in *Remembering Satan: A Case of Recovered Memory and the Shattering of an American Family* (New York: Alfred A. Knopf, 1994), p. 74.

20. Coleman, "Learning from the McMartin Hoax," *Issues in Child Abuse Accusations* 1 (Spring 1989): 68.

Facilitated Communication

The misuse of therapeutic tools has led investigators to many false determinations of child abuse. In Chapter 2 we noted that RMT therapists have implanted false memories of abuse rather than uncovered repressed memories of actual childhood abuse through the improper use of such tools as guided imagery and hypnosis. And, as we have just seen, critics charge that the use of anatomically correct dolls during interviews of children to determine whether they have been abused obstructs rather than aids the process of getting at the truth. The use of another technique, known as "facilitated communication," has also led to false charges of abuse.

FC, as it came to be called, was initially considered a breakthrough for helping developmentally disabled children communicate with others. Some of the most remarkable successes have been seen with autistic children. The technique involves a number of different methods of helping disabled individuals to communicate by pointing at pictures or letters or, more commonly, by using typewriter or computer keyboards. Facilitators offer emotional support and a certain amount of limited physical guidance and restraint. They may gently position a client's hands over a keyboard to initiate communication, for example, or stabilize an arm to reduce the effects of tremor, pull back on an arm or wrist to slow impulsive movement or repetitive gestures, or the like. In some cases the results of such guidance have been spectacular. Children who had never communicated with the outside world suddenly began "talking" to family and caregivers. Autistic children began writing poetry, acing mathematics tests, earning straight A's. The parents and teachers of these children were overjoyed, because FC seemed to indicate that the children were not retarded but, in fact, quite gifted.

Dr. Douglas Biklen, who had observed the technique in use with cerebral palsy patients in Australia, established the Facilitated Communication Institute in Syracuse, New York, where he trained hundreds of practitioners, who, in turn, spread out across the country to teach the methodology to others. Biklen himself called FC "revolutionary, a means of expression for people who lacked expression." Not surprisingly, the story attracted the interest of the popular media. Diane Sawyer reported on ABC's *Prime Time Live* that it was a "miracle . . . a story about hope." Unfortunately, it hasn't been the same story for everyone. Nathan and Snedeker tell the story of an autistic child named Matt Gherardi:

Before he met his facilitator, Matt's vocabulary had consisted of about fifty words. Afterward he was doing well in grammar, algebra, and

141

Shakespeare. His teachers were delighted, but Matt's parents were perplexed. They found it strange that he could suddenly be so literate, and even stranger that he refused to facilitate with his own mother, with whom he was very close.

One day, while working at school with his facilitator, Matt pointed to his keyboard and spelled out these words: "dad herts me." "What happens?" the facilitator typed back. "his balls next to mine," the boy replied. "make me very horney Thursday. Dad give love to my ass and dad give love to my cock with his mouth. the bastard eats cock in mouth then kneel over and — you know."

When Matt's father arrived home that night, there was a warrant for his arrest and orders not to set foot in his house.

Insisting he was innocent, he and his wife began investigating the latest developments in autism education, and discovered two things. One was that researchers recently had begun stressing that the incidence of sexual abuse among disabled children is very high. The other was that with the help of FC, several other autistic children around the country had accused their parents, teachers, and care workers of molesting them.[21]

Because of the strenuous denials of parents who were being accused via FC, authorities began to wonder about the origins of the messages. They conducted tests in which the child and the facilitator were shown two different images, and the child was asked to type what he or she saw. Invariably, the autistic child typed what the facilitator was being shown rather than what he or she saw. Many subsequent tests have been done, always with the identical result: the autistic child always types not his image but the facilitator's. There has never been even a shadow of a doubt about this: facilitators were not giving autistic children their own expression; they were simply using the children's hands to type what was in their own minds. The autistic children were being used as nothing more than sounding boards for the thoughts of the adults who were "facilitating" them.

Researchers concluded that the facilitators they tested had no idea they were controlling the autistic children's communication. It seems to have been a completely "unconscious phenomenon," and when the experiments that showed it to be a hoax were released, facilitators were devastated. "One described the dedication he felt to his autistic students, the overwhelming joy he had experienced at seeing them communicate with FC, and finally, his shock and heartbreak when he learned that the method had

21. Nathan and Snedeker, *Satan's Silence*, pp. 138-39.

never worked at all — that it simply had overlaid his thoughts, and his colleagues' concerns about sexual abuse, onto other people's silence."[22]

Despite these research findings, however, FC still has its defenders. Biklen continues to promote the technique through the Facilitated Communication Institute and to insist that facilitators are dedicated, well-intentioned child advocates. I can understand the desire to cling to an idea that once showed such promise for uncovering hidden skills in the disabled and opening up their lives to their families, but I cannot condone it, given the damage it has done. Some still believe that facilitated communication can be an effective tool if facilitators take pains to avoid influencing their subjects, but it is unclear to me that the technique ever produced any of the good it was said to have produced, and it clearly did bring havoc into the lives of innocent people. It made little difference to Matt Gherardi's father whether his son's facilitator transmitted his ugly accusations consciously or unconsciously; the result was the same. The only actual abuse that took place in that situation was committed by the facilitator, and, as in many such cases, the abuse claimed its victims. The facilitator was guilty not only of falsely accusing Matt's parents but also of helping extend in yet another way the public perception that child abuse is more common than it really is. To that extent, he was helping to fuel the sort of hysteria that would claim yet more victims through such channels as the daycare center prosecutions and RMT.

Hysteria in High Places

Janet Reno came to the Clinton administration from the position of Dade County (Florida) State Attorney with the reputation of being a child advocate. Indeed, it could be argued that precisely that portfolio made her attractive to the Clintons, particularly Hillary Rodham Clinton. Reno has stated that she does not believe in bad people, only bad socioeconomic environments. Some Miami critics called her "Root Cause Reno" because of her insistence that "crime was not committed by bad people but caused by dysfunctional homes."[23] Some of her statements and actions indicate that she believes America is in the grip of an epidemic of child abuse. Some of her prosecutions in Dade County give evidence of the sort of ideological perspective associated with child abuse hysteria, and there is no evidence

22. Nathan and Snedeker, *Satan's Silence,* p. 139.
23. Peter Boyer, "Children of Waco," *The New Yorker,* 15 May 1995, p. 38.

that she abandoned that perspective in her role as Attorney General of the United States.

Reno first went to work for the Dade County state attorney's office in 1973, and one of her first tasks was to organize a juvenile division. She was appointed State Attorney in 1978, and remained in the office through the eighties, during which time she established a reputation for prosecuting cases involving accusations of satanic ritual abuse in daycare centers. The cases closely followed the pattern of the McMartin Preschool incident in California. Parental suspicions led to investigations in which children initially denied that anything had happened, but, after lengthy questioning by child-abuse specialists who employed interview techniques very much like those used in the McMartin case, the children gradually changed their stories until they developed into elaborately detailed tales of bizarre, cult-like, ritualistic activities.

One of Reno's high-profile satanic-ritual-abuse cases involved Bobby Fijnje, a fourteen-year-old boy who babysat children at his church's daycare center in a well-to-do suburb of Miami.[24] The case was opened after a distraught mother took her little girl to a therapist because she suspected that the child had been molested. Law enforcement officials were contacted, and eventually Reno brought in child-abuse specialists to interview other children at the center. Videotapes of these interview sessions show questioning very similar to that in the McMartin case. The children said that Bobby had sexually molested them, that he had killed and eaten babies, and that he had led naked dances around a campfire at night. There were also stories of witches flying through the air and eerie journeys to a cemetery where, one child said, Freddy Krueger came out of a grave. Most of the reported horrors were nocturnal, even though the center was open only during daytime hours.

As in many cases of this sort, it's not clear what criteria the prosecutor used to distinguish valid testimony from false testimony in compiling the long list of charges. Stories involving Freddy Krueger and the witches were easily enough dismissed as fantasy, we can presume, and the stories of midnight orgies around a campfire, baby killing, and cannibalism could have been discounted for a number of reasons, including a lack of any physical evidence and the fact that these activities were all supposed to have occurred during periods of time when the daycare center was closed and

24. For details of the Bobby Fijnje story, see Trevor Armbrister, "Justice Gone Crazy," *Reader's Digest*, January 1994, pp. 33-40; Boyer, "Children of Waco"; and Debbie Nathan, "Reno Reconsidered," *Miami New Times*, 3-9 March 1993, pp. 10-29.

the children were back in the custody of their parents. But the stories of molestation were accepted at face value. Perhaps Reno's office, like many prosecutors' offices, found these charges credible because of a preexisting belief that child abuse is everywhere and that children don't lie about abuse.

In any event, on the morning of August 28, 1989, four policemen came to the Fijnje home with a warrant for Bobby's arrest. The boy's father, Robert Fijnje Sr., was a Dutch national who had brought his family to Miami nine years earlier when he took up a professional position with an international firm. The Fijnjes had been members of Old Cutler Presbyterian Church since their arrival. Robert Sr. had served in the church for three years as a deacon and three more as an elder. His wife, Vivian, attended Bible classes and worked in the kitchen. Bobby and his sister, Nanette, attended Sunday school and had formally become members of the church while growing up there. The whole family was active in church activities. Now, without any prior warning, the police showed up to take the boy away to the Dade Juvenile Detention Center. As it turned out, he wouldn't leave the facility for more than a year and a half.

During the initial police interrogation, Bobby was denied meals, and he nearly lapsed into a coma induced by a blood-sugar deficiency. While he was in that condition, he was coerced into signing a confession — which he recanted as soon as he regained his health. In the end, he pleaded not guilty, and he was scheduled to be tried as an adult on the motion of Reno's office. Pretrial hearings did not begin for a full year, and they lasted until January of 1991. Throughout these hearings, and during the trial itself, the Fijnjes were repeatedly urged by the prosecutors to enter a plea of guilty for their son in exchange for a reduced sentence — and they were warned about what would happen if they didn't: "We were told that he would have AIDS within a week after entering prison," his father wrote later. "We were told what a horrible time he would have in prison, where the jailers are mere administrators and the prison is actually ruled by the prisoners. But we knew Bobby was innocent, and we refused to accept a plea bargain."[25] As the months dragged by, the Fijnjes twice sought to have Bobby released on bond, on the first occasion into their own custody and on the second occasion into the custody of the boy's uncle, a retired Connecticut State Supreme Court judge. The petitions were denied on the grounds that Bobby was "a threat to the community" and a flight risk. Reno added that the child needed to be isolated from his parents because of the likelihood that they

25. Fijnje, "An Open Letter to the American People," posted on the Internet at http://www.efn.org/~srl/bobby.html.

had molested him in the past and would try to prevent him from speaking out about it or any of his own criminal activities.

The trial itself was the longest in the history of Dade County and cost the taxpayers well over $3 million. More than eight hundred members of the church testified on Bobby's behalf, and not a single witness testified to having seen any criminal activity. The jury returned its verdict on May 4, 1991, but the judge delayed revealing it for an hour and a half, waiting for Reno to arrive at the courtroom, because she had said she wanted to be there for the reading. The jury acquitted Bobby on all counts. One journalist reported that Reno stomped out of the courtroom in a fury following the announcement. Soon after, the Fijnjes moved back to The Netherlands, shaken and appalled by the American judicial system.

The Fuster Case

The Bobby Fijnje case was not the first prosecution of suspected child abuse in a daycare facility for Janet Reno's office. Already in 1984, while the McMartin Preschool trial was still much in the news, Reno initiated an investigation of the Country Walk daycare center in Miami.[26] As in the other cases we have reviewed, interviews with children at the center began with denials but eventually produced stories of bizarre and violent acts of ritual molestation. The center's proprietors, Frank and Ileana Fuster, were charged, and Reno, who was then engaged in a tight reelection race for the office of Dade County's chief prosecutor, promised to do "everything humanly possible to see that justice is done." Of course, her idea of justice entailed imprisonment of the Fusters.

The case against Frank Fuster, a Cuban immigrant, appeared espe-cially compelling because the couple's son tested positive for gonorrhea of the throat, and Frank's wife, Ileana, a Honduran immigrant, eventually confessed to charges of child molestation at the daycare center and testified that Frank abused her as well. Prominent feminists and children's advocates made much of the diagnosis of gonorrhea of the throat, insisting that you couldn't get clearer evidence of oral sex between a man and a child than that. In fact, however, the U.S. Centers for Disease Control and Prevention have found the test for gonorrhea of the throat to be highly unreliable: in

26. For details of the Country Walk case, see Pendergrast, *Victims of Memory*, pp. 371-74; Nathan, "Reno Reconsidered"; and Nathan and Snedeker, *Satan's Silence*, pp. 108-10, 169-77, 194-95.

fact, more than a third of children who tested positive did not have gonor-rhea at all but simply a strep infection.

Then there was Ileana's "confession." Arrested in August 1984 at the age of seventeen, Ileana Fuster resolutely maintained her innocence during a period of almost a full year that she was locked up naked in a small, constantly lit cell. In October she received an offer from Reno's office to reduce her sentence significantly if she turned state's evidence and testified against her husband, Frank. She refused to confess to any wrongdoing on her own part or to implicate her husband.

Unhappy with the progress of the investigation, Reno's office called in psychologist Michael Rappaport and his partner Merry Haber, who ran a business called Behavior Changers. Rappaport has since testified that he and Haber visited Ileana in her isolation cell thirty-five to forty times, and that Janet Reno also visited her there. Reno has denied this. The psychol-ogists used threats, inducements, and cajolery in attempts to get Ileana to admit that she had abused the children in her care. She insisted that she had no memories of any such activities, but they eventually managed to convince her that what she and Frank had done was so horrible that she had repressed all memories of it.

Finally, at the urging of Rappaport, who often hugged her, and Reno, who held her hand, Ileana gave a series of "confessions" in court.

> Frequently, when Ileana couldn't answer a question because she couldn't remember, Rappaport would intervene. In one typical exchange, when asked to describe an incident of abuse, Ileana answered, "I couldn't do it. I don't recall." Rappaport interrupted, insisting that "it's not that you can't recall; it's that you don't want to recall. . . ." When she said she couldn't remember, Rappaport would often request and receive "breaks" in which he and Ileana would retire for several minutes in private. They would then return to the proceedings and Ileana would supply an answer. (One of her charges against Frank was that he had put snakes inside her and children's genitals.)[27]

Following the pattern of the children's stories, these confessions gradually evolved into increasingly elaborate descriptions of ritual sex abuse.

27. Pendergrast, *Victims of Memory,* pp. 372-73. Pendergrast notes that "in 1991 Rappaport told journalist Debbie Nathan that Janet Reno had accompanied him on most of these visits. When Reno was nominated for U.S. attorney general and became a national figure, Rappaport retracted his statement. Reno has denied being present during the guided imagery sessions."

Ileana ended up serving three and a half years in a juvenile prison program and then was released and deported to Honduras. In 1994, she recanted her confessions in a sixty-one-page sworn deposition that also described the yearlong ordeal of isolation and intensive interrogation to which she had been subjected. Frank Fuster was convicted and sentenced to serve six life terms plus 165 years; he has been in a Florida prison for over a decade, having survived several attempts on his life.

Sources of Hysteria

We have taken a brief look at some of the overreactions to suspicions of child abuse that have been occurring in increasing numbers in communities around the United States and at all levels of our society, from suburban daycare centers to the offices of our highest law enforcement agencies. What is it that has led us to react in such extreme ways to such questionable charges, that led police investigators to accept fantastic stories unsubstantiated by any physical evidence in the Fijnje case, that led prosecutors to imprison and coerce seventeen-year-old Ileana Fuster, that led otherwise law-abiding parents to attempt to burn down the McMartin Preschool and leave death threats on the Buckeys' answering machines? The short answer would seem to be that we live in fear that our children are at risk. They are more precious to us than anything else, and we are increasingly anxious about their safety. The threat from a thousand ill-defined sources seems almost palpable. We are bombarded by an endless succession of media reports on children tossed out of seventh-story windows, children abandoned in rat-infested hovels, children abducted and raped and murdered by strangers. The world seems to be full of monsters. Similar concerns and reactions are scarcely new, however. The history of Western civilization is peppered with stories about monsters preying on innocent children.

Myths of Ritual Murder

Stories about wicked men and women preying on innocent children are a staple of cultures throughout the world and throughout history. Within Western civilization, these legends go back at least as far as the ancient Greeks, who accused Jews of the ritual sacrifice of infants. During the second century C.E., early Christians were accused of "holding meetings at which babies or small children were ritually slaughtered, and feasts at which

148

the remains of these victims were ritually devoured; also of holding erotic orgies at which every form of intercourse, including incest between parents and children, was freely practiced; also worshipping a strange divinity in the form of an animal."[28] One can see that the originators of these legends were charging the scapegoat groups with the most abominable, disgusting behaviors imaginable: cannibalism, incest, bestiality.

Typically, these legends have come to the fore during periods of cultural change or upheaval, when the social or religious status quo is perceived to be decaying. The threatened majority often lays the blame for the perceived societal chaos on some minority ethnic or racial group within the society. Norman Cohn says that the "essence of the fantasy was that there existed, somewhere in the midst of the great society, another society, small and clandestine, which not only threatened the existence of the great society but was also addicted to practices which were felt to be wholly abominable, in the literal sense of anti-human."[29] Since most cultures view the abduction and abuse of children as the most abhorrent behavior imaginable, it is often a central component of these ritual abuse and murder myths. Society appears to be at risk. The future is threatened by change, and children are the future.

During the twelfth and thirteenth centuries, Jews again came under fire: they were accused of abducting and ritually murdering Christian children — the so-called blood libel myths. These rumors spread through Europe so rapidly, and so many Jews were burned at the stake, that Pope Gregory X found it necessary to extend papal protection to Europe's Jews in 1272. "Most falsely," he wrote,

> do these Christians claim that the Jews have secretly and furtively carried away these children and killed them, and that the Jews offer sacrifice from the heart and blood of these children, since their law in this matter precisely forbids Jews to sacrifice, eat, or drink the blood, or to eat the flesh of animals having claws. This has been demonstrated many times at our court by Jews converted to the Christian faith: nevertheless very many Jews are often seized and detained unjustly because of this. . . . We order that Jews seized under such a silly pretext be freed from imprisonment, and that they shall not be arrested henceforth on such a miserable pretext.[30]

28. Norman Cohn, *Europe's Inner Demons: An Enquiry Inspired by the Great Witch-Hunt* (New York: Basic Books, 1975), p. xi.

29. Cohn, *Europe's Inner Demons*, p. xiii.

30. Gregory X, quoted by Jean Bethke Elshtain in "How German Was the Holocaust?" *Books & Culture*, March/April 1997, p. 35.

After the Reformation, during the sixteenth and seventeenth centuries, belief in satanic rituals and sexual orgies arose again in the form of the great witch craze. The most famous example of community hysteria in American history is, of course, the Salem witch hunt of 1692. Among the charges made against the "witches" during that hysteria were some of sexual predation. But there have been other, less well-known instances of community demonizing in U.S. history. During the great waves of European immigration to America in the mid-nineteenth century, a strong anti-Catholic prejudice came to prevail in this country. Several popular books were published that claimed to offer the confessions of "ex-nuns who had escaped from convents where they witnessed orgies, torture, witchcraft, and the slaughter of infants."[31]

Urban Legends

The spirit of the subversion myth is evident in a variety of modern urban legends about threats to children. One hoary example is that of sadistic people trying to kill young children by poisoning their trick-or-treat candy or inserting pins and razor blades in fruit. Fear of that threat was rampant for some years but seems to have faded more recently.[32] Other legends in this category include kidnappings at Disneyland or Disney World (there has never been one at either place, according to Anaheim and Orlando police). As with other urban legends, these stories of children at risk are characteristically embellished by the teller, who gives them a special immediacy and plausibility by saying that they happened to a friend or relative. The stories serve the same function in modern society that the old fairy tales and folk tales from the Brothers Grimm and Hans Christian Andersen did for earlier generations: they give credence to parents' anxieties about the safety of their children.

Seventy percent of American parents say that their greatest fear is that a stranger will abduct their child, but the threat of it actually happening is

31. Nathan and Snedeker, *Satan's Silence*, p. 32.
32. See Joel Best and Gerald T. Horiuchi, "The Razor Blade in the Apple: The Social Construction of Urban Legends," *Social Problems* 32 (June 1988): 488; Nathan and Snedeker, *Satan's Silence*, pp. 30, 259. The Best and Horiuchi research covered twenty years — the 1970s and 1980s — and turned up only two deaths as a result of Halloween candy tampering, both of which were traced back to a member of the child's own family. Only a handful of other incidents were ever documented, none of which resulted in serious harm to children and most of which were found to have been done by children themselves to get attention.

very small. On average, in a given year only about 200 to 300 children in America are kidnapped by strangers and held for as long as overnight, and about 100 of those are actually killed. Contrary to popular perceptions, these numbers have not been rising in recent years. We are more fearful of the crime largely because it looms so large in media reports — but one of the reasons it makes the news is that it is so rare and brutal. The relative rarity of the crime is, of course, scant consolation to the parents of Polly Klaas and Megan Kanka and others who have suffered this horrible loss, but it should inform our perception of the problem and help to determine reasonable responses to it. We might reasonably seek to tighten regulations surrounding the release of known sex offenders back into communities, for instance, and teach our children as we always have about the dangers of accepting gifts or invitations from strangers. But if we succumb to paranoia and poison our own intimate family relationships with distrust and suspicion, then we are yielding too much to the handful of sociopaths that make it onto the evening news.

In general, blood libel myths and urban legends give evidence of our historical need as humans to demonize the Other — to find a scapegoat outside ourselves for the evils we perceive to be threatening us. Hysterical fear of ritual child sacrifice still exists in America today, but the identity of the Other, the force to be demonized, has changed. Some communities have pointed the finger at underground networks of satanists running the nation's daycare facilities. Radical feminists demonize all men. The clients of RMT therapists look yet closer to home, to the members of their own families.

The Urge to Protect and the Rush to Judgment

Our perception that the world is an increasingly threatening place has heightened our natural concern for the safety of our children. Foreign observers have long viewed Americans as a peculiarly child-oriented society, and it is probably more so now than it is has ever been before. The growing concern for the welfare of children is such a dependable feature of the American psyche, in fact, that it has become a kind of mother lode for politicians. Bob Dole launched his bid for the Republican nomination for president in 1995 by attacking Hollywood for undermining the moral foundation of the nation's youth with lurid movies, hate-filled rap music, and violent video games. Bill Clinton made initiatives associated with children the centerpiece of his second presidential campaign. In an assessment of the 1996 Democratic convention, Richard Stengel wrote, "Policies were constantly formulated in terms of tots. *E. coli* bacteria doesn't just kill people, it kills 'children.' The problem with pollution is that it poisons 'playgrounds.' The reason to fight crime is so that 'children's lives are not shattered by violence.' Look at President Clinton's initiatives: literacy for all eight-year-olds, extra money for child care, adoption tax credits, flex time and family leave."[33] References to kids redeem discussions of virtually every political issue. During his campaign for the presidency, Dole consistently spoke of the national debt in terms of the threat it posed to the nation's children. In his 1996 State of the Union speech, President Clinton proudly declared that "for the first time since the dawn of the nuclear age there is not a single Russian missile pointed at America's children." As Jean Bethke Elshtain has noted, "In American politics in recent years, this sentimental simplification has become the bipartisan platitude of choice, not least because the mention of kids has a way of disarming criticism."[34]

Our feelings about the issue of protecting our children run so deep and are so powerful that they make an effective lever that others can use to push us in one direction or another. Politicians are not alone in making use of this lever. Child-abuse activists have used it to disarm their share of criticism, too, by imploring us to "believe the children." But appeals to strong emotions of this sort without some counterbalancing appeals to reason can help to promote hysteria. There is a considerable danger of deception here — including self-deception. In the McMartin Preschool investigation, the investigators who sounded the call to believe the children did not themselves believe the children when they all initially protested that they had not been molested. The investigators were not prepared to believe the children until the children started saying the sorts of things they expected to hear, telling the sorts of stories that the facilitators, using a variety of contaminating interrogation techniques, induced them to tell. And even when the investigators started hearing the sorts of stories they expected to hear, they believed them only to a point. In the Bobby Fijnje case, for instance, they were willing to believe the children's reports of molestation but not the stories of witches and cannibalism.

Charges of child abuse inevitably inflame our emotions, and it is frequently difficult to determine the facts in such cases with any certainty. Any right-thinking person longs for justice in these situations, but we should not let our natural inclination to protect the children rush us to

33. Stengel, "Carried Away with Kids," *Time,* 9 September 1996, p. 34.
34. Elshtain, "Suffer the Little Children," *New Republic,* 4 March 1996, p. 34.

judgment when that judgment can be so devastating to so many people. False determinations of guilt harm not only those who are wrongly accused but also the children on whose behalf the charges are brought. The prosecutors in the McMartin case not only squandered millions of dollars on the investigation and trial, ruined the lives and livelihood of the accused, and tore apart a community; they also implanted memories of bizarre sexual abuse in the minds of the children they were ostensibly protecting — in effect committing their own kind of child abuse.

Suspicion of the Parent

Another factor that has helped build our anxieties concerning the vulnerability of our children is connected with changes in our society that have affected the ways in which we perceive ourselves, our children, and our families. Some of these changes have been purely economic; others involve our acquisition of new attitudes associated with a variety of post-Freudian psychotherapies that have entered the national consciousness by way of popular culture.

The generation of middle-class Americans that came after World War II is pretty much the first one in which children's primary relationship to the family is no longer significantly economic. Throughout most of the country's history, children in farming communities were expected to begin working early. One of the stories in my extended family is of my grandfather's response when, while working with some of his sons in the field, he was interrupted by one of the women from the house to inform him that his wife had just delivered their fourteenth child. He inquired about the newborn's gender, and, when informed that it was a boy, he replied in his thick Dutch accent, "Goed. Anudder veeder. Ve need more veeders." He didn't love his children any less than any of today's parents, but he wasn't sentimental about the role the new child would have to play in the family. Even in the industrialized cities (certainly up through the Depression), most children went to work after the eighth grade to help support the family. Among the urban poor, children were routinely put to work well before that age.

That economic structure has changed radically — and with it the role of children within families. Parents and children once more typically had to work as partners in a struggle to survive. In the postwar generations, the increasing affluence of the middle class has allowed many parents to provide for their children's needs without requiring them to contribute financially.

To a greater degree than was formerly the case, then, parents have become the providers and children the recipients of the security and comforts afforded by material goods. To the degree that these children associate unhappiness with unmet wants and needs, they are more inclined than those of previous generations to associate their parents with the source of their unhappiness.

That association has been validated and amplified by a variety of post-Freudian psychotherapies that have gained considerable influence in American culture in the postwar period. Once the prerogative of the wealthy few, therapy is now ubiquitous in our society. Airline companies now keep psychologists on retainer so that they can quickly be dispatched to crash sites to comfort survivors and the grieving families of the victims. School systems routinely send counselors into the classrooms after traumatic events such as the death of a student in a car accident. Radio and TV channels are awash with self-styled therapists offering advice in an endless variety of flavors. Bookstores stock shelves full of self-help books. Every weekend the local Marriott hosts a new therapeutic seminar, and twelve-step programs have proliferated to heal victims of virtually every imaginable debility. Almost all of this popular fascination with and reliance on therapy has emerged in the past thirty years. Significant for our discussion here is that many of these therapies have had dark things to say about the family.

An overwhelming anti-parent bias is evident in many of the most popular schools of psychotherapy. The key assumption is that if we as adults feel depressed, inadequate, anxious, or tense or generally have difficulties with relationships, it is because our parents did not give us adequate nurture and freedom when we were growing up. Some of this animus is already evident in Freud's work, as in his formulation of the Oedipus complex — the intense hatred between father and son presumed to be integral to the "formation of all male personality." Today, the mother also comes in for her share of attributes inimical to the child: she is dominating, castrating, controlling, manipulative, seductive, emotionally dependent.[35]

Thomas Harris, author of the exceedingly popular *I'm OK — You're OK* book and dictum of the 1970s, teaches that together the two parents thwart the child's full development by producing "parent tapes" that condition the child through repetition to believe he or she is not good enough or smart enough, thus laying the foundation for failure and unhappiness as adults.

35. See Paul Vitz, *Psychology as Religion: The Cult of Self-Worship*, 2d ed. (Grand Rapids: William B. Eerdmans, 1994), p. 60.

On the one hand, [the child] has the urges (genetic recordings) to empty his bowels ad lib., to explore, to know, to crush and to bang, to express feelings, and to experience all of the pleasant sensations associated with movement and discovery. On the other hand, there is the constant demand from the environment, essentially the parents, that he give up these basic satisfactions for the reward of parental approval. This approval, which can disappear as fast as it appears, is an unfathomable mystery to the child, who has not yet made any certain connection between cause and effect. The prominent by-product of the frustrating, civilizing process is negative feelings.[36]

We received similar messages from other popular therapeutic gurus of the period — Abraham Maslow, Carl Rogers, primal scream therapists, and the like: children are born innocent, creative, free, expressive, and whole, the gurus said, but external forces shackle, smother, and stunt these virtues. As the single most important external force in the lives of most children, parents naturally get the lion's share of blame for their ruination.

Many have pointed out the holes in this cheery view of human nature. Paul Vitz, for one, has suggested that "the myth of the intrinsically good and happy child . . . , with negative influences all coming from the outside, is a form of sentimentality almost touching in its naiveté." For one thing, it completely ignores positive parental influences on the child such as "love, food, music, playmates, dances, nursery school, games, travel, crafts, stories. Such events not only give the child great joy; they are also the common, positive, observable, sustaining activities of a normal child's daily life." Harris also appears to be oblivious to any negative characteristics of children, such as "the ease with which [they] learn the concept 'mine' and the difficulty they have in learning 'yours'; children's extreme self-centeredness; their remarkable capacity to become totally demanding tyrants." Vitz concludes by asking that we call the current psychotherapeutic prejudice against parents by its real name — " 'scapegoating.' When will psychological theory be honest and large enough to allow us all the dignity of accepting that the fault is not in our parents — any more than it is in our stars — but in ourselves?"[37]

Another force that bolsters the idea of the innocent child and malevolent parents is the vastly popular concept of the "inner child." A mainstay of the recovery movement — equally popular with feminists, the

36. Harris, *I'm OK — You're OK* (New York: Harper & Row, 1967), pp. 48-49.
37. Vitz, *Psychology as Religion*, pp. 61-62.

men's movement, and the great host of those recovering from dysfunctional families and codependency — the inner child represents not only the natural goodness and freedom trapped inside the adult but also the vulnerability and fragility of that true inner spirit, oppressed by a hostile and insensitive parental world. At the urging of their therapists, some people cuddle, hug, and talk to their inner child; some even set aside a separate room in their house for it. This bespeaks a powerful attraction to the myth of lost innocence. And any sort of real-world human relationships measured against this sort of idealized innocence will of course look tainted, imperfect, dysfunctional.

I well remember an "alternative school" that was established in the community where I lived in the early 1970s as a protest to the way these seventies parents perceived their own upbringing. The school's organizers remembered having had altogether too many stultifying rules when they were growing up, and they wanted to establish a much freer learning environment. They wanted *their* children to live by their "natural" desires and inclinations. I asked one of the advocates of this alternative education what would happen if my child were suddenly to get a natural inclination to bop his child over the head with a two-by-four. There would have to be a rule about that, he conceded. Pushed a bit further, he acknowledged in the end that there probably would have to be a good many rules. That's because children's impulses, like those of their parents, are not always governed by sweetness and light. What some current psychological theorists denigrate as "negative" — civilization — has always implied a code of rules designed to rein in our darker impulses. My friends, the new educational philosophers, were utopians. Unfortunately, the history of America is strewn with the wreckage of utopian societies.

But the longing for utopia persists. Regardless of whether we have actively subscribed to any of the post-Freudian therapies, the thinking of those of us who belong to the postwar generations has inevitably been affected by them to the extent that we have been exposed to the popular media, which have disseminated their basic concepts in countless subtle ways. And insofar as we have gotten comfortable with the psychological model of the child as a pure spirit and the parent as stultifying and corrupting force, we are that much closer to accepting the basic tenets of RMT. We are that much closer to accepting the possibility that ostensibly loving fathers might in fact have preyed on their innocent daughters during childhood and that those daughters might have buried all memories of the activity during the process of being socialized into their parents' version of civilized society.

Postscript

We have undertaken this consideration of the changing perspective on the problem of child abuse in this country because the ways in which we view this problem significantly affect the ways in which we view RMT. A person who believes that child abuse is epidemic in our society, for instance, will be more inclined to believe that it might have occurred in a specific case reported by an RMT client. On the other hand, a person who believes that investigators elicited false memories of abuse from children in daycare centers will be more inclined to believe that RMT therapists might elicit false memories of abuse from their clients. Given the degree to which our awareness of the problem of child abuse has increased in recent years, virtually everyone has some sort of presuppositions about the subject before encountering RMT. It is important to look at the ways those presuppositions can color our assessment of the validity of RMT.

The passage of CAPTA in 1974 almost immediately brought about a huge increase in reports of child abuse in America. The legislation compelled all public servants and associated professionals to report suspected abuse or face fines and imprisonment; it also granted legal immunity to anyone who reported abuse. It led to vastly greater numbers of both genuine and spurious accusations of abuse, which swamped the social service agencies assigned to deal with the reports. A profusion of reports on the topic in the popular media led to a widespread public perception that child abuse was common, even epidemic. As I have already suggested, this perception not only makes it easier to believe the claims of RMT clients but also makes it easier for the RMT clients themselves to overcome initial doubts about the validity of the memories that they ostensibly recover in therapy.

We also noted that as social service agencies scrambled to handle their exploding caseloads immediately following the passage of CAPTA, they were forced to hire additional investigators. There were few experts in the field of child abuse at the time, and many of the agencies hired individuals who had been specializing in cases of violence against women. Most of these new investigators brought with them assumptions about the nature of abuse that were associated with their former work — including feminist convictions about the prevalence of abuse and male aggression. As we saw in Chapter 4, these convictions were also influential in helping to legitimate and foster the spread of RMT. In addition, the new child-abuse investigators directed the bulk of their resources toward middle- and upper-middle-class environments rather than toward the impoverished settings in which earlier child-abuse experts such as David Gil had said most abuse actually takes place. Most RMT clients also come out of middle- and upper-middle-class families.

We saw evidence of this narrowing of the investigative focus to middle- and upper-middle-class settings in the series of sensational trials involving daycare facilities around the country that took place during the eighties. There are a number of important parallels between these investigations and RMT.

1. The investigators in the daycare cases began with a strong presumption that the facilities' operators were guilty of abuse. They pressed cases on the basis of questionable testimony, ignored the fact that there was no significant corroborating physical evidence, and dismissed the initial denials of wrongdoing by all of the witnesses involved in the cases — including, most importantly, the presumed victims of the abuse. Similarly, RMT therapists often arrive at a diagnosis of repressed memories of childhood abuse on the basis of the most nonspecific sorts of symptoms. In many cases they overrule clients' objections that they have no recollection of abuse, reject the protestations of family members that the remembered abuse could not have happened, and make no effort to look for any other evidence to substantiate the clients' "memories."

2. Prosecutors in the daycare trials typically relied on facilitators to get the children to relate what had happened to them. Critics charge that the interrogation techniques used by these facilitators invariably contaminated the testimony of the children by encouraging them to fantasize and by providing specific sexual images with which to confabulate their recollections (e.g., by presenting them with the so-called anatomically correct dolls). Similarly, critics contend that many of the therapeutic techniques commonly used in RMT render the clients highly suggestible. When used by an untrained or poorly trained therapist, such tools as hypnosis and guided imagery at the very least encourage confabulation and have been shown to have the potential to implant false memories.

3. The testimony of most of the children in the daycare trials followed a three-stage pattern that is often seen in RMT as well: initial denials that any abuse occurred were succeeded by hazy and sometimes contradictory recollections of sexual molestation, and these recollections gradually grew more elaborate until they incorporated details that were clearly beyond the realm of possibility, often involving incidents of satanic ritual abuse. Stories of the ritual sacrifice of animals and

humans (often babies), of being forced to drink blood, and of cannibalism are common to the third stage of recollection in both the daycare and RMT contexts.

We might add to this list another similarity between the daycare prosecutions and RMT: in both settings, the protestations of innocence from the accused have for the most part fallen on deaf ears. This is partially attributable to an inclination on the part of many in our culture, after a generation of exposure to therapeutic concepts by way of popular culture, to view adults (and especially parents) as an inherently corrupting influence on innocent children. In effect, the accused in cases of recollected child abuse start out with at least this strike against them.

We also took brief note of the historical link between periods of social and religious change and the formation of subversion myths and urban legends about children at risk. Scholars contend that the purpose of these archetypal stories about monsters preying on children is to alleviate our anxieties about the unsettling changes taking place around us by codifying our worst fears and assigning the blame for the perceived evil to a convenient scapegoat. Is it possible that RMT is a sort of recapitulation of this phenomenon on a personal level? Many RMT clients first enter therapy with little more than complaints of generalized anxiety, depression, or powerlessness. A diagnosis of repressed childhood sexual abuse can itself be traumatic, but many people find it liberating in some sense because it identifies a very specific cause for an ill-defined collection of symptoms, and it provides a path to recovery through exacting revenge on the scapegoat-incester by way of anything from abreaction to litigation.

Child advocates draw on our natural desire to protect our children and our natural concerns about their vulnerability in issuing the call to "believe the children." Proponents of RMT draw on a similar desire for justice on behalf of adult victims of childhood sexual abuse when they issue a call to "believe the victim." Their appeal is compelling because it reaches us at a profound emotional level. Who is not sickened by thoughts of sexual predators molesting our children? Who does not want to see such individuals brought to justice, regardless of whether the crimes were committed yesterday or twenty years ago? But we have an obligation to everyone affected by such accusations to assess them very carefully. For if the memories of abuse that underlie the accusations are false, then our willingness to believe the accuser — and to accuse and perhaps prosecute people on that basis — will not only ruin the life of the accused but will also further damage the accuser. For in believing the accuser, we are affirming the reality of the abuse. If we endorse the validity of false memories, we simply make it that much more difficult for the accusers to cast them off or move beyond them. In effect, we are helping to condemn people to live with memories of abuse — and that in itself constitutes a definition of abuse.

CHAPTER 7

Pauline

Liz: Our daughter, Pauline, was born the day after Christmas, 1955; her brother, Edward, was born April 2, 1958. Edward was born with diabetes, and Pauline developed asthma at the age of three, which gave me a full-time job just getting through each day without an emergency. Talking about the growing-up years is important to me because I was the care-giver — that is, I was the one who was there twenty-four hours a day taking care of two sick kids while Roger was working three jobs to pay all the medical bills.

When they were growing up, we had a functional/dysfunctional family: in other words, we were normal. Roger and I had grown up in the Depression years, so we tried to give our children everything we did not have — and then some. Pauline even had a pony when she was thirteen or fourteen. We boarded the pony at her uncle's place in Wisconsin, and she'd go up there and ride her pony whenever she wanted. This was typical of our generation: we spoiled our kids. Our son had a mini-bike, and our daughter had guitar lessons — you know, the whole nine yards. When your children are sick, you go twice as far to make life as easy as possible for them. You never know how long you're going to have them.

Pauline had a lot of friends while she was growing up. They were always welcome at our home, and they came often. She still sees them to this day.

We took the children on vacations during their growing-up years. We went to Wisconsin and Colorado, and we did side trips every fall to see the changing colors of the leaves. We didn't have a lot of money, so we tried to do things close to home. Life went on, and Rog and I did what we had to do every day of every year to take care of our children the best

161

we knew how. On December 20, 1969, my mother passed away suddenly, and that threw me into such a depressive state that I started drinking daily. Over the next nine or ten years I was drinking at night to ease the pain of losing my mother, and I was on Valium during the day to stop shaking. I won't pretend that those were good years for Pauline and Edward. They weren't. Those were Pauline's high school years, and I was not there for her. I was there physically, but not mentally and emotionally. Edward suffered through those years too. I did take him to school every day and to work. I did whatever I had to do to get through the day and to take care of my children.

Pauline met George (who was to become her husband) one day while riding her bike at a local park. She had known him in high school, but they were only casual acquaintances at that time. When she ran into him at the park, she brought him home to see us. They started seeing each other often. George was attending Lowell Institute of Technology in Massachusetts. They married in 1978 and moved out to Massachusetts while George finished school. They were gone for two years, and I missed her terribly. It was the first time we had been apart.

We were close, super close — at least I thought we were. During the year following their marriage, I decided to get my life together, and I entered a program to stop drinking. Pauline and I talked often during my "drying-out" process. I have been sober and drug-free ever since then (for almost seventeen years now).

When Pauline found out she was pregnant with our first grandchild, we were thrilled. They had returned to Illinois, and I had helped her find an apartment. After finding out about the baby, they moved from the apartment into a home, and we helped them move again. When our grandson was born, he and I bonded immediately. We were very close and still are, even though we do not see each other now.

Pauline was depressed after the first baby. I stayed with her to help her (as my mother had stayed with me). I remember seeing Pauline shaking as she was giving the baby his baths. When he'd wake up from a nap, she would get really nervous and not know how to handle him. I felt really sorry for her, but I had to leave for home and my own responsibilities. I feel that she had postpartum depression and never really got over it.

Two years later, our beloved granddaughter was born, and we were once again thrilled. We took care of the grandchildren often during the next few years and loved having them with us. Often we would go to their home for dinner or they would come to ours. We were a good close family. Edward had married also, and we had many dinners together.

Roger: I came from a big family, and they became part of that family. When we all got together for holidays at my parents' house, there were five of my brothers and sisters and twenty or more children, all enjoying themselves.

Liz: For the first ten or eleven years of George and Pauline's marriage, everything was fine. But in 1988, her attitude started to change. She had begun to act different: she became quiet and withdrawn and angry with her father whenever he would call her. Rog and I talked about her being angry with him, and I told him he was just being too sensitive and not to worry about it. Then she called me and told me she was depressed. We talked about it, and she said she was going to go to a therapist.

"I don't understand," I said. "You have a beautiful home, two beautiful kids — why are you depressed?"

"I don't know," she said. "I just don't feel right about being on this earth. . . ." Things like that. I hated to think she was having emotional problems. I told her I was sorry she was having difficulties and that I was glad to hear she was getting help with them.

Roger: Shortly thereafter, I retired, and the company I worked for gave me a retirement party. When we talked to Pauline about the party, she did not want to commit to attending. I told her I really wanted her there, that it was important for me to have my whole family there. So she did attend, although she was quiet.

Then, suddenly, Pauline said she thought she had been sexually abused when she was about four years old by a janitor in a church. She and two little neighbor girls had gone to a Bible school kind of thing at a local church that we were not affiliated with (one of the other little girls went to church there). They attended for three hours every morning for a couple of weeks or so. Pauline was a thirty-three-year-old woman now, and she was supposedly just remembering this abuse that occurred twenty-eight years earlier.

Liz: Nevertheless, we believed her. I called the pastor and tried to find out who the janitor was at that time. I wanted to know; I wanted to go after him for touching my daughter. But Pauline told us to stay out of it, that she would handle it. By this time she had seen a minister who ran a sexual assault survival group on the side. She was also seeing a Christian counselor, and together they visited that church, where she now said animals had been killed and children had been molested in satanic rituals.

163

Roger: Not long after that, she accused the nuns and priests at a local school where she had been in first grade — of sexual abuse.

Liz: Pauline was in therapy full-time at this point. We were still very much in touch, and she and I talked about her "memories." I told her I was glad she was seeking help. Her Christian therapist had been recommended by her church.

Then, shortly after that, she abruptly told us she was going to be hospitalized for a while. She chose a leading hospital in Milwaukee, which, she told us, "handles things like this." Of course, I didn't know what "things like this" meant at the time, but I figured that the doctors knew best. (That was our first mistake.)

Roger: The head psychiatrist at the hospital where my daughter became a patient/guinea pig gave her her first sodium amytal interview. Little did we know it was to be the first of many.

Liz: I went to baby-sit her children while she was hospitalized. I cooked their meals, washed their clothes, took them to school, and so forth. When Pauline came home a week later, I returned home. Within a month, I got a call that she was hospitalized again. So I returned to baby-sit the grand-children again. All the while, she was accusing more and more people of abusing her when she was a child.

When she came back from the hospital the second time, something was different. She and George would talk quietly in the kitchen so I couldn't hear what was being said. At that point, I figured it had to be her father that she was about to accuse. Who else was left? She had accused practically everybody else we knew. It was as if everyone that we ever knew had been put on this earth to molest her. Our lives were about to change forever, and we didn't even know it.

Suddenly, after that second hospitalization, we both received letters in the mail. She had already said she was going to write and tell us a few things about her childhood that she didn't like. I remember the day we received those letters. We were sitting at the kitchen table. It was March 1989. I jokingly said to Roger, "Now don't get upset by what's in these letters. Pauline's blowing off steam. She's letting us know what was wrong with her life and what she didn't like about us when she was growing up. It's called confronting, and they are encouraged by the therapist to do this." And I was smiling when I said it.

So we opened our envelopes and started reading through the letters, and I got to the place where she said, "Dad touched me inappropriately." I grabbed Roger's letter out of his hand and looked through it, and it said the same thing. I said to him, "Did you do this?"

And he said to me, "No, of course, I didn't do that."

I said, "If you didn't do that, why is she saying this?"

Roger: Of course, she has never accused me to my face of sexual abuse or rape. She has made these charges to others but never to *my* face. At the time I was supposedly abusing my daughter, I was working approximately a sixteen-hour day or better — not counting travel time — which made the whole thing very far-fetched.

Liz: I don't remember much after reading those letters, except that I started to scream at him. Then I remember calling my son-in-law at work and asking him, "What's going on here? What does this mean? What's happening?"

"You got the letters," he said. "You know what it means."

"George, this isn't right," I said. "What's going on?"

He wouldn't discuss it with me at all. Pauline would not talk to us either. Our life as we knew it was coming to a painful end. I remember that I had promised a friend of mine that I would go to the doctor with her that afternoon. I didn't want to go, but I had promised to go with her for moral support, and I had to go. I remember just sitting there in the waiting room and crying. I remember feeling that my whole life, everything I ever stood for as a mother was ending, and I could do nothing to stop it.

That night I went to our church to talk to a priest, but he was on his way to a wake and did not have time to talk to me. Nor did he assign someone else to comfort me, even though I was sobbing. I have not gone back to church since that time.

Roger: I was reading the letter, but I didn't get beyond the point where she said, "He touched me inappropriately," and I put the letter down and said, "This is a bunch of crap." Later, as time went by and things did not get better, I went upstairs and I packed up everything Pauline owned in this house. Then I met George near Elgin, Illinois, and I gave him everything I had collected. I didn't want anything to do with her. That was how bad it hurt.

Liz: I believed Roger, then I believed Pauline. Then I believed him, then I believed her. I hated him because I thought he had done some horrible things to his daughter. I didn't at that moment put together *all* the accusations that she had made about other molestations. I simply didn't think about them then. I just thought he had done it — and I believed it on and off for the next nine months. It was terrible: I was going to divorce him, I was going to leave him, I was going to kill him. It was just a horrible time for both of us.

Finally, Pauline agreed to talk to me, and I said to her, "What's going on here?"

She said, "It's true, Mother, it's all true. But I still love you guys. I still love Dad, and I still want you in my life."

I said, "How can you love someone who molested you?" She just kept saying to me that she would always love us, and that she would eventually like to discuss this with her father. But she never has — not to his face anyway.

Then she started writing Roger letters, which said, "Dad, I know what you're trying to do, but it's not going to work." I asked him whether he was harassing her. This was after the initial accusations. And he said, "No, I'm not harassing her." Roger and I fought constantly. As it turned out, I had sent her a Christmas card in 1989 (Roger has never even seen the card) that had a wreath pictured on the front of it. Well, evidently someone informed her that a circle (the wreath) was a satanic symbol, and that we were trying to tell her to commit suicide. It was pure madness. (I also found out at that time that she was reading *Satan's Underground,* a book by Lauren Stratford, whom she had met.)

Roger: I knew I was innocent, and I wanted to do whatever I could to prove it. So I immediately volunteered to take a lie detector test. What with delays, the test was not completed until May. The results were negative. We didn't try to keep it mum at all. We told everybody in our families and among our friends what was happening. And I'm convinced to this day that that's the reason I've never been approached by any law enforcement people or the Department of Children and Family Services. From day one, I did not keep my mouth shut. I told everybody what I was accused of and that I did not do it. We went and talked to the police in the town where Pauline lives, and we have gone to the police in our own town also. I even called the FBI and informed them of what was happening.

Everyone was sympathetic but offered no help. We filed a complaint with the Wisconsin Psychiatric Ethics Committee against the psychiatrist and the "Christian" therapist. The board met with us, but they decided that the psychiatrist had done nothing wrong. We were considered third party, and our daughter would not open her records, so there was nothing they could do.

Pauline's third hospitalization was in January 1990, and it was then that satanism came into the picture. It was also when my father became part of the story: he was supposedly the leader of a satanic cult. According to my daughter, my father would come to our home at midnight to pick us up, and we would go to cemeteries and meat lockers to hold sacrifices. (The term "meat locker" appears in the book *Satan's Underground*.) I was supposed to have drugged my wife, Liz, so that she wouldn't know about these rituals. Not only that, but my grandfather allegedly was the one who got me into this satanic behavior when I was a child and stayed on his farm every summer.

Liz: We called and asked for meetings with Pauline, but she and her "Christian" therapist kept turning us down flat. We tried reaching her pastor, but he refused to see us also. Nobody wanted to see us or talk to us. We begged and begged for a meeting with her and her therapist, and with George. All to no avail.

Finally, when she was once again hospitalized in Milwaukee, she called and said, "All right, we'll have a meeting between Dad and me and the head psychiatrist" (who was to function as the "disinterested," or impartial, party). I made up my mind that this was the day that Roger would admit that he had done it. It was to be the first time he would have seen Pauline since her allegations, and I expected him to admit it when he saw her. Admit what he had done and say that he was sorry. Then I was going to get a divorce and get out.

Pauline and her dad and the "mental health professional" were in the meeting for about a half hour — I was sitting in the hallway outside — and Pauline came out and told me to come in because, she said, "Dad thinks that you ought to hear this." When I entered the room, the psychiatrist, sitting there with his cowboy boots and his brass stirrups, said, "Do you want to sit over here by your husband, or aren't you speaking to him?" And he laughed, thinking he was being funny. I said, "I don't think this is funny. This is my daughter's life we're talking about!"

Roger: Then Pauline said, "Dad murdered so many babies I lost count. He made *me* murder three. One time you, Mom, were being raped on an altar, and I had to murder a baby to make them stop gang-raping you." That was, of course, when Liz knew it was all made up. But the whole time Pauline was talking, the psychiatrist's exact words were: "I believe you believe what you're saying, Pauline." It was as if she was in a trance, she was so drugged up with whatever she was receiving from the doctors at the hospital. She was staring with a blank stare, like a zombie, clutching a Bible to her chest.

Liz: She just sat there talking about the horror, the killing of babies, and that I was there as an unwilling participant. She "remembered" little Edward being there too. She said she saw us all at the ritual.

I said, "Pauline, this isn't true," and I got up and hugged her. She was like a limp doll; there was no response. She was like a stranger.

Roger: On the way out of the room, the psychiatrist motioned me aside and whispered in my ear so nobody could hear it, "You know, your daughter's crazy." He also made a statement that day that the people on the floor of the hospital tended to believe Pauline at the beginning, but now they were starting to doubt her.

Liz: Roger and I left the meeting and went to the cafeteria to wait for Pauline. She had a session planned with her "Christian counselor" after the confrontation meeting with her dad and me. His office was just down the hall from the psychiatrist's office; they were now working together. The "Christian counselor" had moved his practice from our daughter's town to the hospital in Milwaukee. Even more bizarre: the therapist Roger and I had engaged in Niles, Illinois, to help us get through this nightmare has also joined this psychiatrist in Milwaukee. Now I ask you, is that an unholy alliance, or what?

We waited for Pauline in the cafeteria until her session was over. But when it was, she wouldn't let us come to her room. She turned and said to me, "Why are you being so nice to me when I've said such terrible things about you?" I said, "Because we love you, and we want you to get better." But she still wouldn't allow us into her hospital room. So we hugged her and said good-bye. If we had known then what we know now, we wouldn't have left her there.

Roger: This was her third hospitalization — it was a year after her first hospitalization — at a thousand dollars a day. And that's not counting doctor's fees. Each time she was an in-patient for about ten days to two weeks. There was probably some insurance cut-off at that amount of time, otherwise they would have kept her in there indefinitely. You can bet they got Pauline's husband's insurance company for a ton of money. They have everything figured out to make sure they get every dollar allowed by the insurance companies. When one diagnosis runs out, they come up with a new diagnosis. They're not only evil, they're very clever. A dangerous combination, especially for Pauline.

Liz: In the intervening summer and fall, I was allowed to go see the grandchildren. It was heart-breaking. I was in such a state: it was like being in a nightmare and never waking up. The pain and disbelief were constant — twenty-four hours a day, every day.

Pauline also allowed me to view some of ten or eleven hours of videotape of her being interviewed under the influence of sodium amytal. In those tapes she talked about how her father came into her room when she was small and what he did to her. She said that she could hear him coming up the stairs, and when the doctor asked her how she felt at that moment, she said that she felt "scared."

I sat through all that in her family room. I was so distraught that I contemplated suicide a lot. I kept saying, "Why would she say these things if they weren't true?"

Roger: During the time of "recovering her memories," Pauline called us and asked her mom for a photo album of when she was little. Thinking this would help her get better, we gave her an album of ours that had pictures of her and Edward as they were growing up. She had the album for about two months, and she told me that she remembered one outfit she was wearing when she was molested by me (there was a picture of her in that outfit in the album). There was also a picture of my grandfather's farm in the album, and she said that that was where I was taught satanism.

It was all so bizarre. Every time we did not hear from her for a while, she would come up with different accusations when we did happen to have contact with her. A few years later, when we were comparing notes with other parents who had been falsely accused, they all said that their children had asked for a photo album of their childhood during their therapy.

Liz: I still did believe that Pauline could have been abused . . . somewhere in her childhood. I didn't know about "memory implantation" or "brainwashing" by psychotherapists at that point. I didn't know what was wrong, just that something was terribly wrong, and that the life we knew had been destroyed.

We also found out that Pauline had been a hypnotism subject; it was confirmed on a videotape that she allowed me to see. She trusted me to view only certain parts that she had preapproved. I did exactly as I was told:

I didn't want to cross her in any way. Her therapist finally did agree to see Pauline and me together. He knew that I was watching the videotapes and was going back to watch more of them. He said, "You'll see in this upcoming part that I lay my hand on Pauline's forehead. That is to bring back things we talked about in the office." Now that was hypnotism, but I didn't realize it then because I was still believing her, and I was so distraught.

When I thought about what she was saying about me being an unwilling participant in satanic rituals, I called her and really got into it with her: "You know very well that I haven't done anything unwillingly in my life. I was always the one who told anybody to go to hell if it was something I objected to. . . ." She knew that.

She said, "Well, maybe they just told me it was you there on the altar being raped." She didn't say, "Maybe I was wrong," but, "Maybe they told me it was you."

I said, "No, Pauline, no."

"Well, maybe that part isn't true," she said finally. "But that doesn't mean the rest of it isn't true."

"Yes, it does," I said. "If you realize part of it may not be true, then why not question all of it?"

Then, all of a sudden, Pauline allowed both of us to see our grandchildren. It was as if she abruptly wanted a relationship with us. Very bizarre. She sent Roger gifts occasionally, on Father's Day and Christmas, for instance. She also sent Bible verses or sometimes a personal sentiment. "Always know you're loved . . ." is how the last one read. It was truly baffling.

Roger: She sent me a Bible one Christmas. She still seems to be a part of that fundamentalist Christian outfit in her area, though she is no longer with her original "Christian" therapist. She now has another "Christian" therapist. She would quote Bible verses every time she'd write us, so that was ongoing.

Liz: But more accusations were always forthcoming. For example, we had traveled to Colorado when the kids were little. Roger had a friend he had met and got to know when they were in the army in Korea together. Well, they had maintained their friendship, and this friend, who was a photographer, even took the pictures at our wedding. He later moved out to Colorado, and we stayed with him and his mother on a couple of occasions when we were on trips with our children. Pauline was now saying that she was molested by Roger's friend, and that he took pornographic pictures of her at his home. She also said that he gave Roger money to let him take Pauline away and use her for pornography.

Roger: My friend had a three-bedroom home. Liz and I stayed in one of the bedrooms, our kids stayed together in another, and our friend's mom stayed in the third bedroom. Our friend stayed in the basement. Pauline says she remembers asking me, "Why are you doing this, Daddy?" (i.e., giving her to him for pornographic pictures), and that my reply was, "Because we need the money, Pauline." None of this happened, so where was it all coming from?

Liz: So I played detective and investigated our friend's past: I called his childhood and high school friends. He had always been a photographer, even in high school. I asked his friends if they ever saw any pornography, and they all said, "No, none at all." I called everyone I could find that knew him. I was calling for help, doing everything I could to find out what was going on.

Even after that session in the hospital in Milwaukee when the satanism charges came up, I still wasn't sure. I continued to be confused, wondering, and very torn up about it. Our life together was still not very good . . . not for a long, long time. I still had doubts.

Roger: I was convinced from day one that they wanted me out of Liz's life. That was one of their goals.

Just to give you an idea of how this all escalated, and how brainwashed Pauline was, one day she called and said to Liz, "Guess what, Mom, I've got something else . . . something new."

"What, multiple personality disorder?" Liz said.

"Yes, how did you know?" Pauline asked.

"Because it's the next thing in the book," Liz replied. She was reading *Satan's Underground* and *The Courage to Heal* because she knew Pauline was reading them. Supposedly, Pauline had come into Chicago to a well-known hospital and was diagnosed with multiple personality disorder. Naturally, she went back home with a sure knowledge that she was a certified MPD victim.

Liz: She told us that she had been depressed from the time she was five years old. We used to go to Grandma's in Skokie (Roger's mother) every Christmas Eve. It was a huge gathering of twenty-seven family members where everybody exchanged gifts and had a wonderful time. Pauline told me, "I used to sit there so depressed . . . because I knew what was going on."

I said to her: "You know, you're one of thirteen grandchildren. Why

171

aren't any of the others coming forward with any of this?" Her reply, of course, was, "Because they are all in denial."

The meeting with the psychiatrists, when Pauline made the accusations of satanic ritual abuse, was in January 1990. About six months later, the multiple personality disorder diagnosis came up. But she had started allowing us to come out to see her and her family because, she said, she wanted a relationship. On New Year's Day 1993 we were allowed to come out and play with the grandkids and have a nice time. But then we would be prohibited from seeing them again — with no explanation. It was like being torn in two for both us and the grandchildren. We felt like criminals: we were afraid to hug the kids or to be alone with them in any room.

Roger: The grandkids wanted me to go upstairs with them, but I didn't want to go up with them without Pauline being along, because I was afraid of more accusations being made.

Liz: Pauline herself has been here in our home, the home she grew up in, only once in six and a half years. When my sister, her aunt, passed away, I asked her why she didn't come to the funeral. "I didn't want to be with you people," she replied. "You people" meant her mother, father, and brother Edward.

Roger: Pauline's in-laws passed away, and we weren't even told of their passing. The funerals were right here near our home, but we didn't find out about them until months later. They didn't call us to let us know because they didn't want to see us. We knew George's parents well and liked them, and we had called them about this problem with Pauline. But they just didn't know what to do to help us. They said that they did not believe the charges our daughter was making against us.

Liz went to the church Pauline now belongs to; she also called and wrote letters all the way to the top of the church's hierarchy. Not one person from the church has talked to us or agreed to see us. If they claim to be a "Christian" church, I don't understand why they wouldn't be willing to help us restore our family. Isn't that what God's love is supposed to be all about?

Liz: We were in touch with other parents who were falsely accused of abuse and satanism by children involved in an off-the-wall church group in Evanston, Illinois. The group is engaged in so-called Christian counseling. They're splitting families apart and doing it in the name of God . . . and calling themselves "good Christians." I don't think that children making false accusations against their parents is what God has in mind for the definition of the word "Christian." Pauline's pastor has refused to see us or talk to us to this day. What kind of "Christian" is that?

Pauline's current "therapist" is an unlicensed social worker (having dropped her license in 1988 or 1989) whose shingle now reads something like "Marriage and Family Counseling." And Pauline claims she's happy now. She's lost her entire family — her parents, her brother and sister-in-law, her cousins, her aunts and uncles, everyone who was ever involved with her life up to the age of thirty-three — and she tells me she's happy. All of her current friends are (self-proclaimed) victims too. Her husband told his parents before they passed away, "All we do is hang around with her sicko friends." He said that at least two years ago; we don't know what he's saying now. He knows that all of her terror did not happen, but he's been no help at all.

Roger: Our son Edward has basically stayed out of it. We found out that when Pauline did talk to him and his wife, he kept it from us. He does not believe his sister's accusations at all. Of course we see him and his family, but he doesn't want anything to do with the subject. He just would rather not talk about it. He and Margot have their own health problems, so maybe it's understandable. But Liz couldn't accept it for a long time — that Edward wouldn't help us get his sister back. It hurt a lot to get no support from our son.

Liz: I asked Roger's sisters — we were all close — to help me get our daughter back, but they wouldn't help me either. The oldest sister did try to help: she wrote Pauline a letter saying that these accusations couldn't possibly be true, that everything she said was wrong, that everything she had been led to believe about her family was a falsehood, and that she should rethink all of it. All she got for her efforts was a nasty letter back from Pauline saying, among other unprintable insults, "I appreciate your concern for my parents, but I was there, you weren't."

Roger: We have kept records of every bit of communication from our daughter and anyone else connected with her, her therapists, her church people (what little there was), everything — we have stacks of it. We intend to give it to our grandchildren someday, when they are old enough to understand what has happened to their mother and old enough to know that we tried with all our hearts to right this wrong.

Liz: Our grandson, Mark, is not quite thirteen, and he and I were very close. He told us not to move so that he could find us as soon as he gets his driver's license.

You see, Pauline took her children — our grandchildren — to the same therapists, and then they too had "recovered memories" of being molested at Grandma and Grandpa's house. It was really sick!

I was there at her home during one of the infrequent visits I was allowed to make, and Pauline said to me, "I know I'm not crazy now because Mark is remembering things in therapy too."

"What!" I said. "That does it, Pauline. You are no longer my daughter, and I am not coming back here again!" We did not know that Mark was standing in the doorway and heard us and started screaming, "No, Grandma, no!" I had to calm him down and convince him that I would come back to see him.

A short time later we found out that our granddaughter, Mary, was having memories "in therapy" of going to "Grandpa's church" and sitting in a circle for Satan worship — our own parish, right here in town. She wouldn't know our church from the Basilica in Rome; she's never been there.

When Pauline brought the children into it, there was no way I could deal with that. What are they going to grow up remembering about grandpa and grandma? Once we've passed away, there will be no one to make sure they know the truth. So we have to fight this fight for their sakes and hopefully for the sake of our daughter that once was.

Our lawyer kept saying, "No matter what, you see those grandkids anytime you can." I knew he was right, but the heartbreak of seeing them sitting on the curb and waving good-bye with all of us crying was just too much. I just couldn't take it anymore. It wasn't fair to them or us to be pulled in two directions. I thought it would be kinder to them for us to stop seeing them altogether.

Roger: We did at one time think about suing our daughter's therapists, and our lawyer agreed to take the case, free of charge, because he is so concerned about psychotherapists' implanting false memories. But in the end we decided not to sue because it would mean putting our daughter on the stand, and we didn't want to hurt her any more than she had already been hurt. We feared that she might commit suicide. But, in retrospect, we probably should have sued: it may have contributed to stopping this nonsense a lot sooner.

Liz: As for the argument that suing your daughter's therapist would drive her further away — well, she couldn't be further away. We've asked ourselves, What's the worst thing they could do to us? They've taken our daughter away, and they've taken our grandchildren away; they've already done the worst thing they can do to us. I told my daughter that it would have been kinder if she had just killed us outright.

Roger: We both said essentially the same thing: we decided to cut off the relationship at that time. Pauline told me that I owed her $350,000 for her therapy. Our last contact with her was in March 1993 — two years ago. I don't know if it was the right thing to do, but we just couldn't stand the pain any longer.

There are people in my daughter's town who claim that I am a cult leader. People I don't even know. My picture was reportedly passed around in a local hospital, branding me a cult leader, so that people would know what a "cult leader" looks like. Our daughter did not even go to this particular hospital. It was a network of "repressed memory" therapists promoting their evil throughout the city. (Note: This hospital has since been closed.)

Liz: After I realized what a travesty this whole business of child abuse and satanism was, I called Pauline's husband, George, and told him that we were going public. I promised him that we would not stop until this was straightened out.

"We're going on TV," I said, "and we're going on the radio. We'll talk to anyone and everyone who will listen."

"I wish you wouldn't do this," he said. "If you would have just kept your mouths shut about it, this would have all been over by now."

We were on the Sally Jessy Raphaël program, and then the *Chicago Tribune* did a feature on us in May 1993. And there have been a lot of public and media appearances since then. When Cardinal Bernardin of Chicago was accused of sexual abuse, we were on almost all the major news stations.

I'm a black-and-white personality: something is either right or it's wrong. And this scenario was wrong. Once I realized that our daughter had been duped by supposedly "Christian" counselors and "mental health professionals" and that Roger was not guilty as charged, then I got mad. You go through this process: first disbelief, then grief — the kind of grief that never goes away. You live each and every day in a state of shock, waiting for the nightmare to end. Then, when the pain can get no worse, anger starts to take over — anger that anyone who takes an oath to *do no harm,* whether it be an oath to God or an oath to the medical profession, could screw up so badly and destroy families without any conscience at all.

175

Even if our daughter comes home, the wound would always be there. It will be hard to trust our love for each other again.

Roger: A friend I talked with recently said, "Your daughter's an adult, and you can't change her mind. You can't be the parent anymore. You have to look at her as another adult, not as your child. This is how she feels, and you can't change it. So you have to stop being a parent and trying to make her better — as we parents do. That's the reason we're all in such pain. We're not looking at this as one adult to another; it's a child-parent relationship, and you dare not tell a child to go to hell. If anyone else — say, a stranger — called you a satanist or a pedophile, you'd probably punch them out, but not your own child." It made a lot of sense to me.

Liz: I feel that a mother's emotions run a lot hotter than a dad's. Especially in my case, because my children were ill, and they were my entire life to me. I always told Pauline that if she was going to accuse *anyone* of abuse, it should have been me, because I, not her dad, was the principal caretaker.

Never in our lives could we have believed that something like this would happen to our family. We treasured our children all their lives, and we double-treasure our grandchildren. How dare someone come into our child's life and take away all the love we have given her! How dare they! I would like an answer!

I have this love-hate relationship with life and with God now, because I don't understand all this. I don't feel I should have to defend my parenthood or my husband's parenthood to anyone. We are in our sixties now. All we wanted was to be a family as close as our parent-families were. We just want to have our children and grandchildren over for dinner on Sunday afternoons. It just isn't going to be that way, I guess. That's very hard to accept. Our daughter seems to know who and where God is. But wow, if it's God who's influencing her critical thinking, I don't understand his reasoning. What "God" would be so cruel? Our daughter never hurt anyone in her entire life. The daughter we knew loved us with all her heart. What a shame to give her such pain for no reason at all. How can these "mental health professionals" look at themselves in their mirrors every morning and still sleep well at night?

Postscript: Months Later

Roger has been deeply depressed and not feeling well physically for a very long time. Liz suspects that it is more than a simple depression that an

176

antidepressant can cure. Numerous tests are completed, and Roger is found to have a large tumor on his pituitary gland. At first it is not known if the tumor is malignant or benign, and the doctor suggests surgery as soon as possible. Fortunately, Roger gets a second opinion, and the new doctor is trying to shrink the tumor with medication.

Pauline is informed of her father's condition by her brother, and she calls her father on the phone. Roger becomes very emotional on the phone with his daughter; he sobs and has feelings of great tenderness toward her. But Liz, despite what she has always said to others about nonconfrontation and despite her best intentions, gets angry. When she gets a chance to talk to Pauline, she says, "Where does it say in your Bible that you can flush your parents of thirty-three years down the toilet and then call with concern when one of them gets seriously ill?" Liz feels that Pauline is only doing what in her mind would be the "Christian" thing to do and that she will abandon them again in the near future.

Pauline, for her part, says her mother is too controlling and she only wants to talk with her father (whom, of course, she accused of horrible acts of satanic abuse and murder). And she is not — in this hour of need and crisis — backing off from those accusations against her father. She is simply calling to tell him she is concerned and she loves him. Pauline says that her mother has never had appropriate "boundaries" concerning her. Liz feels that the word "boundaries" is a therapist's concoction and that all that she ever felt for her daughter was love.

"For the death of the daughter we knew," says Liz, "we hold responsible the unethical, incompetent, and evil 'mental health professionals' — both licensed and unlicensed — as well as the self-proclaimed 'Christians' who are destroying families in the name of God. The name of the game is money, power, and greed. If insurance companies would stop paying for 'recovered memory therapy,' our daughter would become well and whole again."

Once it was determined that Roger's illness was not life-threatening, phone calls from Pauline diminished to a trickle. She says she wants to "keep in touch." They feel this is a step in the right direction, but they are afraid of being hurt again. They are both planning to go on with their lives without their daughter. They pray that their grandchildren will come to them when they are old enough to realize the truth.

"These adult children of 'therapy gone astray' have to take responsibility for what they believe," says Liz. "Their beliefs do not come without consequences. Do we have to die to get our children back? I'm afraid that our death certificates will read, 'Died of a Broken Heart.'"

CHAPTER 8

Multiple Personality Disorder
and Satanic Ritual Abuse

Sybil said, "Well, do you want me to be Helen?" And I said, "What do you mean?" And she said, "Well, when I'm with Dr. Wilbur she wants me to be Helen."

— *Dr. Herbert Spiegel*

In 1973 the book *Sybil*, which the jacket copy described as the "true and extraordinary story of a woman possessed by sixteen separate personalities," shot to the top of the bestseller lists and became a paperback industry phenomenon. The Sybil of the story was a young woman who suffered from an exotic mental disturbance known as multiple personality disorder (MPD).[1] The ailment is said to be brought on by severe emotional trauma

1. Many books, articles, radio interviews, and public television documentaries have dealt with the subject of multiple personality disorder. For examples of positive treatments, see Frank W. Putnam, *Diagnosis and Treatment of Multiple Personality Disorder* (New York: Guilford Press, 1989); Ralph Allison (with Ted Schwarz), *Minds in Many Pieces: The Making of a Very Special Doctor* (New York: Rawson, Wade, 1980); Colin Ross, *Multiple Personality Disorder: Diagnosis, Clinical Features, and Treatment* (New York: John Wiley, 1989); and Ross, *The Osiris Complex: Case Studies in Multiple Personality Disorder* (Toronto: University of Toronto Press, 1994). For more critical views of the troubling nature of MPD, I am indebted to the following sources in my preparation of this chapter: John Taylor, "The Lost Daughter," *Esquire*, March 1994, pp. 76-87, the best exposé of the MPD craze in the popular literature; Mark Pendergrast, *Victims of Memory: Incest Accusations and Shattered Lives*, 2d ed. (Hines-

178

(typically sexual) in a person's youth. In response to the trauma — some say as a coping mechanism — the person's psyche is said to shatter into pieces like a china vase dropped on a stone walkway. Each fragment becomes a separate personality, a distinct alter ego (or "alter") within the subject. The alters of a given person may speak with different voices and dialects, reflecting the experiences of individuals of different ages, races, backgrounds, and genders. The various alters can come forward either with or without the subject's volition.

According to Dr. Cornelia Wilbur, Sybil's tortured MPD was brought on by her mother, who, according to Sybil's recovered memories, copulated with her husband in front of Sybil, sexually molested the girl, shoved objects up her vagina, forced her to watch as she defecated on the neighbor's lawn, and engaged in lesbian orgies with young girls in her presence. The book tells the story of how Sybil "dissociated" into several personalities because of that abuse and how Wilbur helped her deal with her abused past and disturbed present. Wilbur did not write the book herself; she engaged an English professor, Flora Rheta Schreiber, to write a novelization of the story and infuse it with re-created scenes and dialogue. After the book had become a notable publishing success (reaching the number one slot on *Time* magazine's bestseller list), it also became a popular movie starring Sally Field as Sybil and Joanne Woodward as Dr. Wilbur. The popularity of *Sybil* helped pave the way for the publication of similar stories during the next decade. Not insignificantly, the number of reported cases of MPD shot up dramatically after these stories entered the popular culture.

In more than a hundred years of psychotherapy preceding the publication of *Sybil* in 1980, there was a total of about two hundred reported cases of the sort of mental disorders that today would be classified as MPD (the earlier diagnosis was typically "hysteria," which denoted a variously defined category of psychoneurotic complaints). That relatively small number included a brief flurry of diagnoses and claimants to the disorder following the publication of Robert Louis Stevenson's classic story *The Strange Case of Dr. Jekyll and Mr. Hyde* in 1886. Generally speaking, the symptoms in these cases tended to follow the pattern of maladies such as hysterical blindness and hysterical paralysis, in which no physical causes

---

burg, VT: Upper Access Books, 1996), pp. 151-96; Paul McHugh, "Multiple Personality Disorder," *Harvard Mental Health Letter* 10 (September 1993); McHugh, "Psychiatric Misadventures," *American Scholar* 61 (Autumn 1992): 497-510; McHugh, "Psychotherapy Awry," *American Scholar* 63 (Winter 1994): 17-30; and Debbie Nathan and Michael Snedeker, *Satan's Silence* (New York: BasicBooks, 1995), pp. 45-50.

for the problems were evidenced. The onset was typically abrupt, following some sort of acute emotional trauma. But following the publication of *Sybil,* both the symptomology of the disorder and the frequency with which it was reported began to change. By 1984 the number of reported cases had jumped to a thousand, and by 1989 to four thousand. In the 1990s, some psychiatrists and psychologists specializing in the treatment of MPD have estimated that twenty to thirty thousand people are currently suffering from the disorder; Bennett Braun, perhaps the best-known MPD specialist, has claimed that the actual number may range as high as two hundred thousand. And the reported complexity of the disorder has tended to grow along with the estimates of its prevalence. Stevenson's Jekyll/Hyde persona had but two personalities, in the 1950s Eve had three faces, and Sybil weighed in with sixteen alters. These days, MPD specialists frequently describe patients with as many as a hundred alters; one claims to have found four thousand personalities in one person.

The publication of *Sybil* clearly influenced the perception of MPD both inside and outside the psychotherapeutic community. Sybil's Dr. Wilbur became something of a celebrated and charismatic figure for a group of therapists who made MPD their specialty. Eager followers spoke of "the Wilburian revolution" and the "post-Wilbur paradigm";[2] whole schools of MPD thought cropped up, and specific treatment units were set up in major hospitals by MPD specialists, such as Bennett Braun, Richard Kluft, Colin Ross, and Judith Peterson. They have argued that MPD is commonly associated with childhood sexual abuse and that it is much more prevalent than had been previously thought. Given the signal importance of *Sybil* in all these developments, it is worth noting that the validity of Wilbur's original diagnosis of MPD in this case has been seriously called into question.

At one point in her treatment of Sybil, Wilbur sent her patient to a colleague, Dr. Herbert Spiegel, a practicing psychiatrist who had once been her professor at Columbia Medical School. Spiegel was well known for his facility with hypnosis, and Wilbur hoped that he could use this tool to effect some progress in Sybil's case. As soon as Spiegel interviewed Sybil, however, he began to question Wilbur's diagnosis of MPD. Spiegel relates this conversation:

> Sybil said, "Well, do you want me to be Helen?" And I said, "What do you mean?" And she said, "Well, when I'm with Dr. Wilbur she wants me to be Helen." I said, "Who's Helen?" "Well, that's a name Dr. Wilbur

2. Taylor, "The Lost Daughter," p. 84.

gave me for this feeling." So I said, "Well, if you want to it's all right, but it's not necessary." With me, Sybil preferred not to "be Helen." With Wilbur she felt an obligation to become another personality. That's when I realized that Connie [Wilbur] was helping her identify aspects of her life, or perspectives, that she then called by name. By naming them this way, she was reifying a memory of some kind and converting it into a "personality."[3]

Further investigation revealed that Sybil's mother was a schizophrenic, but Spiegel found no evidence to suggest that she or anyone else had ever sexually abused Sybil. He found Wilbur unwilling to consider modifying her diagnosis, however. He was puzzled by her intransigence on this point until some time later, when he was contacted by Flora Schreiber, the writer who was working with Wilbur.

After Sybil had stopped treatment, Schreiber came to see me and asked me to cooperate with her and Wilbur on a book. I agreed and said I would open my files. Schreiber said as she was leaving my office that she was calling it multiple personality disorder. I said she's not; she doesn't have the key figure of MPD, spontaneous switching between personalities. These came up during therapy. They were hysterical, imitative. What gave it away was [Sybil] telling me that Wilbur requested certain personalities.

I said I would work with Schreiber if Sybil was diagnosed as a hysteric or as a dissociative disorder. Schreiber said that publishing companies wouldn't be able to sell it unless it was MPD. I said that was a hell of a reason for a medical diagnosis. She got mad as hell and left the room in a huff. She wouldn't talk to me after that and neither would Wilbur. Their goal was to do something to capture the imagination of the public. They succeeded.[4]

Spiegel was willing to investigate the possibility that Sybil was suffering from a dissociative disorder — an umbrella term for a number of different conditions marked by a dissociation from or interruption of a person's fundamental aspects of waking consciousness. Specific complaints in this category range from a sense of detachment from one's personal experience, body, or self to a variety of different levels of amnesia about past experience. MPD is essentially an extreme form of dissociation in

3. Spiegel, in an interview with Mikkel Borch-Jacobsen, "Sybil — The Making of a Disease," *New York Review of Books*, 24 April 1997, pp. 61-62.
4. Spiegel, quoted by Taylor in "The Lost Daughter," p. 85.

which an individual's sense of personal identity gets lost amid a jumble of other personalities. Spiegel found evidence of a dissociative disorder in the fact that Sybil was extremely suggestible. About one in ten people is susceptible to hypnosis, and the small number within that tenth who have a dissociative disorder, says Spiegel, are extremely easy to hypnotize. In fact, dissociating is essentially what happens when one goes into a hypnotic trance, and people who dissociate easily can go in and out of such trances frequently, often without being aware that they are doing so. Spiegel found Sybil to be "a hypnotic virtuoso": she was extremely easy to hypnotize — which is to say that she was extremely suggestible. If individuals of this sort "pick up a premise — are told or infer that there is a Communist plot to take over the media or that they've been sexually abused by their fathers — they can fill in the details on their own," says Spiegel. They are prime candidates for the implantation of false memories, and they are able to embellish these false recollections so naturally that careless or uninformed therapists can easily be convinced of their validity.[5]

The fact that Sybil failed to exhibit the classic symptoms of MPD such as spontaneous switching of personalities, the fact that she preferred to discuss her problems without resorting to speaking through other personalities (and was quite able to do so), and the indications that the different personalities that had emerged in her therapy sessions with Wilbur had been summoned at Wilbur's request all suggested to Spiegel that Sybil was not suffering from MPD. There was a simpler explanation for her symptoms: she was an extremely suggestible individual who was uniquely qualified and willing to supply the sorts of behavior and "recollections" that her therapist was looking for.

Spiegel subsequently had a fair amount of contact with MPD specialists, and he became skeptical of many of their practices and beliefs. He has found that many of them have received little substantive training beyond their area of ostensible expertise and hence are ill-equipped to recognize alternative explanations for the symptomology they observe. Many have received no training at all in hypnosis and are unaware that highly suggestible patients like Sybil may be entering hypnotic states without knowing it. Given the recent profusion of MPD, the special suggestibility of the patients involved, and the questionable credentials of many of the therapists, Spiegel has come to the conclusion that most of the currently reported cases of MPD are *iatrogenic* — that is, imagined illnesses induced in the patient by the therapist's words or actions. Many others in the medical and psychiatric

5. Spiegel, quoted by Taylor in "The Lost Daughter," p. 85.

communities concur. It is unlikely that a disorder historically so rare should suddenly be turning up in tens or hundreds of thousands of individuals. It is far more likely that well-meaning therapists and suggestible clients are unwittingly collaborating in the production of symptoms fitting a pattern that has been popularized in the culture.

Paul McHugh, director of the Department of Psychiatry and Behavioral Sciences at the Johns Hopkins University School of Medicine, is similarly skeptical of most diagnoses of MPD. He contends that in most cases the reported disorder actually resembles what was formerly referred to as *hysteria* — a condition in which an individual exhibits symptoms of a medical illness as a way of obscuring a genuine psychiatric problem. The imitative behavior of hysterics was observed over a century ago by the famous nineteenth-century neurologist and psychiatrist Jean-Martin Charcot, director of the Salpetriere Hospital in Paris. Work being done at the hospital had necessitated placing some patients who had been diagnosed with hysteria in the same ward with a group of epileptics. Almost immediately the hysterics began to display behaviors that looked like epileptic seizures but were just different enough so that Charcot thought he had discovered a new mental disturbance. He called it "hystero-epilepsy" and devoted resources to observing the patients exhibiting it. Curiously, the more he studied them, the more agitated these patients became; they began presenting "progressively more intriguing kinds of fits." French doctors and members of the Parisian intelligentsia came to Salpetriere to view the phenomenon. But several of Charcot's younger students felt that he was fooling himself, setting up the conditions he was studying. One assistant, Alex Munthe, later wrote, "These stage performances were nothing but an absurd farce, a hopeless muddle of truth and cheating."[6] Eventually, one of the students asked the famous psychiatrist whether it was not possible that he had brought on this behavior "out of his own authority and enlarged it through his interest." To see if this could be true, Charcot isolated the hysterics from the epileptics and gave them indications that he no longer found their condition to be so fascinating. They soon ceased presenting the pseudo-epileptic symptoms, and the staff began to focus on the conditions and behaviors that had brought them into the hospital in the first place. Says McHugh, "MPD is an iatrogenic behavioral syndrome, promoted by suggestion and maintained by clinical attention, social consequences, and group loyalties. It rests on ideas about the self that obscure reality, and it responds to standard treatments."[7]

6. Pendergrast, *Victims of Memory*, p. 410.
7. McHugh, "Multiple Personality Disorder," p. 567.

Charcot showed that suggestible patients can convincingly manifest the symptoms of illnesses that they do not in fact have — and that therapists can facilitate and amplify the manifestation of these symptoms whether or not they are aware that they are doing so. McHugh contends that the same sort of thing is going on in most reported cases of MPD today. I would argue that it is going on in RMT circles as well. Many MPD specialists assume that the source of the disorder can usually be traced back to sexual abuse in a patient's childhood, and, in exploring this possibility with their patients, they inevitably introduce the possibility of therapeutic contamination. We noted that Dr. Wilbur elicited ostensible memories of various forms of sexual abuse from Sybil — and that Dr. Spiegel subsequently found no corroboration whatsoever for the recollections. And beyond the possibility of contamination originating with the therapists, there is also the possibility of clients picking up symptoms from other patients. Clients of RMT are often encouraged to join incest survivor groups and read the movement's literature, so they are immersed in detailed descriptions of the whole range of symptomology reported by victims of abuse.

Charcot observed that no hysterics recovered so long as they remained in the company of epileptics or other pseudo-epileptics and continued to focus on their symptoms and the attention of the attending physician; indeed, in such an environment, they tended to decline, presenting increasingly more elaborate symptoms. The same sort of progression is evident in RMT. Clients who devote increasing amounts of time to therapy tend to become increasingly dysfunctional and to recall increasingly elaborate kinds of past abuse. Recollections of particular kinds of abuse (e.g., such sensational things as satanic ritual abuse, child sacrifice, cannibalism, and the like) often pass through therapy groups and spring up on a widescale basis after the publication of a given book or the airing of a TV movie. It is sadly ironic that the continuation of the therapy perpetuates the suffering and prevents the client from dealing with the problems that initiated the condition in the first place, just as Charcot's fascination with the hystero-epileptics subjected them to rounds of increasingly elaborate symptomology and prevented the hospital staff from attending to the problems that had brought them into the hospital in the first place. The lesson from Paris for RMT is that it is crucial to differentiate between the genuinely incest-injured and those who are burdened with false memories of abuse.

Popular Culture and the Therapeutic Community

Paul McHugh has expressed concern that the problem of therapists tending to find whatever syndromes they are looking for is compounded by the susceptibility of the entire psychotherapeutic community to the influence of the *Zeitgeist* — what he has more starkly called its "thralldom to the gusty winds of fashion." He notes that the practice of psychiatry, like all medical endeavors, has produced its share of mistakes, but he suggests that this inevitable problem has proved to be serious in the case of psychiatry because new ideas in that discipline are more likely to be broadly discussed and adopted. Questionable therapeutic techniques, jargon, and assumptions can spread quickly through the popular culture, influencing laypeople and professionals alike. Trendy new therapies may appeal not only to troubled individuals but also to a whole range of marginally educated, unlicensed therapists and counselors who may quickly adopt new concepts and practices without fully understanding their subtleties, shortcomings, and dangers.

> Psychiatry is a rudimentary medical art. It lacks easy access to proof of its proposals even as it deals with disorders of the most complex features of human life — mind and behavior. Yet, probably because of the earlier examples of Freud and Jung, a belief persists that psychiatrists are entitled to special privileges — that they know the secret of human nature — and thus can venture beyond their clinic-based competencies to instruct on non-medical matters: interpreting literature, counseling the electorate, prescribing for the millennium. . . . [In teaching about] what psychiatrists actually do and how they do it, I am often aware that I am drawing [residents and medical students] back from trendy thought, redirecting them from salvationist aspirations toward the traditional concerns of psychiatry, which is about the differentiation, understanding, and treatment of the mentally ill. . . .
>
> Part of my justification for corralling their enthusiasms is the sense that the intermingling of psychiatry with contemporary culture is excessive and injures both parties. During the thirty years of my professional experience, I have witnessed the power of cultural fashion to lead psychiatric thought and practice off in false, even disastrous, directions. I have become familiar with how these fashions and their consequences caused psychiatry to lose its moorings. Roughly every ten years, from the mid-60s on, psychiatric practice has condoned some bizarre misdirection, proving how all too often the discipline has been the captive of the culture. . . . Psychiatry may be more vulnerable to such errors than other

185

clinical endeavors, given its lack of checks and correctives, such as the autopsies and laboratory tests that protect other medical specialties. But for each error, cultural fashion provided the inclination and the impetus. When caught up by the social suppositions of their time, psychiatry can do much harm.[8]

The current popular fascination with MPD is a case in point. McHugh believes, with many others, that the preponderance of the cases being reported today are iatrogenic. The sensational aspects of the disorder have captured the imagination of the therapeutic community as well as the general public. The idea of the shattered psyche fits in well with the spirit of our depersonalized and future-shocked times. Moreover, the belief that the disorder is typically the result of childhood sexual abuse both appeals to popular concerns and renders the diagnosis more resistant to objections: as we have already noted in the context of RMT, it is difficult to question accusations of past abuse without becoming susceptible to a host of accusations oneself. "Major psychiatric misdirections often share this intimidating mixture of medical mistake lashed to a trendy idea," says McHugh. "Any challenge to such a misdirection must confront simultaneously the professional authority of the proponents and the political power of fashionable convictions. Such challenges are not for the fainthearted or inexperienced. They seldom quickly succeed because they are often misrepresented as ignorant or, in the cant word of our day, uncaring."[9]

Genuine cases of MPD appear to be very rare, and they clearly call for careful professional help. But a lay familiarity with the disorder has so deeply entered the popular culture that it has actually become a subject of magazine questionnaires. C. W. Duncan, author of *The Fractured Mirror: Healing Multiple Personality Disorder*, promised in one magazine article to "give you the facts, the good and the bad, so you can judge for yourself whether or not you have MPD." Appended to the article was a seven-point checklist entitled "Are You a Multiple?" which Duncan assured his readers was endorsed by the "experts."

One of your friends in the incest survivors group is MPD, but it never occurred to you that you might be one too, or has it? "Possibly," you thought, but quickly dismissed it as an unlikely notion. Oh, you had heard about MPD from books, movies, TV soaps and talk shows. "But surely, I am not like them." You buried the hunch deep inside until now.

8. McHugh, "Psychiatric Misadventures," pp. 497-98.
9. McHugh, "Psychiatric Misadventures," p. 509.

"The doctor said that I may have MPD." "No, I don't!" "Yes, I do!" "That's ridiculous!" "No, it's not!" The internal argument continued, but the question hovered in the air like a stubborn mosquito.[10]

So it is that MPD has moved from the footnotes of textbooks to the pages of the Sunday supplements. I suspect that few professional therapists would countenance encouraging the self-diagnosis of a rare and devastating psychological disorder in this fashion, but this is not to say that their own perceptions of the disorder have not been shaped in subtle ways by its popularization. Duncan complains that the psychiatric community still won't accept MPD as a valid diagnosis, but that is increasingly not the case. A number of clinics have been devoted solely to treatment of the disorder, and many therapists have chosen to specialize in such treatment. One of the more prominent of these facilities is part of the psychiatric unit at the well-respected Rush–Presbyterian–St. Luke's Hospital in suburban Chicago. The staff there, headed by Dr. Bennett Braun, the director of the dissociative disorders unit, has made a critical connection between MPD and satanic ritual abuse — a connection that has become increasingly widespread over the years among therapists specializing in treatment of the disorder.

Satanic Ritual Abuse

Widespread interest in satanic ritual abuse took flight in America just a few years after the appearance of *Sybil*, when another book about a woman suffering from MPD hit the paperback stands and captured the imagination of MPD enthusiasts and therapists. By this time the connection between MPD and childhood sexual abuse was firm in the minds of many people. The new book, *Michelle Remembers*, made the same connection but added a new twist: the sexual abuse was linked to satanic rituals. Combining notions of spiritual warfare and talk of demons roaming the earth with the MPD themes that had made *Sybil* a bestseller, *Michelle Remembers* became a supermarket rack phenomenon.

Perhaps it was inevitable that somebody would eventually blame the devil for the symptoms of MPD. In any event, *Michelle Remembers*, co-written by thirty-year-old Michelle Smith and her psychiatrist (later her husband), Lawrence Pazder, was the first public document to do so. (Pazder coined the phrase "ritual abuse" in a paper he gave at the American Psy-

10. Duncan, "The Truth about MPD," *Changes*, October 1993, pp. 79-84.

chiatric Association's annual meeting in 1981.) The book is Michelle's first-person account of having been tortured by a satanic cult (of which she says her mother was a member) that imprisoned her for several months when she was five years old. It is full of graphic details of the tortures to which she was subjected in mausoleums and cemeteries, of "being raped and sodomized with candles, being forced to defecate on a Bible and crucifix, witnessing babies and adults butchered, spending hours naked in a snake-filled cage, and having a devil's tail and horns surgically attached to her."[11] These grotesque torments went on for a full year, until Michelle's "indomitable Christian faith discouraged the satanists, and they set her free." Then, she reports, she completely forgot the experiences for more than twenty years, until she entered therapy with Pazder after suffering a miscarriage. Most of the memories were recovered under hypnosis.

As Debbie Nathan and Michael Snedeker found in doing investigative research for their invaluable book *Satan's Silence*, the problem with Smith's "memories" is that, as is typical of survivor stories,

> there is no independent verification for them; indeed, there is much to contradict them. Smith is from Victoria, British Columbia, and residents of the neighborhood where she was raised say her father was an alcoholic, but that otherwise, there was nothing remarkable about her family. A neighbor and former teacher recall that Smith started first grade in 1955, attended school regularly, and was photographed for the yearbook — at a time when *Michelle Remembers* has her locked in a basement for months.
>
> Further, Smith has no records of childhood hospitalizations, and, while Pazder has documentation that she was treated for dental and dermatological problems as an adult, neither condition has any particular relationship to the tortures she claims she suffered. . . .
>
> A more likely explanation for Smith's "memories" is that they resulted from therapeutic suggestion.[12]

Despite the fact that there was no substantiating evidence for any of the events described in *Michelle Remembers* — no remains of the cult's supposed victims ever turned up, for instance, and the police received no reports of missing infants that might have matched those that Michelle says she saw sacrificed — many people were convinced that the book faithfully

---

11. Nathan and Snedeker, *Satan's Silence*, p. 45; see also Pendergrast, *Victims of Memory*, p. 138.

12. Nathan and Snedeker, *Satan's Silence*, p. 45.

described actual events. It not only spurred popular interest in satanic cult conspiracies but also gave credence to the concept of massive (or robust) repression, the belief that an entire clandestine life story could be buried deep in the unconscious, awaiting the persuasive, caring guidance of a "believing" therapist. It is worth noting that Pazder is a devout Catholic who has long had an interest in "possession states" and exorcism.[13] Michelle could produce on command a rash on her neck, and Pazder interpreted this as a form of stigmata, a welt left by the tail of the devil.[14]

Soon after the publication of *Michelle Remembers*, other women began to report to their therapists, the media, and the police that they too had suffered satanic tortures as small children. Stories of abuse at the hands of satanic cults — stories involving cannibalism, human sacrifice, and blood rituals — became fairly commonplace in newspapers and magazines. *Ms.* magazine featured a lurid cover showing a baby wrapped in the tentacles of an evil octopus-like creature with the tag line "Believe It! Satanic Ritual Abuse Exists — One Woman's Story." The associated article was written by an RMT client who claimed that her children had been sacrificed by a cult of which her mother was a member.[15]

Virtually none of the reviewers of *Michelle Remembers* questioned the validity of Smith's story. Many of those who encountered the book (and others like it) may have considered it unseemly or, as we have seen in connection with RMT literature, professionally dangerous to question the claims of an ostensible victim of abuse, particularly when the abuse was as horrific as that claimed by Smith. Some in the mass media may have had an interest in accepting the stories at face value — or even in presenting them in as lurid a light as possible. Geraldo Rivera captured the highest ratings of his career with his 1988 special on satanism. San Francisco's Channel 2 (KPIX-TV) tried to boost ratings with a sensationalistic four-part series on satanic ritual abuse (SRA) called "Significant Others." The anchormen kicked it off in this way:

Dave: It's one of society's dirty secrets, and the only way to clean it up is to talk about it.

Bob: Twenty years ago it was alcoholism, and nobody wanted to talk about it; then we found out it was everywhere. Ten years ago it was incest, and nobody wanted to talk about that. Then we found out how wide-

13. Nathan and Snedeker, *Satan's Silence,* p. 50.
14. Pendergrast, *Victims of Memory,* p. 138.
15. Elizabeth S. Rose, "Surviving the Unbelievable," *Ms.,* January/February 1993, pp. 40-45.

spread that was, and tackled that too. Well, the lid is off a new Pandora's Box, and it will really shock you. Ready for it or not, we're standing on the brink of one of society's worst secrets. This may be the hardest pill you've had to swallow.

The report went on to show a little girl of three who, according to the narrator, had eight distinct personalities. What led to the MPD? "The answer lies deep in her past," said the narrator. "Her first years of life were spent in a world of abuse, inside a satanic cult. It's a connection that may help to explain one of the most complicated psychiatric disorders of our time. In fact, in the last five years, doctors have treated more multiples than ever before. . . . Experts are finding that three-fourths of the MPDs they treat were ritually abused in cults."

Betty S. was one of them; she claimed to have 386 different personalities. "They are born out of the mind the way a baby is born out of the womb," she explained to the reporter. "And that part of you that's born out of the mind to take on the pain and the abuse and the punishment encapsulates and compartmentalizes that piece of the abuse of that person's life."

Narrator: Victims say the rituals include rape, murder, mutilation, even cannibalism. And these reports are popping up nationwide. . . . Police say that they see evidence of cults in every community, but that they are very hard to track down and crack open because they operate so far underground. But their signs and symbols are all around us.

At this point a detective was shown pointing to upside-down crosses, three sixes, and a strange, complicated circle spray-painted on the underside of a highway overpass to prove the existence of these cults all around us.

Narrator: But the strongest evidence of SRA are the victims that live among us. Spotting them is very difficult because multiples are very good at burying the abuse.

The report went on to establish the existence of MPD and the MPD-SRA connection by introducing us to Caryn Stardancer, an artist, author, wife, and mother. Caryn, who said it was "a miracle that I got this far," recalled being tortured in sadistic rituals as a child. She could not get away physically, she said, so she fled mentally, into multiple personalities. She claimed to have fifteen alters, but she spoke for the reporter in only five of them — two adults and three children. The voices all sounded pretty much alike, some in a slightly lower register, some higher and squeakier. If she was merely putting on an act for the camera, the performance was not very convincing.

Another segment of the "Significant Others" report showed footage of a small child merrily throwing plastic figures into a tub of water. The therapist attending the child related that he had suffered abuse at a very young age when he was thrown out of a boat into the ocean and almost drowned. He was working out the terror and rage associated with the event by throwing the toys into the tub of water. But there was no evidence of terror or rage in the child's face; he simply seemed to be having normal childlike fun, splashing things in the water. Against this benign backdrop, the narrator went on to say, "The torture, the killings, each act of violence . . . the child breaks into pieces, and a new personality is formed. Some say that a new child is born, an alter, with each act of violence. And that's why you hear about people with five hundred alters."

The report also featured an interview with Pamela Hudson, a social worker described as an SRA expert, who asserted that children don't bring up their abuse voluntarily, because the abusers have threatened them: "We've put this bomb inside you," she said. "If you are asked what happened, it will start ticking. If you are ready to say anything, it will blow up." Hudson said that she had treated some thirty children who had been ritually abused, most of them in daycare centers. She explained that play therapy with the children could be very revealing. "They take the dolls, and they reenact the trauma right in front of you." She illustrated this by showing how an affected child would pick out a devil figure if presented with a selection of twenty or so toy figures. In the selection she showed, the devil figure was strikingly different from any of the other toys, the sort of thing that would naturally catch a child's eye first. "The sandbox is where the children act out the conflict between good and evil," said Hudson, as the camera showed a sandbox with a child playing in it. "The children act out their anger by letting the forces of bad people win." She then took the ugly green devil figure, put it in a cage, and buried it in the sand, explaining to the child that now the bad person was gone and couldn't hurt the child anymore. "And the child will say, 'Yes!' It's a moment of triumph for the child." Hudson noted that she also uses the sandboxes in treating adults, encouraging them to reenact their abuse. She calls forth the alters, she said, and asks them to lead her through the memories. "Piece by piece, the truth is revealed," she said. "Some alters were developed to hold the pain, others to hold the guilt."

Both the "Significant Others" report and an independent documentary entitled "Children at Risk," written and produced by Dale and Bruce McCulley, which covers the same sort of territory, end with interviews with Dr. Roberta Sachs of the Rush–Presbyterian–St. Luke's dissociative disorders clinic. Sachs and her colleague Dr. Bennett Braun, who heads the facility, have gained significant reputations from their work in treating people for MPD and for making a connection between MPD and SRA. Braun, who has gone on record with the estimate that as many as two hundred thousand Americans suffer from MPD, is also convinced that SRA is rampant throughout the country and around the world. "We have seen over a hundred people who report satanic ritual abuse in their background," says Braun. "If 10 percent of what I hear about SRA is true, then we have a major problem on our hands." Sachs adds that "the issue of SRA stands where child abuse did twenty or twenty-five years ago. By that I mean, nobody wants to believe it . . . nobody wants to hear it. The judicial system is not prepared for it. If we say too much, then people will shut down completely — because it's just too much to believe. I can understand that . . . because it truly shattered all my belief systems. . . . We have to go somewhere with it so that people will listen and where the justice system will change in a way . . . that children can be protected."

The closing video of the "Significant Others" report showed Sachs working with a patient at the Rush–Presbyterian–St. Luke's facility, a woman referred to as Mary S. Her story has been featured elsewhere, and it has a good deal to tell us about the nature of the treatment being given to suspected victims of MPD/SRA by Braun and Sachs and other therapists who have trained under them and view them as experts in the field.

Mary's Story

The story of Mary S. has been told in a number of contexts to illustrate the dangers of some of the treatment programs for MPD in the United States. She was not able to provide me with a direct interview because she is currently involved in litigation. The quoted material in the following narrative is taken from interviews that appeared in a segment of PBS's Frontline *series entitled "The Search for Satan," produced by Ofra Bikel and Rachel Dretzin, which originally aired on October 24, 1995.*

Mary S. had a loving family and a close relationship with her husband and eight-year-old son, but she had been through a lot in life. While growing up, she struggled with a learning disability, and at the age of nineteen she was the victim of a brutal date rape that produced a child which she gave up for adoption. After marriage and the birth of a son, she had to have a hysterectomy, and after the surgery she developed seizures with associated blackouts. Finally, in 1988, Mary was attacked in a hallway of the school where she taught. After the attack, she fell into a deep depression, started having panic attacks, and lost a lot of weight. Unable to concentrate, she went to a psychiatrist to get medication, and at the same time started sessions with a therapist who had been recommended by a friend. During the next few months her anxiety attacks kept getting worse, and her therapist, who had recently attended a seminar on satanic cult abuse, began to suspect that there might be a darker explanation for Mary's depression than the attack at school and the earlier problems in her life. The therapist sent her to psychologist Roberta Sachs at Rush–Presbyterian–St. Luke's Hospital for an evaluation. Within five minutes of meeting Mary, Sachs diagnosed her as a "polyfragmented multiple."

Unfamiliar with the terminology, Mary had to ask Sachs what this diagnosis meant. "She described multiplicity as taking a vase and dropping it on a cement floor," Mary later recalled. "That's what she said had happened to my personality. It had shattered into that many pieces. And her job as a therapist was to glue those pieces back together into a whole."

Sachs and her colleague Dr. Bennett Braun admitted Mary to the hospital for treatment. The admission form read, "Patient is a victim of satanic ritualistic abuse. Diagnosis of MPD." The vague cult fears that had been intimated by Mary's first therapist now had the stamp of professional certainty. Mary began regular therapy sessions with Braun and Sachs.

From the beginning the doctors seemed to be more interested in larger issues involved in cult membership than in Mary's specific problems. They continually pressed her for the names of other cult members, for the names of people that she and her husband knew, and for details about cult practices. When she couldn't supply any information, they stopped paying attention to her. Despite their constant probing for more information about the cult, though, Mary had the sense that the doctors already knew more about her family background than she did. At one point Sachs told her that SRA victims from all over the country had identified her as a fifth-generation cult member; they had reported that other members of her family were high up in the cult, were in fact cult royalty. She had no memories of such matters herself. They told her that her "cult programming" had been switched on when she was thirty-nine. She asked them how they could know in such detail things about her that she didn't know herself. They told her they were experts, that they'd been studying the phenomenon for fifteen years and had documented evidence of cult activities all over the world. The doctors at Rush were indeed considered the leading national experts in the field. In November 1994, Braun was honored at the annual meeting of the International Society for the Study of Multiple Personality and Dissociation. Most of the leading figures in the field were there praising his contribution to the field of MPD and SRA. His honored peers included Roberta Sachs, Judith Peterson, Richard Kluft, Colin Ross, and D. Corydon Hammond. Gloria Steinem was the keynote speaker at the meeting. So Mary persevered in her treatment despite growing fears and misgivings. They were the experts.

But her condition was deteriorating. Braun had prescribed a variety of medications for her: Halcyon, Xanax, Prozac, and experimentally high doses of the heart medication Inderol. Mary was taking all that medication at the same time and was confused and fearful. Sachs told her that they had found evidence of fifteen developed childhood alters, some of them twins, and a system with seven cult alters. Sachs and Braun encouraged her to cut off all contact with most family members and friends outside the hospital. One of her friends testified that Mary simply disappeared. Her husband told the friends and family members that they could not have any contact with her — doctor's orders. She was warned not to break treatment, because her son's life hung in the balance. She was told that she was the only one in five generations of cult members who had been given the insight to break the chain. If she didn't break free, her son would be doomed to death in the cult.

A turning point in Mary's treatment came when Sachs had her attend a consultation with a respected expert in cult programming techniques, Dr. Cory Hammond, a professor of psychiatric medicine at the University of Utah. Hammond lectured often on the origins and practices of the cult, explaining that a systematic program of brainwashing was being conducted in the U.S. using sophisticated techniques that had come out of Nazi medical experiments and the work of the intelligence community. Hammond hypnotized Mary and asked her if she knew any of the letters of the Greek alphabet. She named a few. Hammond asked her if she knew anything about a "Gamma Erasure Code." She didn't know what Hammond was talking about, but she remembers being told that her Gamma file was still active — meaning that she was still loyal to the cult and thus a danger to the staff and other patients.

Sachs then told Mary that they had determined not only that she was a cult plant and a spy but also that she had ritually abused and programmed her son, and he would have to be evaluated. She said that Mary would have to be deprogrammed so that she couldn't kill her husband, son, or anybody else. The deprogramming, Sachs said, would have to be done by a colleague in Houston, Dr. Judith Peterson. The two therapists often referred patients to each other and had collaborated on several training programs. Mary was sent to Peterson's Spring Shadows Glen facility in Houston, where she remained for the next two years.

"When I look back," Mary says now, "I can't believe this ever happened to me. I had doubts about it all along the way. My journal is full of statements that this can't be true, it's a nightmare, I've made this up. My whole life, my world had been turned upside down at that point. Here I had been a teacher living a normal life and doing normal things — and from there I went to cult royalty. I was told that when you are raised in a satanic cult, as I supposedly was, you abuse people, even the people you love. I was going deeper and deeper into an abyss, a bottomless pit of horrors. I really believed that I would end up in a psychiatric ward for the rest of my life, or that when my insurance ran out, I would live underneath a bridge as a bag lady."

But by then, Mary says, she had begun to believe all the doctors and tried to give them some useful information. The MPD therapists had identified her as a cult perpetrator, and they told her to let the alters who were loyal to the cult come up to the surface to surrender their plan. The doctors told her that she would go to prison because they knew she had abused children and killed people and was part of this international network. Meanwhile, they told Mary's husband that she was in a cult that was intent on killing him — and that Mary's alters had abused their son, Ryan.

Ryan was admitted for MPD evaluation at Peterson's facility in Houston. Although he stayed on the unit right next door to Mary's, mother and son were kept apart. A nurse on the children's unit said that Ryan fit the pattern of many of the children who entered the unit diagnosed with MPD because of SRA. He came in a normal little boy, full of energy and activity, with no knowledge of cults or SRA. But he was exposed along with the other children to a lot of talk about such matters in therapy sessions. The children were also told that they had "parts" inside them, and they were pressured to name these parts; eventually, the parts developed into alters.

Many members of the nursing staff were made very uncomfortable by the activities in the unit. But if they expressed any of their concerns, they faced a great deal of hostility from the psychologists and psychiatrists, who attributed their apprehension to a basic ignorance about what was going on. Peterson wrote in a letter to the administrator of the hospital that no education could occur as long as the objecting nurses insisted on "living in the dark ages." One nurse said, "She let the nurses know that if they objected to the treatments, there would be reprisals. And reprisals

could mean a transfer off the unit, a demotion, in some cases actual termination. . . . People were afraid to object, and yet they knew they had to
object because they feared violating their nurses' practice act."

Meanwhile, Peterson filed a child-abuse report against Mary with the
Child and Family Services Welfare Board of Illinois, stating that Mary had
reported electro-shocking her son and abusing him in different places
around the country. Peterson classified Ryan, who was ten years old at the
time, as "a youngster who is highly programmed as a structured, polyfragmented MPD who has programs for suicide, homicide, and return to the
cult." Peterson then transferred Ryan back to Chicago, to a unit next door
to the Rush North Shore dissociative disorders facility where his mother
had first been hospitalized.

Meanwhile, as Mary's condition continued to worsen, the doctors in
Houston attempted to shock the cult alters out of her, using techniques
similar to those employed in an exorcism. "It was a snake pit, it was like
hell," Mary said. "I was sure that I would die there sooner or later, and
probably sooner. Somehow I had just gotten lost. And no one out there
would even know that I was gone."

After she had spent two years in the Houston facility, Mary's insurance
company began to press for a change in status. Peterson decided that she
should be moved permanently to a nursing home. Somehow, Mary says,
she mustered the strength to resist that move. The hospital agreed to release
her on the condition that she find a new therapist and get a sophisticated
security system to protect her from the cult.

In their second session together, Mary's new therapist asked her if she
liked being a multiple. She said she hated it. The therapist suggested that
she stop working on that problem for a while and focus on restoring her
physical health instead. She was in terrible physical condition at this point
and was going through withdrawal from all the prescription drugs she had
been taking. She followed the therapist's advice, and the change was almost
immediate. "When I stopped working on it," Mary says, "it just dissipated;
the memories disappeared. I found out that I could go outside my apartment and I never got shot at. I could go to the grocery store, and I never
got poisoned. I could make telephone calls, and I wasn't being taped.
Nothing was happening!"

This is not to say that the years of therapy had left her unscathed,
however. When she returned home to Chicago, Mary found that her
husband and son, who were in treatment with Roberta Sachs, still believed
that she was a cult member intent on killing them, and her husband had
filed for divorce. Moreover, she was still listed with the state of Illinois as

196

a child abuser. The years of therapy had stolen a big part of her life from her, and her future was uncertain.

Conspiracy Theories

The evidence from Mary S.'s case is anecdotal, to be sure, but hers is not merely an isolated case of therapeutic excess. Braun, Sachs, Peterson, and their colleagues in Chicago and Houston are far from alone in believing — and acting on the belief — that a massive conspiracy of secret satanist cults has infiltrated every corner of our society, from the CIA to police stations to churches to judges' chambers. Growing numbers of their peers and students are buying into their belief system and interpreting patient symptomology as evidence of the operation of a global network of satanic cults. Moreover, their authority as ostensible experts in both MPD and SRA has enabled them to enlist the support of other psychotherapists as well as police, pastors, prosecutors, child protection workers, and antipornography activists in their war against the satanists. They have convinced many people that the devil worshipers are most active in daycare centers and preschools, where they pose as teachers. In 1988, Dr. Roland Summit of the Harbor-UCLA Medical Center called SRA "the most serious threat to child and to society that we must face in our lifetime."[16]

Interest in SRA also runs high in religious communities — and not just in the fundamentalist circles that in the past have exhibited a conspicuous preoccupation with the activities of the devil. James Friesen, a professor at Fuller Graduate School of Psychology in Pasadena teaching in a seminary-psychology program that has become something of a model of moderate-to-progressive evangelicalism, has expressed views typical of much of this new religious concern about SRA in one of the most popular MPD/SRA books geared to a Christian audience, *Uncovering the Mystery of MPD: Its Shocking Origins, Its Surprising Cure.* Friesen, who claims to have been in "spiritual warfare" against the world of demons even before he encountered MPD, trained himself mainly by "listening to a tape about MPD and by reading the works of [Ralph] Allison and [M. Scott] Peck." He came to believe that most of his clients were multiples, and he held to that diagnosis even in the face of opposition from the clients themselves, citing theories about the nature of memory that, as we have seen, have been unqualifiedly debunked by researchers: "Every life experience must be stored and filed

16. Summit, quoted by Nathan and Snedeker in *Satan's Silence*, p. 230.

somewhere, and no event can be erased. The closest the brain can come to erasing a memory is to become amnesic to what just happened. That involves creating an alternative personality for the occasion."

Friesen's therapeutic approach included cutting off all contact between clients and the family members they had accused. He went so far as to throw away letters from the accused without even having opened them. When questioned about this, he responded, "Jesus said, 'Anyone who loves his father and mother more than me is not worthy of me.' . . . The Christian thing to do is to . . . let go of family members."

Following a familiar pattern, Friesen's clients gradually escalated from symptoms of MPD to stories of satanic ritual abuse. Convinced of the existence of a global satanic cult conspiracy, Friesen is unfazed by the absence of any physical evidence of cult activities. "The perfect way to discredit children's testimony," he says, "is to exhume the remains later, after the children have watched them being buried. Who would believe a child's story when he says he knows exactly where the baby is buried, but no baby is found at the site?" Friesen is one of the SRA enthusiasts who believes that the satanists are "masters at cover-up."[17] Nor does he have any trouble explaining the origins of MPD and cult practices in his patients.

> Information has come to me from a number of sources that cult members are instructed in how to create MPD intentionally in their children. This maintains the secrecy, because the children's host alters will know nothing about the rituals. Electric shock, drugs, and hypnotherapy are skillfully employed by the cult members to program their children to create alters starting when the children are about two. Using brutal brainwashing-type punishments, the cult members train particular alters to behave only in specific ways, and appear only at specified times.[18]

After reading M. Scott Peck's *People of the Lie,* Friesen concluded that many of his MPD/SRA patients were inhabited not just by alters but also by demons, and he began a practice of exorcism.[19]

Other self-proclaimed experts have described plots yet more compli-

17. Friesen, *Uncovering the Mystery of MPD* (San Bernardino, CA: Here's Life Publishers, 1991), pp. 42, 151-53, 175-77.

18. Friesen, quoted by Taylor in "The Lost Daughter," p. 85.

19. Pendergrast, *Victims of Memory,* p. 160. As this book goes to press, Nadean Cool has just won a $2.4 million settlement from her former psychiatrist, Glenn Olsen (another therapist cum clergyman), who diagnosed her as a classic sufferer of MPD/SRA syndrome and performed an exorcism on her.

cated and nefarious than systematic inducement of MPD in children or surreptitious exhumation of the remains of sacrificial victims. In reviewing the case of Mary S., we encountered D. Corydon Hammond, who believes that after World War II, Nazi scientists working with the American CIA developed a sophisticated code that can implant a cult plan of homicide and infanticide into the minds of ordinary citizens. He has further explained that the secret code was originally developed under the leadership of a Hassidic Jew named Dr. Green (a.k.a. Dr. Greenbaum), who escaped from the Holocaust ovens by teaching his Nazi captors the secrets of the *Cabala*. Using Dr. Green's techniques, says Hammond, the satanists are now busy inducing multiple personalities in their occult ceremonies.

> People say, "What's the purpose of it?" My best guess is that the purpose of it is that they want an army of Manchurian candidates, tens of thousands of mental robots who will do prostitution, do child pornography, smuggle drugs, engage in international arms smuggling, do snuff films — all sorts of very lucrative things — and do their bidding, and eventually, the megalomaniacs at the top believe, create a satanic order that will rule the world.[20]

This may sound like paranoid rambling or something from the plot of a B movie from the fifties, but we should not simply dismiss it as harmless nonsense. Recall that Hammond is a professor of psychiatric medicine at the University of Utah, that he has been asked to help determine the course of treatment for patients at Rush–Presbyterian–St. Luke's Hospital, that he was part of the team that hospitalized Mary S., drugged her, destroyed her marriage, took her son away from her, and identified her to the state as a child abuser. More than that, Hammond was instrumental in persuading the governor of Utah to establish a ritual-abuse investigative task force. He proudly reports that as a result of his efforts, 90 percent of Utah citizens now believe that SRA is real.

Another SRA enthusiast, former FBI agent and general satanic cult troubleshooter Ted Gunderson, appeared on *Geraldo* claiming that there were major cult burial grounds in Mason County, Washington. Soon afterward, he went to the area and led a search-team entourage of TV helicopters and private aircraft equipped with heat-seeking mechanisms that were supposed to be able to detect the warmth of decomposing bodies. The governor of Washington, Booth Gardner, approved $50,000 to support

20. Lawrence Wright, *Remembering Satan: A Case of Recovered Memory and the Shattering of an American Family* (New York: Alfred A. Knopf, 1994), pp. 180-81.

Gunderson's investigation. The Mason County sheriff asked the state legislature for $750,000 to buy bullet-proof vests, night-viewing scopes, and electronic surveillance equipment, apparently to protect the posse from any satanists who might be lurking near the mass burial sites. The search didn't turn up evidence of any suspicious activities at all, much less mass satanic burials. Gunderson has also claimed that a demonic element *within* the U.S. government was responsible for bombing the federal building in Oklahoma City. In spite of all that, he has managed to attract support not only from state officials but also from high-profile media people and feminist groups.[21]

Where Is the Evidence?

Those who believe in the worldwide SRA conspiracy talk about huge numbers of people involved in a worldwide network of cults that are continually engaged in sensational criminal activities including large-scale human sacrifice. Victims are ostensibly procured through kidnappings and the serial impregnation of young women known as "breeders." But is there any generally accepted evidence to substantiate these reports of cult activity? We have taken note of some instances in which local law enforcement agencies have acted on the accusations of fearful parents and assertive therapists (e.g., the McMartin Preschool case). But what have *national* agencies been able to uncover in the way of evidence of a pervasive underground culture of satanic cults?

In a word, *nothing*. Investigators have not found one shred of physical evidence establishing the existence of such cults or their practices, despite zealously following up on leads from self-proclaimed survivors. National investigative teams, aided by police departments around the country, have aggressively investigated these reports, questioned thousands of people, dug for bones thought to be left after satanic rites, and searched for ritual locations. What have they found? No remains of sacrificial victims, no photographs or videos of satanic ritualistic sex acts, no scars or other physical evidence on the bodies of people who report having been physically tortured.

In 1994 the National Center on Child Abuse and Neglect, after studying 12,000 reported accusations of satanic abuse and surveying 11,000

21. Wright, *Remembering Satan*, pp. 179-80; Pendergrast, *Victims of Memory*, pp. 192-93.

therapists, social-service workers, and law-enforcement professionals, found that not one single case was substantiated. Later that same year, a research team under contract with the federal government announced, after studying the matter for almost five years, that there was no evidence of any organized satanic cult incursions into public child care. Investigations of the much-publicized daycare cases of the eighties similarly turned up no evidence to substantiate the children's stories of human sacrifice, infant cannibalism, blood rituals, or the like — and it was not for lack of trying on the part of police. Law-enforcement workers in these cases went to extraordinary lengths to locate bones, bodies, pornography, burial sites, clothing — all to no avail. In the McMartin case, 21 houses, 7 businesses, 37 cars, 3 motorcycles, and a farm were thoroughly searched, and a national park in South Dakota where Ray Buckey had camped one summer was excavated. Thousands of pornographic movies and stills were seized from other investigations and carefully reviewed. Investigators visited Europe in search of pictures and enlisted both the FBI and INTERPOL to help them find evidence. Nothing was ever found.[22]

Kenneth Lanning, the FBI's chief investigator of crimes against children, has investigated more than three hundred SRA cases personally and found no evidence of the existence of satanic child-abuse groups. "As someone deeply concerned about child abuse, I didn't take the allegations of victims lightly. Initially I was inclined to believe them. I had dealt with bizarre, deviant behavior for many years," says Lanning. "But as the cases poured in and years went by, and none of them panned out, I became more skeptical."[23] After studying the issue for seven years, the FBI made this official statement: "There is little or no evidence . . . for allegations that deal with large-scale baby breeding, human sacrifice, and organized satanic conspiracies. It is up to the mental health professionals, not law enforcement, to explain why victims are alleging things that don't seem to have happened."[24]

22. Nathan and Snedeker, *Satan's Silence,* p. 88; Pendergrast, *Victims of Memory,* pp. 188-89.

23. Lanning, quoted by Pendergrast in *Victims of Memory,* pp. 188-89. On the failure of law enforcement agencies to turn up any evidence of alleged satanic cult activities, see also Nathan and Snedeker, *Satan's Silence,* pp. xi, 130-33; and Wright, *Remembering Satan,* pp. 86-87. Pendergrast lists three other books on the SRA legend that reach the same conclusion: Arthur Lyons's *Satan Wants You,* Robert D. Hicks's *In Pursuit of Satan,* and Jeffery Victor's *Satanic Panic.* Tales of a global satanic cult conspiracy, says Pendergrast, constitute "a hoax, a fraud, a paranoid delusion fomented by the media, credulous therapists, distraught patients, pressured pre-schoolers, fearful parents, and over-excited policemen."

24. "The Search for Satan," PBS *Frontline* documentary produced by Ofra Bikel, originally broadcast 24 October 1995.

Perhaps Americans suspended much of their normal skepticism about satanism and devil worship after 1978, when Jim Jones's followers engaged in mass ritualistic suicide at the People's Temple in Jonestown, Guyana. They have also encountered stories about self-proclaimed witches (notably the Wiccans), spoof satanists (notably Anton LaVey's Church of Satan, founded in San Francisco in 1966), and similar groups formed as pagan alternatives to organized middle-class religion. The Church of Satan, for example, has publicly staged satanic weddings of celebrities, but it seems to function mainly as a satire of organized religion. More to the point, these groups are very small, do not proselytize among teenagers, and have never been implicated in any criminal activity. During the 1970s, many parents came to fear cults associated with Eastern and New Age religions — and, indeed, a good many young people did disappear for a while (a few for good) into these cults. Though some of these cults practiced strange, purportedly biblical or long-abandoned cultic rites such as polygamy and child sexual initiation (which can certainly be considered a form of sexual abuse), none of them has been criminally implicated in any widespread conspiracy involving rape, incest, infant sacrifice, or cannibalism — the sorts of practices typically featured in the recovered memories of MPD/SRA and RMT patients. The absence of any evidence that SRA exists, however, has done little to stem the increasing conviction that ritual-abuse cases are real and widespread. A 1994 *Redbook* survey found that 70 percent of Americans believe in the existence of sexually abusive satanic cults, and almost a third believed that these groups are being deliberately ignored by the FBI and the police.

Why Do They Believe?

The fact that investigators are unable to turn up evidence of the reported satanic cult activities does not appear to affect the certainty of the true believers. When Dr. Peterson filed criminal abuse charges against Mary S. in the state of Illinois, child protection services investigators were assigned to the case, and they were frankly skeptical of Peterson's sensational charges of SRA. If there really was evidence of such horrific crimes, they wanted to know, why weren't criminal investigators being assigned to the case? "The answer was always that they were gathering evidence to crack into this very secretive and dangerous cult," one consulting social worker noted, "and that the people who had infiltrated the cult in the past were either dead or had become members themselves. The reason why [the cult] was never uncovered was that these people ate the evidence [i.e., the human bones, etc.], so there was no evidence, and there were doctors involved who could do coverups of anything. There were always answers to any questions anybody had." A similar litany of reasons why investigators can't produce compelling evidence of satanic activity appears in *The Courage to Heal*: society is in denial, investigators don't document the stories because they're too unpleasant, prosecutors don't want to take cases they might lose, and satanists not only employ highly refined brainwashing and mind-control techniques but also have supernatural powers to eradicate evidence.

In some cases, the true believers appear to acknowledge problems with their position but then simply ignore them. In an influential paper by Bennett Braun, Walter C. Young, and Roberta Sachs entitled "A New Clinical Syndrome: Patients Reporting Ritual Abuse in Childhood by Satanic Cults," the authors state, "Despite the fact that some patients have discussed ritual abuse with other patients, and the fact that patients have had contact with referring therapists who may have provided information to them, it was our opinion that ritual abuse was real."[25] In other words, they chose to discount therapeutic contamination even though it was quite evident.

In a case similar to that of Mary S., Patti B. was hospitalized by Braun along with her two sons for more than two years at the Rush–Presbyterian–St. Luke's psychiatric facility because he was convinced that she had initiated the boys into a satanic cult and that they had been involved in baby sacrifice, cannibalism, and other vile activities from the time they were infants. Using a system of rewards for the best stories the boys told, Braun elicited a range of bizarre tales. One of the boys reported that he had cut a man's stomach open; he described the intestines popping out and talked about the horrible smell. Braun was greatly impressed, but Patti was not. She told Braun that the boy was simply recounting a scene from one of the Star Wars movies that they had seen together, in which one of the characters cuts open the belly of an animal. Braun ignored the mother's prosaic explanation for the story. Later, while testifying as an expert witness in an SRA trial in California, Braun recounted the boy's story and insisted that it must have been real because it was filled with details that the child could not have picked up anywhere else: "Having done surgery, I know that's exactly what happens. If the anesthesia isn't done right, the intestines pop out just like he said. Here's a five-year-old who can describe to me something I know something about. Where does a five-year-old learn about this? There are no five-year-old boys in operating rooms!" Later, after Patti managed to extract herself

25. Braun, Young, and Sachs, quoted by Wright in *Remembering Satan*, p. 76.

from Braun's care and recover from the massive doses of drugs he had administered, she got a court order and retrieved her sons from the psychiatric unit. Devout Catholics, she and her husband had gone to Rome when their younger son was an infant and had him blessed by the Pope. At one point during her recovery, Patti showed Braun the picture of her son being blessed by the pontiff at the Vatican and asked him to reconcile the religious devotion it signified with his claims that she had been a high priestess in a satanic cult. Braun's response was that her photograph simply constituted proof that the pope was part of the worldwide satanic conspiracy.

Postscript

How can we account for the great divide between those who buy into the whole MPD/SRA phenomenon and those who do not? Most of those who believe that we now have an epidemic of MPD began by accepting the premise that large numbers of adults are burdened with repressed memories of childhood abuse or have managed to recover previously repressed memories of abuse. They infer from this that we must be in the midst of an epidemic of child abuse. On the basis of the testimony of experts, they accept the assertion that some percentage of this child abuse is extreme enough to produce MPD, and, on the basis of the testimony of survivors, they accept the premise that some percentage of the trauma producing MPD is associated with SRA.

Those who are skeptical of the RMT, MPD, and SRA phenomena hold to more traditional assessments of repressed memory — namely, that it is a rare phenomenon usually of limited duration and involving a limited range of experience, as, for instance, a temporary inability to recall the details of an automobile accident or a physical assault. They note that there are extremely few documented cases of massive repression, in which memories of extended periods of time have been repressed, and none in which such memories have been successfully recovered in any significant detail. Given this, they conclude that most "recovered memories" are in fact confabulations of dreams and images introduced through the use of hypnosis, guided imagery, and other therapeutic techniques. They similarly maintain that in the vast majority of cases, MPD is a contemporary manifestation of what was once called "hysteria," a disorder in which people consciously or unconsciously imitate the symptoms of other diseases to divert attention from the real cause of their disturbance. In that sense, skeptics say, the presentation of multiple personalities is either iatrogenic (induced in a patient by a therapist's suggestion) or imitative of a pattern picked up through reading or viewing popular accounts of the disorder. They dismiss recovered memories of SRA as similarly induced or imitated.

*   *   *

Mary S. spent three years of her life in psychiatric wards. Her insurance company paid out about 2.5 million dollars for treatments that pushed her further and further out of touch with reality. Patti B. and her sons spent over two years in a treatment facility, at a cost of more than $3 million. Like many clients of RMT, she was persuaded by her therapists that she had been sexually abused as a child, and she cut off contact with her father and mother for nine years. In the end, however, Patti was more fortunate than Mary: her husband stuck with her, and they were able to rescue their sons and put their family back together; she has also reconciled with her father and mother.

The dissociative disorders unit run by Dr. Judith Peterson at Spring Shadows Glen, Houston, was shut down by the state of Texas in 1992. Peterson continues to see patients in private practice. She is being sued by ten former patients, including Mary S.

As of this writing, Bennett Braun and Roberta Sachs are still operating the dissociative disorders unit at Rush–Presbyterian–St. Luke's Hospital, and the unit remains a nationally recognized center for the treatment of MPD/SRA. Braun is also being sued by several of his former patients, including Mary S. and Patti B.

"Are they evil?" asks Mary S. "I know that many people have stories very similar to my own. This has been going on for ten or twelve years, under these same doctors. I don't know how anyone could know what they know now and see what this 'treatment' has done to families — and continue to do it. Yes, I think that is pretty evil."

CHAPTER 9

Sherri

I am one of many faceless souls lost behind the firefight that currently rages in the helping professions over the theory of repressed memory. What is left for me to do but shout long and loud and hope to be heard over the angry din? I am called a recanter; I am also called a traitor. To some I am a prodigal child returned; to others I am a deluded soul in denial. I shun the names. By my own definition, I am none of these. I have walked down a peculiar path, and I have a tale to tell: it is a tale of therapy, delusion, understanding, and growth.

I do not claim to speak for others who have made the same, or a similar, journey. Although I have met with many who share my attitude and whose experiences are uncannily parallel to mine, they all have their own voices and their own tales. By telling my story and analyzing specific personal characteristics — as well as therapeutic techniques — that contributed to my belief in a delusion, I hope to shed further light on the dynamics that created this situation in my life, and perhaps in some way help prevent someone else from experiencing its inherent pain.

My story begins in 1972, when I was thirteen. A doctor who was treating me for menstrual disorders began to sexually molest me while I was under sedation. I saw him for treatment once a week for several years until I woke during one of these sessions and fled in terror. When I reported what happened to my parents, they dismissed my account as a hallucination because "Dr. B. would never do that." I knew that it was no hallucination, but after continually failing to convince my parents, I shut my mouth like a dutiful daughter and resolved not to think about or mention it again. I managed to keep that resolution for nineteen years, until 1991, when I read in the newspaper that this doctor had been charged with rape by several women patients. Publicity drew out dozens more accounts, including mine, and I was asked to testify in court.

Several weeks before I learned of the charges against this doctor, I was involved in a particularly traumatic car accident. Becoming active in the case against Dr. B. seemed like an ideal opportunity both to redress an old wrong that had never really left me and to divert my mind from the car accident that I was reliving in relentless technicolor detail. I had no name for the grisly replays I was subjected to: they were a mind-riot of every sensory perception, tuned to the highest possible pitch, of the few frozen instants of the impact. I was game for anything that might free me from their grip.

But the attempt was futile: soon I was reliving both the doctor's sexual abuse *and* the car wreck. My condition continued to deteriorate. None of the homegrown, commonsense advice — "get involved in other things, start a new hobby, take a vacation" — worked. I lost weight, did not sleep, could not concentrate, could not complete the simplest tasks; and always, there were the waking, walking nightmares of rape and the accident. I was sure I was sinking, irrecoverably, into madness.

In utter desperation, I sought therapy — as the last hope for sanity. But my expectations from therapy were far too high for any simple human being to bring about: I needed a magician or a god. For the first couple of months I hoped for a miracle, that somehow by magic incantation, or simply sharing the same air as the therapist, I would be cured. He was my last and only refuge, yet trust had always come hard for me, and this was no exception. I kept my emotions safely encased in steel, and I gave him only the most superficial information. I recounted stupefying scenes of horror without a flicker of emotion on my face; I recited the list of symptoms that plagued me with no betrayal of their emotional toll. I hoped that I would find relief without having to plunge into my emotional wreckage in the presence of a stranger. To that end I described in exhaustive detail the symptoms brought on by my emotional turmoil and the events that caused the turmoil in the first place. But I left the feelings out of the picture. When he asked for sensitive details or genuine feelings, he became a sinister intruder rifling through my possessions for the gun and ammunition that could kill me. I tested him continually in the early months: Would he make time for me outside our scheduled appointments? Would he honor his pledge to do all he could to keep me out of the hospital? Would he break the code of silence and divulge some personal information? I wanted proof of an extraordinary commitment on his part and hoped for confirmation that I was "special" to him. Only then would I share with him the emotional frenzy of the abuse and the accident.

Trust was slow to grow, or so it seemed at the time. After about four months of seeing the therapist two to four times weekly, I began to believe his repeated reassurances: "I promise you I will not harm you." And when the barrier fell, it fell in a big way. During the four months I'd been in therapy, my therapist and I had discovered several areas of mutual interest. Occasionally the "therapeutic dialogue" would lapse and we would have impassioned conversations on one of several subjects. His breadth of knowledge was dazzling. His ability to see beyond the most obscure allusions or metaphors into the heart of a reference convinced me that he was an extraordinarily insightful person. The sensitivity he showed to the nuances of every word I spoke, every action and gesture, silenced my old fears. The symptoms that had plagued me began to abate, but I was staggered by the intensity of the emotions that were unleashed, including the depth of the attachment I felt to the therapist. I was thoroughly charmed. And thoroughly frightened of the power of that charm.

A nameless dream, amoebic in nature, lived in me — sliding a piece of itself in one direction, then another. The fear of madness was not diminished, only metamorphosed into a nebulous form that I could not associate firmly with the rapes or the accident. I was terrified and ashamed of the chaos of emotions I felt and far too embarrassed by such adolescent yearnings — more appropriate to a fifteen-year-old than a thirty-three-year-old woman — to confess to my therapist the depth of my attachment to him. My devotion was total; I would do anything to please him. And this paradox was painfully apparent: in therapy our goal was independence and healthy functioning, yet my achieving that goal would mean losing the relationship with the most important person in my life. Ostensibly, I sought to please him, and pleasing him meant "getting better"; but I was well aware of the tension between the stated goal and the longing I had for the attention he gave me.

I made a return visit to my childhood home during a period when my therapy was focusing on my parents' reaction to my telling them about being raped by the doctor when I was a teenager. I found this visit very distressing. My therapist and I had anticipated this, and we'd scheduled three phone sessions for during the trip. In addition, I was free to call if I felt the need at any time between the planned calls. While I was at my parents' home, I began to have a recurrent nightmare that plagued me for several months.

The dream was set in a nightmarish carnival. I was trapped on a racing carousel that spun faster and faster and more out of control as the speed increased. Convinced I would die if I remained on the merry-go-round, I hurtled off the ride and landed in a dusty midway. Garish neon-lit booths lined the pathway, and barkers screamed for me to play their games. I ran down the dirt path while iguana-like demons chased me, flailing at my legs with razor claws. My legs were streaming blood and I was sure I would falter and be torn apart by these hellions when I heard a comforting voice call to me from the other end of the midway. It was my father's voice. I ran toward the sound. When I reached the other side of the dirt path, I realized the voice was coming from inside a hall of mirrors. With the demons still slashing at my legs, I plunged into the building. My father's voice was louder here but still distant; it seemed to be coming from below me. Stumbling, I felt my way around the maze until I fell down a dark chute that opened into a cave. To my left I could see a faint glimmer of light. My father's voice, promising me safety, was very near. I approached the light coming from around a corner in the cave, and coming around the corner, I saw a stone altar in the center of the room. Beside it a huge creature — half man, half reptile — stood in attendance. He was completely naked with an enormous erection. Darting out of the shadows, two smaller creatures grabbed me and threw me on the altar. They pinned me down, one on my left side and the other on my right. Somehow through all this, my clothing disappeared. The large reptilian man said, "I'm glad you've come." His voice was my father's. He stepped forward very ceremoniously and raped me. As he entered, his penis turned into a sword and I felt myself being eviscerated. At that moment, I awoke.

It was a provocative dream that could easily be interpreted on a superficial level as an "incest dream." I recounted the dream to my therapist but declined to discuss it further.

After I returned from this visit to my childhood home, my emotional turmoil deepened, and my preoccupation with my therapist escalated to near-obsession. I lived exclusively for therapy. Our sessions revolved around my family of birth, while my days and nights between sessions revolved around my therapist. My level of functioning was on a steady decline. I dropped my classes and quit my tutoring job. I no longer cleaned house or cooked. I had visual hallucinations of rats swarming in my kitchen and giant faces on the floorboard of my car. The slightest things were sources of intolerable anxiety. The phone ringing, the doorbell, a simple question from my husband or daughter was all the trigger I needed to dissociate myself from my body and enter an internal world, wholly removed from external reality. My family watched in impotent frustration as I sank deeper and deeper into a world they could not see, feel, or understand. My therapist's droll response to their concerns — "She has to get worse before she can get better" — offered little comfort. But they deferred to my therapist's expertise and waited in silence for the wife and mother they had always known to return to them. My therapist, claiming confusion over my deteriorating condition, suggested, "There must be something more, some significant trauma in your past that is causing this." When I protested that I had told him everything I knew, he explained that the cause could be something I was unconscious of; when I was truly strong enough to know, my mind would allow it to rise to consciousness.

We continued to focus on my family, especially my tempestuous father, whose rages were frequent and volatile. During one session, after weeks of what I perceived as relentless pressure from my therapist to admit my father did not love me, I collapsed into a fetal ball screaming of my father's love. This was the beginning of my "incest history." My therapist's attention to my hysterics was intense. The gravity of his concern and the depth of his compassion were palpable as he bent close to me and whispered, "You know what you're telling me, don't you? You *do* know what you're telling me." For an instant I did not know what he believed I was saying; an instant later, I did know, and I believed it too.

Now I had a name for the pain. Now, only now, did I deserve all the tenderness and loving attention I had received. The dreams made sense, the emotional turmoil made sense, and the ever-present dread made sense. I was absolved of responsibility because my unhappiness now had a reason and a name.

In the beginning, my conversion to my newfound identity, "incest survivor," was not complete. I still wavered between relief at having an answer for my problems, disbelief that it could have happened, and guilty pleasure over the attention that it brought me. I had no real memory — thus it could not be true. But I could see the havoc it wreaked on my life — it must be true. I needed my therapist — it must be true. My therapist dismissed my doubts by calling my distress a witness to the incest's truth: "You know better than anyone else the kind of pain you're in. Do you really think you'd feel so bad if it weren't true?" Soon I began to say the same thing. Therapy took a mystical spin: mine was a sacred wound, and the gates of hell had opened and revealed its tumult. My therapist was the hierophant of my own Eleusinian mysteries. From this point on, each step was sanctified, and every therapy session was elevated to a ritual that brought me closer to the divine.

I immersed myself in incest. Just as my therapist predicted, the "memories" began to return. Vague at first, they gained in detail as I pondered them. I read all the incest survivor books, watched all the specials on TV about the subject, and I saw myself in every one. I joined a therapy group solely for incest survivors and believed myself to be on a holy quest in the company of fellow seekers. The terror of reliving the abominable memories was mitigated by a deep sense of being cared for and of belonging. The external world and its mundane reality, including my husband and daughter, offended me. I had no patience for its banal demands. All "real" life orbited the therapy-incest duo. If something did not pertain to therapy or incest, at least peripherally, it was not real. Anything or any person that challenged my truth or questioned my path was evil, and I severed all contact with anyone, including family, who was unconvinced of the truth of my "incest." Every activity I pursued revolved around therapy.

I became my own inner child — with teddy bears to sleep with and cuddle, popsicles and lollipops to lick and slurp. The purpose of my day was to care for this child. She was the divine infant, the miracle child sprung from the union of myself and my therapist. Of course, I was too embarrassed to tell him that. The brutal accounts of incest that I was reading in books and seeing on television played through my mind, over and over in stark relief, until the features melted and the faces and bodies became my own. I poured myself into the homework that was assigned in group therapy. I was tallying all the facets of my life explained away by incest, feeling through the memories that grew like pearls around the vague sensations that were disturbing me. My journal was a treasure chest filled with gems from a past I had never known. My husband and daughter complained about my withdrawal; they said I was getting worse, not better. I discounted their comments and concerns. My holy quest required a descent through the seven circles of hell. My family was trapped in mundane reality, while I consorted with demons and gods.

*   *   *

Later, in coming to terms with this head-over-heels involvement, I spent a great deal of time and effort trying to understand how it came about. What was my contribution? What was the therapist's, both as a person and as a professional? What role, if any, did therapeutic techniques play in contributing to — or facilitating — my delusion? There was no simple explanation. I could not point to my therapist and say, "It's all his fault"; nor could I say that of myself, even though assuming all the responsibility myself would have been satisfying in its simplicity. I could not indict therapy itself as the progenitor of the madness. It might have been more satisfying if that were so. The truth, at least in my case, was not nearly so simple or satisfying. The seeds were dormant within me. They germinated in the benign environment of therapy like seeds in fertile, loamy soil, and a field of illusions grew.

The essence of my seed-hood, so to speak, brought several personal characteristics to therapy that, I feel, contributed to the growth of this delusion. My self-sufficiency was my greatest prize: I proudly proclaimed that I needed no one, and I believed it with all my heart. To ask for help was not only to fail but also to acknowledge that failure, which was worse than the failure itself. It was a defeat of my being and it was a confession — "I am existentially insufficient." Madness and death were the same to me, and seeking therapy was the admission that my path led to these twin terrors and that this was my last chance to avoid them. Given my despair, my expectations of therapy were the same as hoping for a miracle. The therapist was the little god who would work the miracle. The desperation I felt led me to look for desperate answers, including incest.

I had always been a high achiever, always strained to excel. It was not enough to be good; it was not enough to be superior to most of my peers; I wanted to be the best. Of course, I frequently did not achieve that goal, but I never quit trying for it and never was free of the guilty resentment I felt for those who outperformed me. Once I overcame my initial difficulties in trusting my therapist, I brought that high-achieving attitude into therapy as well. I worked hard to be his star client and resented the attention others received.

Genuine intimacy had been a rare — and seemingly dangerous — commodity for me. I had one close friend and a gaggle of acquaintances. I feigned a friendliness and self-assurance I did not feel to elicit people's acceptance. Between the resentment I felt toward competitors and a deep fear of rejection, I rarely risked anything approaching a real exchange. And when I experienced the intimacy that I had always feared, yet yearned for, in therapy, I was appalled at my greediness for more and disgusted by the depth of dependence I felt.

I took great pains to keep my therapist from knowing how dependent I had become, expressing to him only a very diluted version of the truth. Although my neediness was a common topic of our discussions, I was too ashamed to let him know that what he perceived as dependence was only a pale reflection of my real dependence. I also felt guilt for the care I received from him, as though my problems did not merit special attention. I longed to be more than a client. Sister, wife, lover, daughter, friend, protégé — I wanted to be any of them, all of them. But in the absence of that possibility, I would settle for being his star patient. And if it took incest to be that star, then incest it would be.

One more thing: I lived predominantly in my dreams and fantasies, where I always achieved the excellence I longed for and the stunning successes that eluded me in reality. There was an adolescent quality to these dreams, a grandiosity that embarrassed me as an adult. I knew they were exaggerated beyond the possibility of fulfillment, so I kept them strictly private, even from my therapist. I also had some artistic proclivities that lent themselves nicely to fantasies of grandeur, but I lacked the self-confidence to exercise them in the real world. When my therapist encouraged me to pursue those fantasies and took a passionate interest in my productions, he unwittingly became a mentor, a wise sage in my secret dream. We were allies in a spiritual art against the banal truths of the mundane. Creativity, art, therapy, and incest intertwined until they were indistinguishable from each other. All these factors combined to form a potential that was inchoate in my veins. Therapy and the therapist were the keys to unlock that potential.

I am not qualified to address the motivations of my therapist; that is another narrative altogether. But I can comment on my reactions to his methods. There were several techniques in particular that he used which I feel contributed to the growth of my delusion, specifically: *inner child work, guided visualization, dream work,* and what I call "mysticization," for lack of a better term. While these methods may have been benign in themselves, the way they were used in my case helped to create the delusions I came to believe as truth.

In *inner child work* the therapist encouraged me to keep the "little wounded girl within" in the forefront of my mind, to feel and to act on her emotions, her needs, and her wishes — in essence, to *be* that child. Consequently, I spent a great deal of time feeling and behaving like a five-year-old. Though I knew, rationally speaking, that my inner child was a metaphorical concept, experience told me otherwise. It was rather like knowing that the earth is round, yet my eyes see and my feet walk a flat surface. As a result of my therapy's urgings, my inner child was no metaphor; she was me. I resented it when banal reality forced me into my adult skin — to renew my driver's license or take my flu-stricken daughter to the doctor. I missed my inner child and could not wait to complete the task so I could return to her. As often as not, I did not bother with adult responsibilities; I simply ignored them until someone else took care of them. That sanctioned selfishness was seductive. The more inner child work I did, the more self-indulgent I became. As I functioned more and more on a child's level, when circumstances called for an adult response, I was unable to provide one. Total panic would overwhelm me. I lost the reality of myself as an able adult and became an overgrown, ludicrous child. There was no capacity in me, as a five-year-old, to question the truth of the incest.

Guided visualizations were especially potent for me. I had taught myself the technique many years before. I used it in painting or drawing to visualize the scene; I used it whenever I had to write a story in school; and I used it for pleasure and relaxation. It was a simple step to apply the same technique to the quest for memories. But this time I was using the technique with the belief that the experience unfolding around me was a piece of objective reality from my past. And now the horror that I searched for and found was every bit as compelling as the pleasure I had derived before from the visualization technique: I would sweat, my heart would pound, my body would feel battered, and my stomach would revolt. In therapy I learned that even my ability of visualization itself — to create in my mind an alternative reality that I experienced as real and vivid as the world around me — was an indication of the "incest" I had suffered as a child. I would not have persisted in my belief without that confirmation of memories, most of which I recovered through the guided visualization technique. When my therapist cited the intensity of my reactions to the memories as proof of the "truth" of the incest, it did not occur to me that the *pleasant* reactions I'd had when using this method for enjoyment were just as intense. There was no difference in the level of emotional intensity, only in the content.

Once I accepted my "incest history" as true, I expected to discover traumatic truths encoded in dreams. I expected them, and I got them — scene upon scene of incest in stunning detail. My therapist interpreted dreams that were not overtly incest dreams in a fairly traditional manner, while he accepted dreams that depicted incest at face value. I did not consider the possibility that the dreams were a subjective representation; he never mentioned that that was possible. The focus on dreams, as well as the guided visualizations, made it difficult to distinguish between reality and the unreal. The edges blurred between waking and dreaming. Often the dream's actions repeated themselves during the day in a flashback. And vice versa: flashbacks that accompanied the memories retrieved through guided visualization and other techniques reappeared in my dreams. My states of consciousness became diffuse, and I was not certain where reality left off and fantasy and dreams began.

Furthermore, the introduction of a mystical element redefined therapy into a religious experience — beyond simply a strategy for achieving emotional stability. By creating and using rituals at home, with the encouragement of my therapist, I extended the therapy session indefinitely. I was constantly submerged in a mystical undertaking, which was one way to stay connected to the therapist at all times. My goals and images in therapy had a religious ring to them: nirvana, bliss, paradise, communion with the gods. There was little motivation to "get better" when a psychotic episode was defined as the "dark night of the soul." I was on a holy path, and the seven circles of hell were a part of it. Convinced that I was undergoing a profound mystical experience, rare and privileged, I had no incentive to try to change it. Quite the opposite, I was inspired to descend as far as I could go.

I feel that, in addition to the more general techniques described above, some of the therapist's specific actions and comments contributed to my creation of and belief in a fictitious past. In my first or second session, I told the therapist about my earliest memory of being bathed by my father when I was about three. He asked if there was any sexual element to that memory. I was shocked by the question, pretended that I hadn't heard it, and then asked him to repeat it. He responded, "Never mind. We'll know very soon." If I had not heard his question, his response would have been enigmatic; as it was, it was not enigmatic at all, and what echoed through my mind frequently was the question, "Does he think I was abused by my father?" Combined with the authority I invested in him, the question took on the shape of a statement.

While I was talking about the doctor who had raped me, my therapist told me in graphic detail of one of his client's attempts to discourage her father's sexual advances. It may have been meant as a casual anecdote, to be heard once and forgotten. But nothing said in therapy was heard only once; I replayed every word over and over again. By the time the next session would arrive, I had meticulously scrutinized the previous session a hundred times. I amplified and analyzed every shadow of meaning, the nuances of every gesture. And my intense scrutiny was not limited to the time between sessions; it was ongoing. When my therapist rubbed his legs to smooth the wrinkles in his pants and his mouth relaxed, I would notice and know that I had his unbroken interest. When he stifled a yawn with a short, quick breath between clenched teeth, I would notice. I knew when he was bored, displeased, touched, tired, excited. I watched him very closely. His body language, facial expressions, and changes in voice cued me that he experienced some sort of satisfaction when the subject was incest.

The therapist's frequent compliments and emotional statements helped create in me a belief that I was special to him, even extraordinary, far removed from the usual client. In fact he had me hoping that I was so appealing that I transcended "client" and was becoming something more personal. When he emphasized his presence in my life as the only "genuinely loving man," the "only person who loved me simply for myself," and used the word "love" to describe the therapeutic relationship, it increased the already significant distance I felt from my family, my husband, and my friends. The banality of my relations with them stood in very sharp contrast to the emotional intensity I experienced in therapy and its related activities. My therapist's phone calls to see how I was feeling, his willingness to accept my frequent calls for anything I felt I needed him for, his special arrangements made for contact during his vacations — all these reinforced my fantasy of having special significance to him, and contributed to the lackluster comparison with my own family. None of them made themselves available to me in the way he did.

To say that I loved the attention would severely understate the situation. I was driven by it beyond any compulsion I had ever known. At one point I told my therapist that his lungs drew my breath and his heart pushed the blood through my veins. It was an apt description of the ferocity of my need: therapy and therapist were transfigured into a vital organ; separation was vivisection. Anything that threatened its continuation, including "getting well," was life threatening. His response to my torment may have been born of very human compassion at the sight of my pain; nevertheless, it constituted his participation with me in a genuine *folie à deux*. His was the warp, mine the weft, that wove together a cloak of incestuous illusion that covered our eyes.

*   *   *

Fifteen months after I began therapy, my sacred world imploded. My therapist had begun to talk of termination about three months earlier. At first, it was not to be so much a termination as a change in relationship. We discussed the terms of a friendship that we would pursue after my therapy was over. I looked forward to the lunches, the long, intense conversations, and the joint pursuit of our common interests that we planned. As the agreed-on transition/termination date approached, my therapist withdrew further and further from the relationship we had been so carefully planning. He was sullen when I would mention the future. A fear, dark and unspoken, came into spindly bloom, that there would be no friendship, no lunches, no long conversations, a fear that he would cut himself from me cleanly —

216

and deep. I turned away from the fear with the magical thought that if I didn't acknowledge it, it didn't exist. I deluded myself into believing it would not happen — that there would be no last day. There would be a change, a metamorphosis, but not an end. There could not be an end, because the end of my therapy with this therapist would mean the death of my world — with me in it.

When I could no longer ignore the raw truth of that termination, I tried to kill myself. I washed down a full bottle of antidepressants with a tumbler of cognac. I phoned my therapist ten minutes later to tell him what I had done, thus departing with a scenario in which I could not lose: either he would see his mistake and return to save me or I would be dead anyway and he would know that he had scripted my death. As we spoke on the phone, the steady rhythm of my heart dissolved into an arrhythmic flutter that felt like a butterfly's tickle in my chest. My hands and feet grew cold, then numb. When I tried to move my arms, they did not respond. My therapist phoned the paramedics. When they arrived I was slipping back and forth between a twilight world, dimly perceived, and a suffocating grayness, like wadded cotton, that blotted out all my senses. By the time we arrived at the hospital, there was only the grayness.

My heart stopped for eleven seconds, but responded well to the resuscitation efforts of the emergency room staff. I remained unconscious until late the following day. I spent three days in ICU and an additional five days in a psychiatric facility.

Immediately after I was discharged, I returned to therapy with a different therapist. However, I quit seeing her after only a few sessions. I was numb. For months I simply waited for my body to catch up to my inner feeling. I missed living but did not remember how to do it. Eventually I returned to therapy with a third therapist.

For a long time I was dissatisfied: my new therapist neither showed nor encouraged the degree of intensity my first therapist had. She kept the focus on the present. When I would wander back to my "incestuous" past, she would pull the subject back to today. She discouraged me from the excessive dependence that I both feared and craved. She never questioned my "incest survivorship," but she did not focus on it either. She maintained my concentration on a here-and-now level at which I wanted to function. I couldn't see that this therapy was of much help at the time, because it was inconceivable to me that any therapy could take place without severe emotional upheaval. I was too polite to tell my therapist all that, but I did tell family and friends.

"But," they protested, "you're so much better. You're functioning better than we've ever seen you." It was a long time before I could see what they were seeing.

I left therapy almost two years later — a mutually agreed on, gently attained termination. Although I still considered myself an incest survivor at that time, I had expanded so far from that narrow identity that my "incestuous past" was only a small facet of my self. I inhabited a world grown full and lush that did not revolve around incest and therapy. I had new friends, a fledgling career, hobbies and interests that sparked my imagination. Incest was no longer my totality; it was, in fact, an ever-diminishing part of my identity.

Some months later, while writing a scene in a short story, I noticed a resemblance in the method I used to construct the scene in my mind and the "incest memories" I had retrieved in therapy. Intrigued, and not a little appalled, I began to research how memory functions. The more I learned, the more I doubted my recollection of incest. The significant difference in my mind between my recall of incest and my recall of abuse by the doctor contributed to my uncertainty. At first, I actively fought my doubts; the implications, if they proved to be true, would be too enormous to face. I would have to see my weakness, my suggestibility, my neediness, my manipulation, all the ugly faces in my own darkness. But the day came when I had to face them. There was no way I could turn my back on reality any longer. My doubts had grown into certainty.

Coming to this realization did not herald my immediate and joyous return to the bosom of my family. I was humiliated by what I had seen of myself. Thoroughly sickened, I anticipated complete rejection by everyone: husband, daughter, mother, friends, and therapists. I prepared myself as best I could to bear the words I was certain I'd hear — "You're not worth it. Stay away from us." One at a time, over the course of a couple of months, I told my family members, friends, and therapists the truth: I was not an incest survivor. Every person I told was a new ordeal as I resigned myself to the contempt I expected from each. I was astounded when no one responded with the expected contempt. Instead, I was welcomed with such an outpouring of love and support that the self-disgust I felt began to fade, and I began to grow once again.

CHAPTER 10

Religion and Psychology

Mass movements can rise and spread without belief in God, but never without belief in a devil. Usually the strength of a mass movement is proportionate to the vividness and tangibility of its devil.

— Eric Hoffer

It looks like the fin is going to come early this siècle.

— Anonymous wag

We are a society dedicated to the pursuit of happiness. But the rush of the technological age, conflicts at work and within our families, and our general feelings of powerlessness to affect the course of our lives make it difficult for us to achieve that happiness. During a period that has seen the decline of the family, the church, education, and many community-binding institutions, as well as what Ellen Herman calls "a collapse in the rational appeal and workability of democratic ideology and behavior," where can individuals gain a sense of security, self-worth, and connection to other humans? What avenues remain for us to travel in our pursuit of that elusive sense of happiness? In recent years, American society has increasingly turned to the therapeutic community for comfort and answers.

Not that many years ago, people who sought treatment for psychological problems tended to keep quiet about it. The talking cure may have had a certain cachet, thanks to romantic images from books and the movies, but institutional care often bore a real social stigma. People whispered about acquaintances and family members who had suffered nervous breakdowns or been locked up in asylums. Comparatively few people were familiar with therapeutic practices. It is estimated that during the 1950s fewer than one in eight Americans underwent therapy; today the number is closer to one in three. And today people are much more ready to discuss their problems; many view it as fashionable to be in therapy. Psychological problems and treatments are not only freely discussed in American homes, schools, churches, and the media but have become staples of television and radio talk shows. Moreover, virtually no judicial proceeding of any significance takes place today without the input of psychotherapy in one way or another.

There has been an astounding proliferation of therapists during the period since World War II. Membership in the American Psychiatric Association increased 760 percent between 1940 and 1970, from 2,423 to over 18,000. Membership in the American Psychological Association grew 1,100 percent during that same period, from 2,739 to 30,839. And in the two and a half decades since 1970, membership in both organizations has more than doubled again. When we add to those the number of clinical social workers, which more than tripled (from 25,000 to 80,000) between 1975 and 1990 alone, we are looking at a very large number indeed. Add to that a growing number of untrained or marginally trained "wounded healers" (such as the health food and bookstore manager who facilitated Steven Cook's false memories of sexual abuse at the hands of the late Joseph Cardinal Bernardin), and it is difficult to estimate the number of people now engaged in trying to heal North Americans in emotional distress.

The therapeutic impulse has grown strong in American religion as well. Jewish and Christian clergy are now routinely expected to provide some sort of psychological counseling as part of their ministry. Current seminary curricula reflect the new demands being placed on the ministers-in-training. The traditional core disciplines of the seminary education — Scripture, church history, systematic theology, ethics, and homiletics — have been shrinking in most seminaries, while courses in pastoral counseling have ballooned. Courses such as "Ministering to the Alcoholic," "Ministering to Codependents," and "Counseling in the AIDS Community" have become so popular as to suggest that at least some of the students consider it their ultimate purpose not to preach the gospel but to minister to those in emotional distress.

While in some ways this evolution is laudable, it has its drawbacks.

From the perspective of the historic orthodox church, it raises the problem of pastors who are not as well trained in exegetical-homiletical methodology and depth as their counterparts were in the past; this is not a happy prospect for those who believe that penetrating interpretation of Scripture and meaningful worship are essential to the church's health and stability. From the perspective of historic and scientific psychotherapy, the prospect is no less disturbing: pastors who emerge from seminaries with a smattering of courses in trendy psychosocial "issues" have no real grounding in scientific and methodological psychology (to offer those courses, the seminaries often hire psychologists and social workers from outside the seminary or even outside the confessional body whose connection to the pastoral setting is tenuous), and their insights and methods often reflect what is most popular among the plethora of facile recovery and self-help books and videos now flooding not only the religious market but also the pastoral counseling course reading lists. One is beginning to hear much about the "inner child" from the would-be therapists who are studying at the seminaries these days.

The therapeutic/recovery culture has made inroads into virtually all confessions — Jewish, Catholic, Lutheran, Reformed, Wesleyan, and the like — and across the spectrum from liberal to conservative bodies within these confessions. Even churches that have self-consciously held to traditional, historical ways and eschewed the spirit of the age have tended to show a new openness to therapeutic concerns in recent years. Take, for example, the Christian Reformed Church, a Protestant denomination so conservative that it just recently ordained its first female minister after decades of intra-church wrangling over the issue. But even before it took that step, in 1994 the denomination established a churchwide child abuse prevention office after surveying a sample of its adult members and finding that as many as 28 to 32 percent of them reported that they had experienced some form of physical, emotional, or sexual abuse as children. The new office was established to "address the problem of abuse, promote healing, and work to prevent future abuse." The administrator of the office announced, "It takes a whole church to heal a survivor." The survey results, which stunned many in the denomination, were based on self-reporting questionnaires returned by 643 of the 1,000 people to whom they had been distributed. No effort was made to assess or corroborate the claims made by the respondents. To a large degree this survey and response are typical of church efforts in this area. The survey itself defined abuse broadly enough so that most people would be likely to have experienced it in some form — it included "spreading gossip" as a form of emotional abuse, for example, and specified that "kissing and hugging . . . can be considered sexually abusive acts" — and it focused principally on the respondent's feelings as opposed to any objective assessment of the behavior in question. Though the results of the survey can scarcely be characterized as "facts," that is how they are touted: "Facts don't lie" says the booklet that reported the survey results to the denomination.[1] The establishment within this conservative denominational body of an office to deal solely with the problem of abuse gives some indication of the extent to which all aspects of our culture have been sensitized to the problem and open to therapeutic responses to it. This sort of openness is a sine qua non for accepting the plausibility of RMT.

Victimization as Religion

To the extent that the traditional religions are opening themselves up to the therapeutic impulse, they are also opening themselves up to — and in some cases incorporating outright — the axioms of some of America's *secular* religions. I have in mind here principally the basic assumptions of the nation's vast recovery movement, with its twelve-step programs, its unique creeds, pledges, and de facto priests and supplicants. It is an essential part of the self-perception of vast numbers of Americans today that they are in recovery from one thing or another — an eating disorder, a bad childhood, or an addiction to any of a host of things such as alcohol, drugs, gambling, sex, cigarettes, shopping, the Internet, chocolate, and the like. Additional hosts of people fill out the ranks of codependents, enablers, and parents and adult children of the afflicted. To some degree, all of these people are invested in the belief system of the recovery movement. They first of all view themselves as recovering *from* something — the source of their pain. But they are also trying to recover *something* — a lost innocence that they believe they knew as children, before they were victimized by their problem. This belief in a mythic innocence is a key tenet of many of America's secular religions, and it is being subtly imported into many traditional religions along with the rest of the therapeutic worldview, despite the fact that it is incompatible with the belief structures of many of those traditional religions.

In the past, traditional religious leaders taught that an excess of any-thing — alcohol, food, sex, gambling, or the like — will do you in. They

---

1. Beth A. Swagman, *Too Close for Comfort* (Grand Rapids: CRC Publications, 1994), pp. 8, 11, 12-13.

counseled moderation in all things and asserted that the human will is capable of making right decisions but prone to make wrong ones, for which there are consequences. Many in the recovery movement disagree with this view. They characterize addiction not as sin but as disease, and they contend that it is wrongheaded and even perverse to talk about people being responsible for their diseases. This view of the matter has in fact become so pervasive in our society that few Americans today would publicly assert that addicts are responsible for their addictions. A further sign of the triumph of the therapeutic perspective can be found in our views on guilt in this connection. Even in traditional religious contexts, many counselors now hold that guilt of a religious nature for one's addictions is unhealthy and should be purged.

Aspects of the secular religion of recovery have entered traditional confessions not only in subtle ways but also explicitly in some contemporary theological reflections. At the liberal end of the ecclesiastical spectrum, some feminist theologians have suggested that historic Christianity is steeped in patriarchy and the mythos of the traditional family and as such is intrinsically abusive of women and children and has turned them into victims. Some have even charged that the doctrine of atonement is a doctrine of child abuse.

Joanne Carlson Brown and Rebecca Parker, for example, have asserted that "women are acculturated to accept abuse. We come to believe that it is our place to suffer. . . . Christianity has been a primary — in many women's lives *the* primary — force in shaping our acceptance of abuse. The central image of Christ on the cross as the savior of the world communicates the message that suffering is redemptive. If the best person who ever lived gave his life for others, then, to be of value we should likewise sacrifice ourselves. Any sense that we have a right to care for our own needs is in conflict with being a faithful follower of Jesus."[2] Brown and Parker go on to claim that this view of discipleship is borne out particularly in women's roles in the church, where they have been assigned the "suffering-servant" role.

> Our full personhood as well as our rights have been denied us. We have been labeled the sinful ones, the other; and even when we are let in, so to speak, we are constantly reminded of our inferior status through

---

2. Brown and Parker, "For God So Loved the World?" in *Christianity, Patriarchy and Abuse,* ed. Joanne Carlson Brown and Carole R. Bohn (Cleveland: Pilgrim Press, 1989), pp. 1-2.

language, theological concepts of original sin, and perpetual virginity —
all of which relate to sex, for which, of course, women are responsible.

The women who stay [in the church] are as surely victimized and
abused as any battered woman. The reasons given by women who stay
in the church are the same as those coming from women who remain in
battering situations: they don't mean it; they said they were sorry and
would be better; they need me/us; we can fix it if we just try harder and
are better; I'd leave but how can I survive outside; we have nowhere else
to go. . . . This Christian theology with atonement at the center still
encourages martyrdom and victimization. It pervades our society. Our
internalization of this theology traps us in an almost unbreakable cycle
of abuse. Our continuing presence in the church is a sign of the depth
of our oppression. . . . This glorification of suffering as salvific, held
before us daily in the image of Jesus hanging from the cross, encourages
women who are being abused to be more concerned about their vic-
timizer than about themselves. . . .

Is it any wonder that there is so much abuse in modern society when
the predominant image or theology of the culture is of "divine child
abuse" — God the Father demanding and carrying out the suffering and
death of his own son? If Christianity is to be liberating for the oppressed,
it must itself be liberated from this theology. We must do away with the
atonement, this idea of a blood sin upon the whole human race. . . . This
bloodthirsty God is the God of the patriarchy who at the moment controls the whole Judeo-Christian tradition. . . .

We do not need to be saved by Jesus' death from some original sin.
We need to be liberated from the oppression of racism, classism, and
sexism, that is, from patriarchy.[3]

Another feminist theologian, Rita Nakashima Brock, puts it this way:

I believe that patriarchy is the encompassing social system that sanctions
child abuse. Theologically, the patriarchal family has been and continues
to be a cornerstone for christological doctrines, especially father-son
imagery and in the unquestioned acceptance of benign paternalism as
the norm for divine power. . . . The basic social structure of the patriarchal family, a structure that socializes women for domestic responsibility
and men for dominance and aggression in public arenas, represents an
important element in Christian theology. Christological doctrines . . .
assume the unquestioned norm of the patriarchal family. Hence, I believe

---

3. Brown and Parker, "For God So Loved the World?" pp. 3, 26-27.

such christological doctrines reflect views of divine power that sanction child abuse on a cosmic scale and sustain benign paternalism.[4]

Brock goes on to interpret Alice Miller, the Swiss object-relations therapist who has been very influential in the recovery movement. (In her book *For Your Own Good: Hidden Cruelty in Child-rearing and the Roots of Violence,* she speaks of the "soul-murdering rules" by which "soul-murdered parents" unconsciously "soul-murder" their own children.) Miller, says Brock,

contends that virtually all child-rearing in our culture is control oriented. The use of control takes away a child's sense of distinct identity and subsumes it as an extension of parental will. Whether parents use techniques such as positive reinforcement or physical abuse, the parents shape the child into a being who reflects the parents' needs or wishes. . . . The use of control and punishment of any sort abuses children, producing lifelong damaging effects. Children learn to bury their feelings and needs, to rely on false selves that mirror their parents' feelings and needs, and to respect the powers of authority and dominance, rather than their own feelings and needs. Without direct access to one's feelings and the ability to express them, intimacy is impossible. . . . One of the most devastating combinations of elements in child-rearing described by Miller is the loving-punitive parent. The child receives both painful punishment and loving support from the same parent. In doing so, the child links the two together, confusing abuse with love. As an adult, a child so reared will be unable to give a healthy, nondestructive love. . . .

In patriarchal systems self-acceptance and intimacy are difficult achievements. We find instead a legacy of dominated and abused children. . . . To break free of and be healed of patterns of abuse, we must find the metaphors that lead us back to the Child, the vulnerable center of ourselves that carries our demons and wounds and that is the center of our power to connect. . . . Because we have believed in a divine being capable of such destructive power, we have made ourselves in that image. To continue to rely on such power will not see us out of our morass. To trust in the fragile Child, to challenge the powers of destruction with love, interdependence, care, and compassion, we must be courageous. But it is absolutely necessary — and a little Child will lead us.[5]

---

4. Brock, "And a Little Child Will Lead Us: Christology and Child Abuse," in *Christianity, Patriarchy and Abuse,* pp. 42-43.

5. Brock, "And a Little Child Will Lead Us," pp. 46-48, 59.

Capitalization notwithstanding, I do not think that Brock is referring to the Child Christ when she uses the word *Child* here. The defining clause following her initial use of the term ("the vulnerable center of ourselves that carries our demons and wounds") suggests a greater debt to pop psychologist and media personality John Bradshaw, champion of the concept of the abused inner child, than to anything from traditional Christian theology. In fact, she demonizes christological doctrines, charging that they are contaminated by patriarchal imagery and an "unquestioned acceptance of benign paternalism."[6]

Sympathy for the basic assumptions underlying RMT has thus entered the church through a general openness to the therapeutic community, and it has entered churches at the liberal end of the spectrum more explicitly through the writings of feminist theologians. But in recent years it has also made inroads in the churches at the conservative end of the spectrum in a dramatic way, through the popularization of belief in the threat of satanic ritual abuse.

Believers in Satan

Conservative Christians began to emerge as a political force in America during the 1970s. During the past two decades, the liberal mainline denominations have experienced a slow but continual loss of membership, while conservative, fundamentalist, and Pentecostal confessions have consistently grown, in both numbers and prominence. Religious sociologists continue to argue about the numbers and characteristics of the new conservatives. Broadly speaking, they tend to work in suburban America, worship in large suburban churches, and practice what appears to be a squeaky clean American religion. They work hard, they support "family values," they pursue the material benefits of the American dream with a clear conscience, they don't have any problems with patriarchal overtones in their religion. They profess belief in the inerrancy of scriptural norms for their lives, they condemn abortion and homosexuality as unqualifiedly evil, and large numbers of them are convinced that satanic cult activity is widespread throughout the world.

Their acceptance of the reality of multiple personality states and satanic ritual abuse is not connected to a sentimental belief in a state of

6. Brock, "And a Little Child Will Lead Us," p. 43.

childhood innocence corrupted by adult intrusions. Quite the opposite: it is connected to a strong belief that fallen and unregenerate human beings are intrinsically evil from the point of conception and that the devil literally stalks the world, seeking whom he may devour, working in everyday human lives to ensnare those created in God's image and to turn them from the truth. In not a few cases, they believe, the devil is successful, and any number of people have been induced to worship Satan and do all manner of unspeakable acts in his name.

Many fundamentalist beliefs about the nature of the devil and his activities are associated with views of the end times. One of the most popular of the end-times worldviews among conservative Christians is the millenarianism first espoused in this country by the nineteenth-century British divine John Nelson Darby. Drawing on a few verses in the biblical books of Daniel and Revelation, Darby argued that the world is preordained to be taken over by the Antichrist at the consummation of history before Christ's return. He believed in the inexorable decline of society and the emergence of the Antichrist from a newly revived Roman Empire. Darby taught that immediately before the Antichrist begins his global reign, Jesus Christ will return and "rapture" all believers out of this world to be with God. The unbelievers left on earth (the chaff, the goats) will attend the celebrity coronation of the Antichrist, who will establish a single world government and rule for seven years. At the end of seven years, God will depose the Antichrist, judge all those who aligned themselves with him or her, and inaugurate a thousand-year reign of Christ.

If all of this sounds a bit too close to something out of Hieronymus Bosch or Federico Fellini, consider that a recent candidate for president of the United States, Pat Robertson, not only believes in this scenario but espouses it publicly and often in books and on his own television program. Robertson spoke with trepidation about the formation of the European Community in his 1991 book *The New World Order,* anticipating that the emergence of a "possible United States of Europe" would presage the formation of the single world government that would quickly usher in the Apocalypse. Similar fears of a world government are evident in all corners of our society, from radical militia groups to conspiracy theorists fretting about the United Nations, the Trilateral Commission, and an international Jewish banking cabal. Books popularizing the end-times worldview have become hugely popular as we approach the third millennium after Christ. The best-selling book in America after the Bible is Hal Lindsey's *Late Great Planet Earth,* with more than nineteen million copies in print. Historian Grant Wacker observes that "Darbyite premillennialism proves to be one of the most resilient and widely held belief systems that has ever gripped the American imagination."

Millenarian expectations are nothing new. Such views have tended to heat up at the end of every century during the Christian era, and we might well expect a little extra fascination at the end of a millennium. The important factor for us here is the associated rise in interest in the activities of Satan and Satan worshipers, which appears to be amplifying or focusing concern among conservative Christians about the prevalence of satanic ritual abuse in our society. And, just as a common concern about the threat of pornography led to the curious coalition of radical feminist Catharine MacKinnon and conservative Attorney General Edwin Meese during the eighties, so a common concern about the threat of child sexual abuse — and specifically satanic ritual abuse — has made curious bedfellows of radical feminist theologians and fundamentalist preachers. Indeed, the concern is very widespread: a recent poll indicated that fully 70 percent of the American public now believes in the existence of a worldwide satanic cult conspiracy involving animal sacrifice, the ritual abuse and murder of children, cannibalism, and other horrors. And belief in SRA is closely connected with belief in MPD and the validity of RMT.

From the Michigan Militia and Montana Freemen to the more than five million Americans (including at least one Harvard University professor) who apparently believe that space aliens are routinely abducting humans and subjecting them to sexually abusive experiments, a vast number of Americans have shown a disturbing susceptibility to all manner of outlandish conspiracy theories. The willingness of people to believe such implausible stories in the absense of any credible supporting evidence — and, indeed, to accept elaborate and equally implausible theories explaining the disappearance of such evidence — suggests something bordering on clinical paranoia. As we have seen, even people grounded in traditional belief systems, both liberal and conservative, have been willing to accept at face value the stories of widespread satanic cult activities. Perhaps this is because they are immersed not only in an orthodox faith culture but also in the popular culture, joining fellow believers not only in traditional houses of worship but also in the audiences of Jerry Springer, Geraldo, Sally Jessy Raphaël, and the rest of the daytime talk-show constellation. They listen dispassionately to the sensational stories of an endless stream of people who claim to have blown the lid off government coverups, seen the insides of UFOs, taken part in satanic rituals. They are not so much credulous as they are desensitized to the extravagance of all the claims, open to the notion that pretty much anything is possible, and in the end swayed more by the emotional testimony of self-proclaimed survivors of the conspiracy du jour than by a critical examination of the evidence in the case. And so, in communities across the nation, when the tocsin of SRA is sounded, there is often a sympathetic crowd waiting to listen to the details.

The Ingram Case

One of the most bizarre and famous cases involving claims of repressed memories and satanic ritual abuse at the nexus of fundamentalist religion and psychotherapy is that of Paul R. Ingram. Ingram was the chief civil deputy of the sheriff's department in Olympia, Washington, and a local Republican party chairman. Along with his wife, Sandy, and their three sons and three daughters, Ingram was a member of the Church of the Living Water, an affiliate of the International Church of the Foursquare Gospel founded by Amy Semple McPherson in Los Angeles. A Pentecostal group, they believe that the gifts of the Holy Spirit — prophecy, healing, discernment, speaking in tongues — are essential to salvation and available to all who believe. The church sponsored an annual retreat for teenage girls called "Heart to Heart," and, in 1988, Ingram's daughter Ericka attended. One of the speakers was Karla Franko,

> a charismatic Christian who believes she has been given the biblical gifts of healing and spiritual discernment. Before going to Bible college, she had been a dancer and a stand-up comic as well as an actress, and had parts in several sitcoms and TV commercials, which added a note of celebrity in the minds of the young girls in the audience. Often in speaking to youth groups such as this one, Franko would feel herself filled with the Holy Spirit and would make pronouncements that the Spirit urged upon her. Many extraordinary events took place at the 1988 retreat. At one point, Franko told the mesmerized group that she had a mental picture of a little girl hiding in a coat closet, and saw a crack of light under the door. Footsteps were approaching. There was the sound of a key locking the door. At that, a girl in the audience stood up, heaving with sobs, and cried out that she had been that little girl.[7]

---

7. Lawrence Wright, *Remembering Satan: A Case of Recovered Memory and the Shattering of an American Family* (New York: Alfred A. Knopf, 1994), pp. 24-25. I am greatly indebted to Wright and this brilliant study for the lineaments of the Ingram story that follows, and for other insights regarding religion and popular culture throughout this chapter. Subsequent references to this volume will be cited parenthetically in the text.

Franko then reported another vision of a young girl being molested by a relative, and a deaf girl rushed out of the room. She was later found in a bathroom trying to commit suicide. Ericka had been serving at the retreat as a sign language interpreter to the deaf girls in attendance.

On the last day of the conference, Ericka failed to join the rest of the girls boarding buses to return home. Counselors found her in the conference center sobbing. She wouldn't say what was wrong. One of the counselors asked Franko, who was getting ready to leave for the airport, to come and pray over Ericka.

> "What does she need prayer for?" Franko asked. The counselor shrugged. Franko went back to the stage, where Ericka was sitting Indian-style, a portrait in dejection. Franko stood over her and began praying aloud. Almost immediately, she felt the Lord prompting her with information. She stepped back and was silent as she listened to the Lord's urgings. The word "molestation" presented itself to her.
>
> "You have been abused as a child, sexually abused," Franko announced. Ericka sat quietly weeping, unable to respond. Franko received another divine prompting, which told her, "It's by her father and it's been happening for years." When Franko said this aloud, Ericka began to sob hysterically. Franko prayed for the Lord to heal her. When Ericka's weeping eventually began to subside, Franko urged her to seek counseling, in order to get to the memories that were causing her so much pain. (*RS*, pp. 25-26)

Shortly after the church retreat, Ericka and her sister Julie moved out of the Ingram home. About two months later, around Thanksgiving, Sandy Ingram arranged for a meeting with Ericka. Supported by her best friend, Paula Davis, who was to be her advocate in everything that followed, Ericka told her shocked mother that she had been repeatedly molested by her father when she was young. The abuse had continued for several years, she said, from 1970, when she was four years old, until Paul was born again in the Pentecostal church in 1975, when she was nine.

When Sandy confronted Paul with the accusations, he insisted that he was innocent. Later she called the pastor of their church, who had already heard about the allegations from the retreat counselors; he told her that the charges were probably true because children did not make up those kinds of things. Ericka was twenty-two years old at the time. Then the youngest daughter, Julie, who was eighteen, volunteered that she, too, had been molested by her father, and also by her older brother, Paul Ross.

As questions about the abuse arose, both Ericka and Julie began telling different stories to different people. Ericka initially said that the abuse had stopped thirteen years before, when her father joined the church. Then she said it had not stopped until 1987. In the last interview she had with police before they arrested Paul, she said that he had molested her just two months earlier, in September of 1988. Julie told her mother that her father last touched her five years earlier, when she was thirteen, but she told the detectives that he had last assaulted her three years earlier, when she was fifteen. In the space of a single week, both girls changed key aspects of their stories several times.

When the news broke, it made the front page of the local paper. People were shocked, but no one seemed to doubt the allegations. Even Paul Ingram's best friend, Jim Rabie, believed the charges against Paul at first. "It just goes to show you, child abuse can happen anywhere," he said (*RS*, p. 50). That was before he himself was charged with having repeatedly assaulted Julie during late-night poker parties at the Ingrams' house. The associate pastor of the Ingrams' church, John Bratun, who also believed in Paul's guilt immediately, was called in because Paul believed he had a demon in him and wanted Bratun to perform an exorcism. "You don't have a demon, but you've got several spirits," Bratun told him (*RS*, p. 58). The pastor had served for a time in Southern California, where he believed he had developed the ability to discern when people were in bondage to spirits. He called on spirits of sexual immorality, gluttony, and other specific sins to leave Paul, but neither of them was satisfied that he was successful in removing them. Even so, Paul reported feeling "delivered" after their session together, and when he returned to the interrogation room, he had new recollections of abuse against his children that had been committed by his friend Jim Rabie. He now reported that while he had stood helplessly by, Rabie had sodomized his son Chad. Chad, who was then twenty years old, testified that he had never been abused, sexually or in any other way, by his father or anyone else.

One of the things that make this case so interesting is that, after his initial protestations of innocence, Paul Ingram himself became the chief witness to the incidents of abuse. Once the police interrogation began, Ingram retreated from denials that the abuse had ever occurred and said instead simply that he had no recollection that he had ever done anything like what his daughters were describing. The investigators told him it was common for abusers to repress memories of the ugly things they had done, and they asked him why the girls would lie about such a thing. This touched Ingram: at several points, even while he was insisting that he could not remember having abused the girls, he also said, "My kids always tell the truth." The investigators took this as an acknowledgment on his part that the abuse had in fact occurred and assumed that Ingram was simply reluctant to own up to it. In one interrogation session, detectives Brian Schoening and Joe Vukich and psychologist Richard Peterson focused on what they considered to be Ingram's weak point.

> "Why don't you listen to what [your daughter Julie] wrote here, Paul," said Vukich. "She says, 'I was four years old, he would have poker games at our house and a lot of men would come over and play poker with my dad and they would all get drunk and one or two at a time would come into my room and have sex with me.' Now, your daughter wrote that."
> "This is her writing, Paul," echoed Schoening.
> "And you told us that she's honest," said Vukich.
> "Oh, yes, my kids are honest." Ingram was sobbing now. . . .
> "Choose life over living death," Peterson exhorted, lapsing into the religious language that seemed to reach Ingram. "You are as alone as Jesus was in the desert when he was comforted."
> "God's given you the tools to do this," Vukich said. "You've got to show him by what you do and what you say as to whether or not you're worthy of his love and redemption and salvation."
> "Oh, Jesus!" Ingram cried in a frenzy. "Help me, Lord! Help me, Lord!"
> (RS, p. 45)

And then he began to supply the detectives with the details of what he described as pictures being presented to him. Hazy at first, they began to grow in clarity as the detectives told him what to focus on.

> "Is somebody taking pictures?" Vukich asked.
> "Uh, pictures — is there somebody off to the right of me? Uh, it's possible, let me look. I see — I see a camera."
> "Who's taking the pictures?"
> "I don't know. I don't see a person behind the camera."
> "That person's very important," Peterson said. "He's the one who holds the key. . . ."
> "Well, the person that I think I see is Ray Risch," Ingram said. (RS, pp. 47-48)

Risch was a mechanic for the Washington State Patrol. He was only one of many people that Ingram eventually named in interrogation sessions. In response to requests from the detectives, Ingram was consistently able to corroborate the details of his daughters' evolving stories and to supply additional information in whatever direction they pointed him. In fact, his memory became more and more active as the days passed. Helped by visualizations and constant prayer and assurances from Pastor Bratun that God would not allow anything but true thoughts to come into his memory, Paul began to see people in robes kneeling around a fire and one special individual in a red robe wearing a helmet of cloth. "Maybe the Devil," he suggested (*RS*, p. 59). This was new territory for the investigation: his daughters had said nothing about satanic ritual abuse.

Sandy Ingram had believed in her husband's innocence from the beginning, and when he began to confess, it shook her to the core. In her confusion, she went to see Pastor Bratun. Though Bratun was intensely involved in the case and had been passing information freely between the police, members of his church, and the accusing daughters, Sandy said later that she always felt she could trust him. But Bratun agreed with a detective who had said that Sandy either knew about what was going on in her home and ignored it or she participated in it. Bratun told her to her face that she was "eighty percent evil" and that she would probably go to jail unless she made a confession (*RS*, p. 94).

After being informed (by Bratun) of her father's confessions involving satanism, Ericka began to report her own memories of having been involved in SRA. As was the case with her previous memories, this new category of recollections changed from one telling to the next. Over time, she reported that she had been ritually raped and impregnated many times and that the fetuses had been aborted for use in sacrifices. She also reported that she had been scarred in many places by knife cuts administered by her father, Jim Rabie, and the Satanists. Julie reported much the same thing, adding that the scarring had made her so self-conscious that she had never changed clothes in the school locker room, and she never wore a swimsuit without putting on at least a T-shirt over it. In order to document this evidence for use against her father, the police asked that the girls be examined by a doctor specializing in the treatment of abused women. The examinations not only failed to turn up any evidence of previous pregnancies but also failed to find any scarring of any sort on either girl, apart from an appendectomy scar on Ericka. At one point in a series of different stories that Ericka provided after the examination, she claimed that she had never been sexually active — apparently contradicting all of her previous accounts of multiple sexual assaults by her father and his poker-playing buddies.

Frustrated by the bizarre turns and reversals in the case, the prosecution team called in Richard Ofshe, a Pulitzer prize–winning social psychologist from the University of California at Berkeley, to examine Paul

233

Ingram. Ofshe had written extensively about how thought-control techniques used in the Soviet Union, China, and North Korea were being used and refined by various religious cults. But, as he listened to Ingram rehearse the facts of the case, Ofshe grew increasingly skeptical. The way Ingram described his recollections was out of keeping with the way human memory actually worked. For example, at one point in the police interrogations, one of the detectives asked Ingram if he knew what time of day one of the incidents had occurred. With some effort, Ingram visualized the scene and "zoomed in" on the wristwatch of one of the people to read the time. Ofshe knew that nothing of that sort could possibly be valid. In general, he noted a pronounced difference between Ingram's descriptions of the incidents of abuse and his description of more routine events in his life. Ofshe was also concerned about the means by which Ingram was recovering the ostensibly repressed memories of abuse. He described how he would get an image and then pray on it, making use of a relaxation technique he had read about in a magazine. For his part, Ingram was sure that the memories he was conjuring up were real, because Pastor Bratun had assured him that God would reward these efforts only with the truth. But Ofshe noted that Ingram's descriptions of the recollected events were strewn with subjunctives and conditionals indicating that he was depending more on the convictions of others than on his own certainty about what had happened.

As a test, Ofshe told Ingram that his children had told the police that he had forced them to have sex with each other. Ofshe selected this story because it centered on one of the few deviant activities that nobody involved in the case had yet brought up. When first confronted with the false accusation, Paul said he couldn't remember it happening. But he closed his eyes and put his head in his hands, and in a few minutes he said, "I can kind of see Ericka and Paul Ross" (*RS*, p. 137). Ofshe told him to say no more but to go to his cell and pray about it. Two days later, Ingram came back and presented Ofshe with a three-page written confession of the new category of abuse. The experiment, along with other observations, convinced Ofshe that Ingram was a highly suggestible individual with a remarkable ability to create false memories without being aware of it. In Ofshe's opinion, this suggestibility, combined with the fact that Ingram was obviously desperate to please his interrogators, rendered questionable the validity of everything Ingram had "remembered" while in custody.

Ofshe also met with the other principal figures in the case, Ericka, Julie, and Sandy. He got the same sense from each of them that their memories of the ostensible abuse were different from their recollections of normal life. Sandy was by this time explicitly talking about two different kinds of memories: regular ones and those she remembered after seeing Pastor Bratun. Ofshe asked her to describe the memories she was getting with the help of Pastor Bratun, and Sandy detailed several rape scenes with Paul's best friends, plus satanic rituals in the woods. Ofshe noted that whenever she spoke of these events, she clearly slipped into a trance state. He had no doubts that Bratun and a psychologist she was working with were both feeding her images of abuse that she was interpreting as memories.

In the end, Ofshe concluded that all of the testimony from all of the Ingrams was false: the girls' accusations, Paul's confessions, and Sandy's visualizations were all manufactured. His official report dealt a severe blow to the prosecutor's case against Paul Ingram, which was also unraveling on other fronts — an ironic turn, given the fact that it was the prosecutor's office that had called Ofshe in on the case. Later Ofshe urged Ingram to withdraw his guilty plea before sentencing, telling him, "Nobody can blank out as many events as you think you blanked out — it has never happened" (*RS*, pp. 186-87). By this time Ingram was having increasing doubts about what he was supposed to have done, but he still believed that if he could just fill in the gaps in his memory, he could arrive at the truth about his daughters' accusations. And through it all, he was unwilling to create a situation in which his daughters would be forced to testify in court, because he was convinced that the trauma of that experience would damage them for life.

Two months later, however, he had a spiritual experience that he likened to conversion. As he was praying, he heard a voice say, "Let go of the rope."

> A deep feeling of peace settled over him. His mind began to clear. Suddenly, he could see that all the visualizations of rituals and abuse had been fantasies, not actual memories. He no longer believed that he was a Satanist or a child abuser, or even the victim of child abuse himself.... He wrote in his Bible, "PRI DIED TO SELF 7-19-89." (*RS*, p. 187)

He got a new lawyer and changed his plea to not guilty, but it was too late. He was convicted of six counts of third-degree rape. The prosecution had decided not to press any charges in connection with his confessions to having engaged in SRA.

At Ingram's sentencing hearing, Ericka asked the judge to give her father the greatest possible sentence. Failing that, she said, "I believe he will either kill me or Julie. He destroyed me and Julie's life and our entire family, and he doesn't care. He is obviously a very dangerous man." When given his chance to speak, Paul Ingram said, "I stand before you, I stand before God. I have never sexually abused my daughters. I am not guilty of these crimes" (*RS*, p. 188). Most first-time sex offenders in Washington state receive a sentence of six months if they agree to undergo treatment. The maximum sentence for the crimes of which Ingram had been convicted fell in a range from thirty-three to forty-three months. But the judge determined that the severity of the crimes warranted setting aside normal sentencing guidelines, and he sentenced Ingram to serve twenty years in a federal penitentiary. He is still serving time today. Charges against Jim Rabie, Ray Risch, and many others accused by the Ingrams were dropped or never pursued.

For all its sensational aspects, the Ingram case followed patterns evident in many criminal cases based on recovered memories of childhood abuse — initial denials on the part of the accused, a lack of any substantiating physical evidence, a gradual escalation of the charges from claims of molestation in the distant past to bizarre satanic cult activities in the more recent past, and the accusation of increasing numbers of people over time. Ingram's list of participants in the satanic rituals grew to include ten county employees, and, according to Lawrence Wright, "he also named members of the canine unit — the actual dogs, not their handlers — and described a scene in which the animals raped his wife." Ericka Ingram eventually claimed that Thurston County was controlled by thirty Satanists, including Undersheriff Neil McClanahan and Detective Brian Schoening, the men who headed up the prosecution of her father. "How high does this go?" asked Ericka's attorney, Thomas Olmstead, a fundamentalist Christian and former FBI agent. "The governor? Who knows?" (*RS*, p. 189).

And yet, despite the wildness and inconsistency of the claims and the lack of substantiating evidence, countless people believed the stories that the Ingrams produced. Even McClanahan, whom Ericka accused of being a Satanist, still believed in the rest of her story. "Satanic abuse is real," he contends. "This case proves it" (*RS*, p. 190).

As Wright points out,

> Ritual abuse cases have much in common; indeed, this is often taken as proof of the existence of a single, all-powerful satanic network. It can also be interpreted as evidence of the common fantasy life that has been

236

a feature of our culture for centuries. . . . One of the fascinating details of the European witch-hunts, which didn't end until 1700, is that frequently the witches' confessions — like Paul Ingram's — were voluntary and apparently deeply believed in. The elements of sodomy, incest, pedophilia, cannibalism, and the ritual use of human blood appear to be universal elements of demonology in all cultures. They correspond to inherent human fears and taboos.

As for why the satanic-ritual hysteria would appear again in our century, one can point to the rise of fundamentalist religions, the social anxiety about the loss of traditional values, and political uncertainty following the collapse of international communism. In addition, one can't help noticing the repeated theme of abortion. Both Ericka and Julie talked about receiving abortions and having their babies cut up and rubbed on them. This seems to be an element of nearly every SRA account. The imagery of babies being cut up and sacrificed is also a prominent feature of antiabortion protest. It is only a theory, but perhaps the psychic damage done by the abortion debate is reflected in the anguished fantasies of so many young women. (*RS*, pp. 197-98)

While he was in jail awaiting trial, Paul Ingram spent most of his time praying and "visualizing" with his pastor, elaborating his confession. He was a very devout man. Indeed, it is clear that the role of religion was important in the whole Ingram family story. Every member of the family believed in the existence of satanic cults, a belief that logically flows from the Church of the Living Water's doctrine that Satan is real and walks the earth. Their belief system, which includes a view of the world as radically dichotomized by the forces of good and evil, may have helped the Ingrams to imagine that Paul could exhibit a kind of Jekyll-and-Hyde complex, living one life as a county Republican chairman, law officer, and devoted Christian and another as a devil-worshiper guilty of the vilest crimes imaginable against his wife and children. Moreover, Pastor Bratun assured the family that Satan could prevent them from easily remembering any satanic cult activity that they might have been involved in. A number of factors, then, helped them to believe that they might all have been living two different lives, remaining entirely unaware of their monstrous activities as Satanists during the time they spent in the normal world. Others involved in the case, including Ericka Ingram's attorney Thomas Olmstead, seem to have been driven by similar ideological convictions to believe in the validity of the SRA charges as the foundation of the case against Ingram even after the prosecutor's office had abandoned all such charges as groundless and unsupportable.

Talk Show Mania

Wright argues that the willingness of many of the people involved in the Ingram case to believe the sensational accusations arose as much out of their grounding in popular culture as out of their religious beliefs. Tabloid television has done much to turn what once was considered bizarre behavior into everyday fare. It has also served to put the spotlight within reach of people who hunger for it. As talk-show host Jerry Springer puts it, "You are a person with no power, no money, no fame, but you've got something you want to talk about? Get up! There's the stage!" So ordinary people with a taste for notoriety get up and do just that in droves — on more than a dozen syndicated shows being aired daily. Every day brings a new parade of exhibitionists and a live audience to applaud their confessions and accusations, their pregnancies, affairs, petty larcenies, sexual kinks, conspiracy theories, and blood feuds. The line waiting for the fifteen minutes of fame stretches around the corner.

Just before Julie Ingram wrote a note to her teacher charging her father and his poker-playing buddies with having raped her, the Ingram family had watched a Geraldo Rivera special together entitled "Devil Worship: Exposing Satan's Underground." It was one of the most widely watched documentaries in television history, although it was only one of many such shows. The day before, the subject of Rivera's daily program had been "Satanic Breeders: Babies for Sacrifice." Daytime talk shows had become obsessed with SRA since the McMartin case. "No region in this country is beyond the reach of the devil worshipers," Rivera said on location in Nebraska. "Even here in the heartland of America, stories of ritual abuse crop up. The children you're about to meet were born into it. They say their parents forced them to witness bloody rituals and even, they say, to participate in ritual murder." Then he showed a clip of a young girl who testified, "My dad was involved in a lot of it. He's, like, one of the main guys; he's a leader or something. He made us have sex with him and with other guys and with other people" (*RS*, p. 80). At about the same time, former FBI agent Ted Gunderson was looking for funding to finance his search for the mass burial grounds of satanic cults in Mason County, Washington, right next door to the Ingrams' Olympia.

Three years later, after she had seen her father convicted of having abused her and sentenced to twenty years in a federal penitentiary, Ericka Ingram made her own pilgrimage into the limelight. If Geraldo's exposé had served as the prologue to Ericka's accusations, Sally Jessy Raphaël would provide the denouement to the Ingrams' story.

"Today, this woman will come face to face with the man [Jim Rabie] that she says sexually tortured her in satanic rituals for seventeen years. A show you don't want to miss," said Sally Jessy Raphaël to her television audience. . . .

"They were people in the community, like policemen," Ingram said as she described the cult. "There were some judges, doctors, lawyers. Different people in the community that had high political standings."

"What happened at the rituals?" Raphaël asked, her voice full of prodding compassion. "I know it must be pretty awful, but what happened?"

"First they would start with just, like, chanting," Ericka said. "Sometimes they would kill a baby."

"A baby?" Raphaël echoed. "Where would they get babies?"

"Sometimes people in the cult would have them just for this."

"Did this happen to you?" Raphaël asked. "You remember being on a table and people having sex with you?"

Ericka nodded.

"Wow. What else?"

"Sometimes they would drink blood," Ericka said. . . . "One time, when I was sixteen, they gave me an abortion. I was five months pregnant. And the baby was still alive when they took it out. And they put it on top of me and then they cut it up. And then, when it was — when it was dead, then people in the group ate parts of it." A gasp arose from the thrilled audience. Later Ericka asserted, "I spent most of my life in the hospital. And that is true. And, I mean, doctors were just, like, looking at my body, just going — *ugh!*"

This, of course, was not true. Ericka saw a number of doctors, including the expert in abuse assigned by the prosecutor's office to document anything that might be used as evidence against the men the Ingram girls had accused. None of the doctors found anything that might constitute such evidence.

Richard Ofshe also appeared on the show, balancing the views of another guest, radio evangelist Bob Larson, a self-proclaimed expert on satanic cults.

"What is the whole thing about satanism, Dr. Ofshe?" Raphaël asked.

"Right now, there is an epidemic of these kinds of allegations in the country," Ofshe said. "They are totally unproven."

"There's an epidemic of satanism in the country, not allegations," evangelist Larson interjected.

"Why would you say there is this epidemic, as a sociologist?" Raphaël asked.

"In part because it's a way of reasserting the coherence and authority of fundamentalist perspectives in society," Ofshe said.

"All right, let's talk to Bob," said Raphaël. . . . "Bob, you've got a man here saying that in no case — and there have been one hundred court cases, I believe, maybe even more, involving satanic rituals in our country — in no case has there ever been any evidence, hard-core evidence, nor has anyone, except Ericka's father, ever said that they've done that. In other words, there's never been a confession."

"He's only technically correct."

"Technically correct," Raphaël repeated flatly. When Larson cited the enormous number of people in therapy who have complained of satanic abuse, Raphaël asked again, "Why, if there are all these people that are under care, why isn't there one shred of evidence?"

"The difficulty is that the evidentiary basis of the justice system is not commensurate with what you deal with in a therapeutic process," Larson said. "When are we going to start believing people who come forward like this, instead of putting them through some type of legal litmus test?"

"One supposes," says Wright, "that the 'legal litmus test' he was referring to was the need for Ericka to provide credible testimony in order to convict Rabie of the crimes she accuses him of" (*RS*, pp. 190-92).

Psychology as Religion

In a recent book, psychotherapist James Hillman notes that stories of incest and violence against children are archetypal, appearing throughout history in various cautionary contexts. And yet they have attained a special prominence in our time. Why, he wonders, "has this particular syndrome, when there are so many other cruelties and injustices around, seized our white-bread American culture just now at the end of the millennium?"

Stan Passy, in conversation with Hillman, suggests that contemplation of the horror of this sort of victimization of the innocent fills a special need in the Christian imagination. "It's a question of hell," says Passy. "We've lost the place of hell in our culture. . . . We have to have a Hell! We have to have some place where all our monsters can reside, where our doubles and our shadows can act out! Most people don't believe, as they did in the medieval world, in a real, geographical, topological Hell in which they imagine their monsters. We are desperate to rediscover it, and I'm

240

convinced that in modern culture the rediscovery of hell emerges as: Our childhood. . . ."

In delivering people from the remembered trauma of their childhood, so the reasoning goes, therapists are serving as modern-day messiahs, rescuing clients from the contemporary vision of hell. It is a relationship that appeals to both participants: the therapists get caught up in the glory of providing salvation, and the clients are relieved to be able to assign their problems to forces external to themselves — corrupting influences in their past — and to be able to receive deliverance from a messiah on a fee-for-service basis.

"It can't be overstated," says Passy, "that the only way that childhood could *become* Hell would be if we imagine the child as a Christ-innocent nature."[8] That is to say, this view of the therapeutic covenant is based on the assumption that we are all born innocent and that we would remain so were we not damaged by people and events beyond our control. As we have already noted, this sort of thinking is often evident in RMT literature. Clients are urged to look for the source of their adult distress — whatever that distress might be — in a violation of their childhood innocence. All too often, RMT has the effect of magnifying the recovered memories of that violation until they reach literally demonic proportions.

Religion, in its ethical dimension, clearly has something to say about psychology, and vice versa: both participate in the issues of selfhood, family, and values. But, as Wendy Kaminer suggests in her sharp and insightful book *I'm Dysfunctional, You're Dysfunctional,* there has been a kind of unhealthy merger of religion and psychology in recent decades as religion has become enamored of psychotherapy's language and view of the self and as popular psychology has increasingly adopted a religiosity or "spirituality."

> The marriage of religion and psychology has been tentative and episodic, disrupted by Freud, and marked by periods of considerable hostility on both sides for much of this century. Now, we're witnessing not just a truce but a remarkable accommodation. . . . Religious writers would minimize or dismiss the effect of psychology on religion, fiercely denying that it has made doctrinal changes, but it does seem to have influenced the tone and packaging of religious appeals. . . .
>
> Religious writers justify their reliance on psychology by praising it for "catching up" to some eternal truths, but they've also found a way to

---

8. James Hillman and Michael Ventura, *We've Had a Hundred Years of Psychotherapy — and the World's Getting Worse* (San Francisco: HarperSanFrancisco, 1993), pp. 191-93.

make the temporal truths of psychoanalysis palatable. Religious leaders once condemned psychoanalysis for its moral neutrality. Now popular religious literature equates illness with sin (Satan works through personality disorders), which makes psychotherapy a penitential technique, if not a form of exorcism. . . . But whether psychology has caught up with religion, infiltrated it, or been adopted by it, the popular versions of both psychology and religion are becoming less and less distinguishable.[9]

Much current psychotherapy shows a pronounced romanticist tendency to rely on feelings for evidence, on metaphors for reality, on inspiration and intuition for guidance. As new drugs have proved effective in treating such major illnesses as depression and schizophrenia, psychotherapists without medical degrees have increasingly turned their focus to the more nebulous and "spiritual" complaints of North American society — the sense that our lives are not going as we imagined they would, the chasm between our idealized visions of ourselves and the reality of who we are. Whereas earlier generations tended to accept the dictum that life is not fair, many today believe that they are entitled to happiness and resent any impediments to the fulfillment of their desires.

The tension between those emphasizing a scientific, rational approach to therapy (who tend to explore pharmacological solutions) and those emphasizing an intuitive approach (who tend to favor the talking cure) mirrors the empirical/romantic tension that is part of the fabric of our whole society. Put in a more philosophical way, this can be viewed as a tension between objective reality and reality as perceived by the human receptor (i.e., how one *feels*). This existential tension is at the core of postmodern discussions that have been going on for decades in the fields of philosophy, history, literature, and theology. Postmodernists such as the exceedingly influential Michel Foucault deny the modernist assertion that words signify realities in an objective world around us and affirm instead that in a fundamental sense words construct our reality — in fact, that apart from words there is no reality. Some have understood this to mean that whatever we feel or perceive at any given moment constitutes reality. It brings to mind an old saw from a symbolic baseball game: the premodern, objective-reality umpire says, "There's balls and there's strikes, and I call 'em the way they are." The modernist umpire says, "There's balls

9. Kaminer, *I'm Dysfunctional, You're Dysfunctional: The Recovery Movement and Other Self-Help Fashions* (New York: Vintage, 1993), pp. 124-25.

and there's strikes, and I call 'em the way I see 'em." The postmodernist umpire declares, "There's balls and there's strikes, and they ain't nothin' until I call 'em."

This last, the postmodernist view, has so penetrated our culture that we now hear mass media therapists mouthing its clichés as if they were gospel. The following is a conversation I heard on a public radio call-in show in Milwaukee:

Therapist: There is no objective reality. What is or what may have happened is only a construct of words that we have agreed to assign to some objects or experiences.

Caller 1: If there is no objective reality, what prevents mass delusion?

Therapist: Well, there *has* been mass delusion. Look at Germany under the Nazis. I don't want to think about delusion. In my work I don't care about objective reality. I care only about my patient's reality.

Caller 2: What if your patient claimed to have repressed memories of having suffered satanic ritual abuse? Would you feel obligated to check out external evidence for the truthfulness of that claim?

Therapist: It is extremely difficult to check things like that out. Everyone is in denial. You will not get anybody to admit that this sort of activity went on. Even the patient has been in denial. No, I simply go with my patient's reality, and I treat her as though what she says she's experienced is true.

It is clear that, in this view, it doesn't matter whether a patient is confabulating or making up a "memory"; indeed, it doesn't matter if the patient is outright delusional. In order to validate the client, the therapist accepts the delusion, affirms the delusion, and allows the client to continue to embrace the delusion. This approach tends to lock both therapist and client into a diagnosis of repressed memories: if the client accepts the therapist's interpretation of her reality, the acceptance serves as a confirmation of the therapist's interpretation; if, on the other hand, the patient resists the diagnosis, the therapist will interpret the intensity of her resistance as denial of the reality of her condition.

Much current therapy shows the influence of the postmodern ethos in a cognitive/emotive dichotomy: it sends the message that it is harmful to *think* but healthy to *feel*. We can see it in such twelve-step recovery program slogans as "Stinkin' thinkin'" and "Your best thinking got you here" (i.e., into addiction). Critical, analytical thinking is caricatured as arid, cold, bloodless, full of rules and "shoulds"; feeling, on the other hand, is presented as warm, creative, honest, spontaneous, the antithesis of hidebound rules. This sort of dualistic view of the human mind and psyche goes back to the ancient Greeks and St. Paul. But through the centuries most philosophers — and healers as well — have promoted a search for balance between the claims of heart and mind as the ideal. When postmodern therapists deny the validity of any sort of critical thinking on the part of their clients, they are closing the door to a resource that previous generations considered crucial to the process of healing and recovery. As a practical matter, they would also seem to be stripping their clients of a component essential to independent thought and autonomy, thereby helping to promote a new kind of dependency.

Postmodern assumptions are evident in a wide range of new faith-oriented therapies, including specifically "Christian" therapies. A whole entrepreneurship of religious self-help books by writers from Charles Swindoll and James Dobson to M. Scott Peck and Rabbi Harold Kushner has emerged to help people through the shoals of personality development, child rearing/parenting, spouse abuse, and loneliness, along with the search for love, happiness, and salvation. Religious codependency books are practically indistinguishable from the secular codependency books — except for the exhortation to rely on God for strength. "The most effective means for overcoming codependent relationships is to establish a relationship with Christ himself," writes Frank Minirth, cofounder of the Minirth-Meier clinic. Once published by religious houses almost exclusively, these books have such a huge market today that mainstream, secular publishers are bidding for them.

What these authors — pretty much across the theological spectrum — are saying about the self, at least in terms of historical theology, is very interesting. It is a relatively new view of the self: it advances the principle that loving yourself is as important as loving your neighbor (instead of the other way around). It is the basis for a healthy relationship with God, they say, as well as a scriptural imperative. In this new view, says Kaminer,

> low self-esteem is sinful, an affront to God who loves you, warts and all. Evil is a kind of personality disorder . . . which may be a weapon of Satan. Like a bad parent, he deprives you of self-esteem and plays upon your weaknesses.
>
> What is interesting about these familiar messages is their blend of religion, popular psychology, and popular communitarian critiques of American culture. Although . . . [religious books] speak to subcultures

of believers, especially conservative Christians, they partake in prevailing mainstream notions about goodness, health, selfhood, and social relations. . . . And on the margins of denominational religion, from New Thought and Christian Science to New Age, spiritualism has sought credibility in pseudoscience, describing the magic of cosmic energy while borrowing from new theories about the human psyche and the power of imagination.[10]

Self-esteem is hardly an original theme for self-help writers today. It has been a doctrinal plank in the platform of Robert Schuller's Crystal Cathedral for decades. Rabbi Kushner insists that "one of the goals of religion is to teach people to like themselves and feel good about themselves." David Seamands, a Christian psychologist, says, "Low self-esteem is the most powerful psychological weapon that Satan uses against Christians."

Evangelicals and secular seekers alike seem to agree that one of the chief threats to the development of healthy self-esteem is an inclination toward "perfectionism" that arises in "critical" home environments when children seek to appease unpleasable parents with suitable behaviors. The more secular of the self-help gurus have had no compunctions about specifically identifying perfectionism as a part of the disease of codependency. They suggest that Christians are particularly prone to burnout and perfectionism because of their ethic of service, not to mention their high moral standards. Twelve-step programs are full of people bemoaning their drive to be perfect, their low self-esteem, and the "shaming" behavior of their abusive parents. "Christians can be such shamers!" Charles Swindoll says, borrowing the recovery jargon. The underlying axiom of all this thinking is that "God created us all perfect beings, and our parents screwed us up."[11]

But is not the ethic of service the ethic of Jesus? Surrender of the self and selfless service to the other? Considering Jesus' message in the story of the rich man and Lazarus and his admonition in the parable of the sheep and the goats ("as you did it to one of the least of these my brethren, you did it to me"), is there any way to avoid the conclusion of traditional orthodox Christian theologians that a theology that fails to honor and reward doing good to others is a bankrupt theology?

Another message of the self-help/recovery Christians is that you have

10. Kaminer, *I'm Dysfunctional, You're Dysfunctional*, pp. 123-24.
11. Swindoll, quoted by Kaminer in *I'm Dysfunctional, You're Dysfunctional*, p. 135.

to love yourself in order to receive God's grace. In this connection, Swindoll says that "the individual whose track record is morally pure has no better chance at earning God's favor than the individual who has made a wreck and waste of his life." Some people find this reading of the doctrine of grace comforting; others maintain that it cheapens grace to define it this way, that an understanding of grace completely severed from concomitant moral obligations will excuse, encourage, or at least trivialize bad behavior. For their part, the self-help Christians tend to dismiss the concept of a God who requires honor, justice, and righteousness and who shames wickedness as a throwback to Old Testament legalism.

What sort of God, then, is envisioned in the new self-help/recovery religion? Kaminer writes that in this context "God is invariably portrayed as the ideal parent whose love you can never exhaust . . . a cross between a gentle patriarch and a New Age life force. Do our notions of good parenting derive from our relations with God, as religious writers suggest, or is our vision of God shaped by our parents?"[12] We have already seen what sort of answer some feminist theologians are supplying to that question.

Religious dysfunction is attributed to psychological disorders, such as paranoia and low self-esteem, which, in turn, are attributed to dysfunctional families and the work of the devil. Bad relationships with God derive from bad relationships with parents — or, as David Seamands puts it, Christians with "damaged love receptors" can't receive God's love, so they distort his character, presuming him to be untrustworthy, critical, and "unpleasable," like their parents. The belief that one's parents are ultimately responsible for one's woes as an adult, long an article of faith in the secular recovery/therapeutic community, has clearly become part of the new psychotherapeutic gospel of even conservative Christians. To some extent, this is simply an expression of a basic human tendency to look for the source of our problems outside ourselves. But it is a tendency that can also lead to scapegoating and demonizing the Other. To some degree, it was evident in the Ingram case. Once the initial charges were made, most of the people involved in the case seemed to have little difficulty believing that the Ingrams had led a double life, devout Christians by day but slaves to Satan by night. Even Paul and Sandy Ingram accepted the assertions of others that they were unwitting playthings of the devil — in effect demonizing the Other by assigning guilt to alter egos that remained strangers to them in their normal waking lives.

12. Kaminer, *I'm Dysfunctional, You're Dysfunctional*, p. 136.

Kaminer writes that

> popular religion, like a twelve-step group, reminds us that we're power-
> less. What's missing in much popular religious literature today is a model
> for ethical action in the world. Focusing on the individual relationship
> with God, on the state of individual belief, while disparaging individu-
> alism, most popular religious writers offer no thoughtful discussion
> about moral behavior, giving us no basis for community. . . . People
> convinced of their own helplessness as individuals don't come together
> in democratic companionship; they come together as mobs, bereft of
> both self and community.[13]

Widely varying belief systems lead people to widely varying perceptions of the sources of evil in the world and of the sorts of conspiracies
that are spreading that evil by abusing people. There is much evidence to
suggest that belief in a primal innocence and the exaltation of self-esteem
as a virtue can help to produce the same sorts of delusions as a thorough-
going belief in the activities of demonic forces in the world. Both sorts of
beliefs reflect a conviction that our problems are imposed on us by forces
outside ourselves. To the extent that we, as a culture and as members of
communities of faith, continue to cling to this conviction, we will remain
vulnerable to the temptation to demonize the Other, to blame our woes on
individuals who are in fact guiltless. And some among us will be tragically
susceptible to the influence of therapists who are convinced that a vast array
of psychological complaints can be traced back to a history of childhood
abuse.

13. Kaminer, *I'm Dysfunctional, You're Dysfunctional*, pp. 149-50.

Epilogue

Everyone prefers belief to the exercise of judgment.

— Seneca

The trouble with truth is that it is mainly uncomfortable and often dull. The human mind seeks something more amusing, and often caressing.

— H. L. Mencken

During the cold winter of 1691-1692, in Salem Village of the Massachusetts Colony, eleven-year-old Abigail Williams and her nine-year-old cousin Betty Parris spent weeks listening to tales of voodoo, spells, witchcraft, and illicit cultic practices related by the family's West Indian slave, Tituba. Over the course of the winter, as several other girls from strict Calvinist homes gathered at the Parris home to listen to Tituba's alluring stories, they developed perplexing behavioral changes and mental states. They had highly emotional fits and trances; they choked and had body contortions; they fell down screaming and flailing away "at night and at prayer"; they were periodically blind, deaf, and dumb; and they had epileptic-like seizures.

Betty Parris's father asked the village doctor, William Griggs, to examine the girls. Unable to find a physical cause for the girls' strange behavior changes, and as bewildered as everyone else, Dr. Griggs diagnosed the problem as "bewitchment," saying that the "evil hand is on them." The consensus of the clergy and town fathers, who regarded the girls as victims and paid great attention to their symptoms, was that agents of Satan — that is, witches — were at work in the community. Mr. Parris sought the assistance of community leaders to help him deal with these "evil spirits."

Already by early 1692, the evil spirit affliction had spread to about a dozen other girls of the community. The main symptoms were dumbness or inarticulate mumbling, choking, temporary blindness and deafness, muscle spasms, inability to pray, and spells, or trances, during which they saw vivid and frightening apparitions. At first the girls did not reveal who their persecutors were, but after much questioning by the town leaders, they revealed Tituba's identity, as well as a growing list of others in the community, whom they seem to have chosen at random.

On February 29, 1692, the town fathers arrested Tituba and two other women and put them in a Boston jail. But the girls, who now had the entire community in their thrall, continued to accuse others, and by this time the hysteria was in full hue and cry. Previously unaffected citizens came forward to say that they too had been visited by "servants of the devil" in the night, that their crops had been ruined and their livestock affected by the evil spirits. Only three months after the imprisonment of the first three "witches," in April 1692, the witchcraft epidemic had spread to other communities in the Massachusetts Bay colony. Fifty people were accused in Andover, and prominent citizen John Alden, a wealthy fur merchant in Boston, was accused by the girls of being the leader of a group of witches in that city.

William Phipps, governor of the Massachusetts Bay colony, appointed seven distinguished men to preside over the trials of the accused witches. The young girls spoke of pains inflicted on them by the accused and of visits in the night — though all of the accused had secure alibis for the times during which the untoward activity was said to have taken place. Even in the court, during the trials themselves, the girls screamed out that they were being pinched and poked by the accused, as the latter were sitting quietly across the courtroom. The magistrates and judges, who could see the accused sitting at a safe distance from the screaming girls, nevertheless accepted this "spectral evidence" of guilt. People of that time and religious persuasion believed that witches were able to operate in this way. As a matter of practical fact, to be accused of being a witch by the young girls was to be convicted of being a witch.

The magistrates dismissed the denials of the "witches," and in the period between June 2 and September 17, 1692, the court convicted twenty-seven people of witchcraft. Nineteen were promptly hanged, one man was pressed to death with heavy stones, and four died in prison. Ironically, Tituba, who confessed to witchcraft, was neither tried nor convicted — nor were any of the others who confessed their witchcraft and renounced the devil (usually under torture).

Only a week into the Salem witchcraft trials, Judge Nathaniel Saltonstall resigned in disgust over the proceedings, appalled at the conduct of the colony's leaders. He was not the only prominent citizen of Salem Colony who had become uneasy with the proceedings. The Reverend Increase Mather, president of Harvard College and the Massachusetts Colony's ambassador to England, was also deeply disturbed by the events in Salem. He considered the evidence being used to convict people of witchcraft very questionable. "It were better that ten suspected witches should escape," he said, "than that one innocent person should be condemned. . . . I had rather judge a witch to be an honest woman than judge an honest woman as a witch." But his son, Cotton Mather, the famous Puritan divine, was convinced of the guilt of the accused, and he fell in with the hysteria.

Once the trials had concluded and the accused had been executed, one might expect that the accusations would have stopped, but they did not. By October, the girls were accusing a widening circle of prominent citizens, including Governor Phipps's wife and Judge Nathaniel Saltonstall himself.

Finally, on October 26, 1692, after being goaded by Increase Mather, the Massachusetts legislature told the Salem magistrates that they would have to establish much more stringent criteria before they could judge someone guilty of witchcraft. They finally perceived that a prosecution grounded on spectral evidence was capricious: it could not be refuted because it could not be proved. Three days later, Governor Phipps dismissed the court, effectively bringing the witch trials to an end. Eventually, several of the young women admitted that their beliefs had been delusions and that their accusations had been false.

January 14, 1997, marked the three hundredth anniversary of the Massachusetts "Day of Repentance." Five years after they had jailed more than 150 innocent people as witches and condemned twenty to death, the twelve jurors in the witch trials signed a statement of repentance, claiming that they themselves — rather than the children or those accused of being witches — had been misled by the devil. For many years thereafter, the courts and churches of Massachusetts declared days of penance and prayer for the injustices that had been done to innocent people. In subsequent years, descendants of those executed as witches were granted redress for their losses, compensation that in some cases continued until as recently as 1957. The jurors came to believe that they had shed innocent blood, a mortal sin for which they did not expect forgiveness. They composed and signed the following statement, which came to be known as "The Salem Jury's Rule":

We whose names are underwritten, being in the year 1692 called to serve as jurors in court at Salem, on trial of many who were by some suspected guilty of doing acts of Witchcraft upon the bodies of sundrey persons:

We confess that we ourselves were not capable to understand nor able to withstand the mysterious delusions of the Powers of Darkness and Prince of the Air, but were for want of knowledge in ourselves and better information from others, prevailed with to take up with such evidence against the accused as on further consideration and better information we justly fear was insufficient for touching the lives of any (Deuteronomy 17:6), whereby we fear we have been instrumental with others, though ignorantly and unwittingly, to bring upon ourselves and this People of the Lord the guilt of innocent blood, which sin the Lord saith in Scripture he would not pardon (2 Kings 24:4), that is, we suppose, in regard of this temporal judgement.

We do therefor hereby signify to all in general (and to the surviving sufferers in especial) our deep sense of and sorrow for our errors in acting on such evidence to the condemning of any person, and do hereby declare that we justly fear we were sadly deluded and mistaken, for which we are much disquieted and distressed in our minds, and do therefore humbly beg forgiveness, first of God for Christ's sake for this our error, and pray that God would not impute the guilt of it to ourselves nor others. And we also pray that we may be considered candidly and aright by the living sufferers as being then under the power of a strong and general delusion, utterly unacquainted with and not experienced in matters of that nature.

We do heartily ask forgiveness of you all, whom we have justly offended, and do declare according to our present minds, we would none of us do such things again on such grounds for the whole world praying you to accept of this in way of satisfaction for our offence, and that you would bless the inheritance of the Lord that He may be entreated for the Land.

Similarities between 1690s and 1990s America

Some Americans, during the infancy of this republic, learned the lesson of Salem — that great evil can be wrought by those on a crusade to save the children and to deliver the world from evil spirits and evildoers. But it was a lesson not learned well enough — or for long enough. In the early 1950s, much of the nation was again paralyzed by fear of evil spirits among them. Senator Joseph McCarthy identified the threat as Communism, and he worked to expose and punish all who had been seduced by it. Most of the accused were in high-profile positions in government, academia, the arts, and the entertainment industry, and McCarthy took evident delight in bringing them low. At the peak of his power, the senator stood virtually unchallenged, for to question his methods was to invite his devastating charges against oneself. By the time his reign of terror came to an end, McCarthy had left a trail of ruined careers and suicides from coast to coast.

Just thirty years after McCarthy finished his run, a new witch hunt began in this country, focused on the evil of child abuse. Of course the psychotherapists, social workers, child advocates, and feminists who have been swept up in the excesses of this new movement are not much inclined to see many similarities between their crusade and those of their illiberal predecessors. And, indeed, in many respects there is a world of difference between the belief system of a representative proponent of RMT and that of Joseph McCarthy or a typical seventeenth-century Massachusetts Calvinist. But the crusades to which they have devoted themselves are chillingly similar. For evidence of the reactionary elements in the otherwise progressive ideology of the new child advocates, we need look no further than the ease with which they have allied themselves with such conservative forces as Ed Meese, Jerry Falwell, and the ranks of the Christian Right. The two camps have worked together to fight against pornography, to press for investigations of daycare centers, and to uncover the operations of an international network of satanic cults. And, inasmuch as their efforts date back at least as far as the McMartin Preschool case in 1984, their witch hunt has already far outlasted the Salem trials of the 1690s and the McCarthy hearings of the 1950s.

The similarities between the 1690s witch hunt and the 1990s witch hunt are quite remarkable. In Salem, the charges were initially made by children; today, they are made by children under the tutelage of adult facilitators and by adults ostensibly recovering memories of childhood abuse with the help of therapists. In Salem, the witnesses were initially immersed in tales of witchcraft and then coached in their testimony by believing adults; today, clients of RMT are commonly immersed in therapeutic literature (e.g., the bible of the RMT community, *The Courage to Heal*) and subsequently guided in recalling past abuse by therapists who are convinced that it must have taken place. In Salem, the accused were convicted solely on the basis of "spectral evidence"; today, RMT clients are accusing people solely on the basis of what they believe to be recovered memories — which is to say that, then as now, people have been charged and convicted of crimes without any objective evidence of guilt.

Further, doctors have played an important role in both contexts. In Salem, the town doctor examined the girls, found no physical cause for their writhing, choking, and incoherent babbling, and concluded that they must have been "bewitched." Today, doctors of psychiatry such as Diane Humenansky, Bennett Braun, Judith Peterson, Corydon Hammond, and Cornelia Wilbur examine women complaining of depression, insomnia, bad relationships, low self-esteem, and similar broadly defined complaints and conclude that they must be suffering from multiple personality disorder or the residual effects of childhood sexual abuse or satanic ritual abuse.

In both contexts, the hysteria has progressed in waves. In Salem, the hysteria started in the Parris home and spread rapidly throughout Salem Village and surrounding communities, soon reaching the hub city of Boston. In our media-saturated society, descriptions of every conceivable psychological disorder and all manner of sensational behavior associated with such disorders spread so rapidly and in such detail that therapeutic contamination is not only easy to induce but virtually impossible to prevent.

In both contexts, the charges have followed a characteristic pattern of escalation. The individuals making the charges typically describe increasingly bizarre and horrible abuse and identify increasing numbers of perpetrators over time. The girls of Salem did not stop until they had accused one of the judges appointed by the governor, the governor's wife, and other prominent members of the New England society. In the course of the McMartin trial, the children eventually accused not only the preschool staff but the police investigators and prosecutors pressing the case, the judges, prominent people in the community such as the Manhattan Beach mayor's wife, and of course their own parents.

The narratives in this book, especially Kristin's and Pauline's, give an indication of the pattern of escalating accusations typical of RMT. Clients often start by accusing someone like a church janitor or an uncle, then include fathers and grandfathers, then mothers and grandmothers, and then still others outside the family circle. As Pauline's mother put it, "It was as if everyone that we ever knew had been put on this earth to molest her."

Neither the pattern of escalation in general nor the absurdly large numbers of abusers named in individual cases ever seems to undermine the credibility of the testimony in the minds of the true believers; it merely serves to confirm their preexisting belief that abuse is epidemic in our culture.

Common also to the witch hunts of yesterday and today is the notoriety enjoyed by the accusers. In Salem, the children making the accusations had never before enjoyed such attention and power. As long as they kept up a steady flow of accusations, they continued to enjoy the benefits of their allegations. Conversely, they were aware that public recanting would result in significant embarrassment, possible punitive measures, and certainly an end to the attention and notoriety. Many factors, then, including the promptings of the investigators and prosecutors, encouraged the accusers to hold fast to their accusations. We can see the same phenomenon in investigations of child abuse today. In many of the cases we have reviewed in this book, children were clearly coached to produce stories of abuse and rewarded for doing so. They were, in effect, coerced into falsifying their own histories, into believing their own falsifications, and on that basis into helping to destroy their families and send innocent people to prison. We can only presume that if, later in life, they are able to confront the true nature of their accusations, they may well feel such remorse that they will need therapy to deal with it.

Ann Putnam, the eleven-year-old who was perhaps the smartest and most vindictive of the Salem girls, later made a confession of sorts when she was received into the Salem Village church. She expressed her sorrow that she had,

> by such a providence of God, [been] made an instrument for the accusing of several persons of a grievous crime, whereby their lives were taken away from them, whom now I have just grounds and good reason to believe they were innocent persons; and that it was a great delusion of Satan that deceived me in that sad time. . . . What I did was ignorantly, being deluded by Satan.

Even in this apology, though, she still placed the blame outside herself. She added that she was innocent of any "anger, malice, or ill-will," though one of the Salem girls admitted that they had done it "for sport, they must have some sport."[1]

The amazing contemporary witch hunt in the small Washington town

---

1. Cited by John Updike in "Elusive Evil," *The New Yorker*, 22 July 1996, p. 69.

of Wenatchee, an exemplar of child-abuse hysteria in this country (still in progress as I write), provides uncanny echoes of Salem Village. The citizens of Wenatchee have been terrorized by continually escalating accusations of sex crimes within the community, accusations coming from eleven-year-old "D.E.," the foster daughter of Wenatchee's only sex-crimes investigator, Robert Perez. Perez has a record of petty crimes and domestic strife; one police department evaluation conducted before his appointment as investigator characterizes him as "pompous and arrogant," a man who tends to "pick out people and target them." He pressured his foster daughter into accusing more than eighty adults of heinous sexual crimes against children (court testimony establishes that he threatened to punish her if she refused to testify as he specified). At one point Perez was driving "D.E." up and down Wenatchee streets in his pickup, encouraging her to point out the houses in which the satanic activities were supposed to be taking place. She identified twenty-three such houses. On the basis of such accusations, Perez brought 3,200 charges of child sexual abuse against one woman alone.

Perez's biggest quarry in the community was Pastor Robert Roberson and his wife, Connie. "D.E." accused Roberson of leading his entire congregation in ritualistic sex orgies involving the public rape of children and other satanic activities. Perez arrested the Robersons and placed their five-year-old daughter Rebekah in the custody of Child Protective Services. After four sessions with the girl, a therapist concluded that she had been molested. No tapes or transcripts of these interviews were preserved.

By the time the Robersons' case came to trial, "D.E." was unable to testify, having suffered a breakdown and been placed in a psychiatric unit. The only other child witness (besides their daughter Rebekah) admitted under cross examination that she had made false accusations of rape against her foster father and her counselor. That left the prosecution with just one key witness against the Robersons: a repeat sex offender who had agreed to provide testimony against the minister and his wife in return for a reduction of charges in a separate case from first-degree rape to misdemeanor assault. In the end, the Robersons were acquitted on all fourteen charges of child sexual abuse and molestation.

Despite the absurdity of the sensational charges, the universal denials of the many people charged, and the complete absence of any physical evidence, forty adults were arrested and placed on trial in Wenatchee. Almost half of those charged were women — a percentage unprecedented in child abuse cases. Most of those who were able to hire their own lawyers got the charges against them dropped (on the grounds that there was no substantiating physical evidence and the children's testimony had clearly been tainted in interrogations conducted by Perez and therapists) or were acquitted. Of those who had to rely on publicly appointed attorneys, twenty-eight were convicted, sentenced, and incarcerated. Some chose to plead guilty after being threatened with life sentences in case of conviction. A number of them are still in prison at this writing. In all of this we hear another echo of Salem: those who confessed that they were in league with the devil — such as Tituba, the slave who first told the girls voodoo tales from the West Indies — were let off; those who maintained their innocence and refused to plead guilty were executed.

When Washington state attorney Mike Lowry asked Attorney General Janet Reno to intervene in the case of Wenatchee's railroaded parents, Reno refused; Lowry's request also received a "chilly reception" from Hillary Rodham Clinton. That left the accused with no place to turn, given that the federal government grants absolute immunity to those who report or act upon reports of child abuse. Dr. Edward Zigler, former director of the Office of Child Development and chief of the U.S. Children's Bureau, testified before the Senate, "I am very troubled by what I see. In fact, child abuse is the only instance I know of in which the individual is considered guilty until he is proven innocent." Accusations of child abuse, like accusations of witchcraft in 1692, have generated a public hysteria that demanded suspension, or at least weakening, of the twin pillars of common law criminal justice — the presumption of innocence and proof beyond a reasonable doubt.

Hoaxes

But the controlling similarity between Salem Village and the current child abuse hysteria in North America — and the reason we can legitimately call what is happening today a witch hunt — is that the accusations made then and the ones made now are all built on hoaxes.

However difficult it might be for us to fathom today, a belief in the existence of witches arose naturally out of the belief structures of Western civilization for hundreds of years. Nor was it only the uneducated who were susceptible to these superstitions. The best minds of British, Continental, and American culture — people including Luther and Erasmus, Jonathan Edwards and Cotton Mather — believed in witches. When it became agonizingly clear, after far too long, that innocent people were being killed, the powers that be stopped the practice of executing witches. But those powers did not say, "We don't believe in witches anymore." They said, "We still believe in witches, but we have to be more careful in identifying them."

Belief in a worldwide conspiracy of satanic cult murderers invading our daycare centers is as foundationless as belief in witches. There is no evidence that either of them exists. Like the stories of witches in Europe and Salem Village, the modern-day stories of a vast network of Satan worshipers who conduct secret ceremonies, sacrifice babies, drink human blood, and perpetrate an extensive array of additional lurid crimes constitute a hoax that has nonetheless engendered far-reaching social hysteria. We may shake our heads in disbelief at the gullibility of the benighted Salem Village faithful who believed in a conspiracy of witches — and at their viciousness in wanting to kill them — but that is simply because we don't believe in witches anymore. In our day, the crusade against child abuse has gathered near-universal support because it is grounded in things that we believe in — even if, at the fringes of the campaign, people are investing belief in misrepresentations, bad science, utter fictions, or downright hoaxes.

The popular fascination with multiple personality disorder goes back at least as far as the publication of *The Strange Case of Dr. Jekyll and Mr. Hyde;* interest was vastly increased in more recent years by the publication of *Sybil,* which was billed as a true story of MPD but which Dr. Herbert Spiegel has testified was a hoax concocted by Dr. Cornelia Wilbur and author Flora Schreiber. Some scientists and doctors question the validity of any diagnosis of MPD; the vast majority of qualified mental health experts maintain that it is at most an extremely rare disorder and that there cannot be anything like the hundreds of thousands of cases that have been diagnosed in recent years. In the vast majority of these cases, the complaint is most likely an artifact of the psychotherapeutic setting; most people being treated for MPD are actually suffering from a form of hysteria in which they imitate a condition they have observed in other people, read about in books, or seen in the movies or on TV talk shows.

Satanic ritual abuse can be dismissed even more conclusively as a hoax. Even though whole psychiatric units are dedicated to finding it in disturbed people's backgrounds, television "news" shows have aired specials, and TV docudramas have been produced with actors gravely attesting its rampant growth among us, SRA is nothing more than a dark fantasy. A 1994 federal survey of more than 12,000 accusations of satanic ritual abuse failed to find a single instance that could be substantiated with any physical evidence. Not the McMartin case, nor any of the hundred or so McMartin-like cases around the country that prosecuted daycare workers for the ritualistic abuse of their wards, ever produced any physical evidence — and yet many people have gone to prison on the basis of those charges, and some of them are still there.

Facilitated communication, a tiny blip of a satellite in this loony orbiting system, was quickly nipped in the bud after autistic and other mentally disturbed children, with the help of their "facilitators," began accusing their parents of heinous sex crimes against them. All investigators had to do was show the child and the facilitator two different images, and the child invariably typed into the computer what the facilitator saw. The sex abuse charges were revealed to be a hoax, entirely fabricated by the "child advocates" and foisted on the mentally handicapped children they were "helping."

Finally, repressed memory itself, the central star around which these other hoaxes orbit, has itself fallen under a cloud of suspicion. The consensus of virtually all memory researchers and most mental health professionals is that massive repression of memory is either extremely rare or altogether undocumented. In the small handful of cases in which something like massive repression has occurred, it has involved a permanent loss of memories of some extremely traumatic occurrence. There are no documented cases of the recovery of massively repressed memories that are generally accepted as valid by the professional psychotherapeutic community. Freud abandoned his original theory of repression after continued experience with patients rendered it unsupportable. Recovered-memory therapists have not yet produced anything more than anecdotal evidence in support of their theory — and the impassioned tales of "survivors" are often internally contradictory and in many cases falsifiable on the basis of external evidence such as physical examinations. Moreover, in virtually all cases, there are simpler ways of accounting for the client's stories than positing a long history of sensational abuse. Many experiments have demonstrated the ways in which individuals can be rendered extremely suggestible by the sorts of therapeutic techniques typically employed in RMT.

In a survey of literature on the subject recently published in the journal *Psychological Medicine,* Dr. Harrison G. Pope and Dr. James I. Hudson report on their failure to find any valid research demonstrating or supporting the notion of repression.

> We sought studies which have attempted to test whether memories of childhood sexual abuse can be repressed. Despite our broad search criteria, which excluded only unsystematic anecdotal reports, we found only four applicable studies. We then examined these studies to assess whether the investigators: (1) presented confirmatory evidence that abuse had actually occurred; and (2) demonstrated that their subjects had actually developed amnesia for the abuse. None of the four studies provided both

clear confirmation of trauma and adequate documentation of amnesia in their subjects. Thus, present clinical evidence is insufficient to permit the conclusion that individuals can repress memories of childhood sexual abuse. This finding is surprising, since many writers have implied that hundreds of thousands, or even millions of persons harbor such repressed memories.[2]

Memory expert Elizabeth Loftus has stated that "there is no good scientific support for repressed memories. We should not be dragging people through the courts on folklore." And Richard Ofshe says, "The notion of repression has never been more than an unsubstantiated speculation tied to other Freudian concepts and speculative mechanisms. The only support repression has ever had is anecdotal and contributed by psychoanalysts who presume the existence of the repression mechanism."[3]

Since the Child Abuse Prevention and Treatment Act of 1974, we have been inundated with what Dr. Elaine Foster calls the "myth of rampant child abuse." In 1995, Foster told a Congressional hearing that in 1992 alone there were 1,227,223 *false* allegations of child abuse. The National Center for the Prevention of Child Abuse has acknowledged that 61 percent of reports fail the "credible evidence" test. Richard Wexler, author of *Wounded Innocents: The Real Victims of the War against Child Abuse,* believes that 61 percent is too low. He cites a federal study on child abuse and neglect which found that child-protection workers were two to six times more likely to wrongly substantiate a case than to find a case unfounded.[4]

In the latter part of the twentieth century, most Americans would agree that the Salem witch trials were a sham, because they do not believe in the existence of witches and they would not be willing to hazard a judgment solely on the basis of "spectral evidence." Despite compelling evidence provided by experts in the fields of memory research, psychotherapy, and criminal investigation, however, not as many Americans are yet willing to abandon their belief in the validity of repressed memory syndrome, multiple personality disorder, or the operation of worldwide satanic cults. It is perhaps understandable that the general public would be slow to abandon these popular hoaxes, since they have less access to appropriate professional literature than to specious tabloid news stories and shallow

2. Pope and Hudson, "Can Memories of Childhood Sexual Abuse Be Repressed?" *Psychological Medicine* 25 (1995): 121-26.

3. Ofshe and Ethan Watters, "Making Monsters," *Society* 30 (March/April 1993): 5.

4. See Wexler, *Wounded Innocents: The Real Victims of the War against Child Abuse,* 2d ed. (Buffalo, NY: Prometheus, 1995).

movies of the week. But the therapists, social workers, and child advocates who continue to ignore the evidence and base charges of child abuse and social policy initiatives on these debunked theories are like the anthropologists of an earlier generation who continued to defend theories of human evolution based on the Piltdown Man even after it had been exposed as a hoax.

Psychotherapy and the "Etiological Model"

There appear to be a number of reasons why these hoaxes have seized the imagination of people in the fields of psychology, social work, and child advocacy. One factor is what is sometimes called the *etiological* model of contemporary psychotherapy — the popular assumption that psychological distress can always be traced back to some influence outside ourselves, some trauma from our past, usually in childhood and usually associated with our parents. The popularization of this view may have begun with Freud, but it has gained such momentum among the current generation of the practitioners of talk therapy in this country that it has become something of a staple of our cultural thought as a whole. In the contemporary mythology of talk therapy, the therapist and patient courageously face the unknown mysteries of the mind, the therapist locates the cause of the distress in some force in the patient's past, and then the therapist offers the patient what Richard Ofshe has described as a series of "seductive ideas": "1) that there exist specific, identifiable events for every problem or disorder; 2) that those reasons remain in the patient's memory or in the unconscious; 3) that it is possible to make a causal connection between the symptom and cause by talking to the patient; and 4) that digging up and understanding this connection can cure the disorder." In *The Courage to Heal,* one woman is quoted as saying, "Even though it was traumatic for me to realize that everyone in my family abused me, there was something reassuring about it. My life suddenly made sense." A feeling of relief when confronted with a history of abuse is a characteristic response, say Ofshe and Watters:

> The proposition that we are unconsciously controlled by specific events in our histories is a seductive one for prospective patients because it lifts responsibility for seemingly self-inflicted problems off the patient, while at the same time promising to solve problems that may in fact have no satisfactory solution. For those plagued by anything from serious mental disorders that cannot presently be effectively treated to those haunted by

the simple feeling that their lives are not as fulfilling as those of the people around them, the message that they are controlled by subterranean forces carries a type of absolution: the patient is forgiven the sins she appears to have committed against herself. At the moment the patient receives this forgiveness, she is offered the promise that through therapy she can learn to understand the deep currents that move her, and, through that understanding, take a greater measure of control of her life and the events that befall her.[5]

If she is a client of an RMT therapist, she will be directed to rewrite her history and her family's history — that is, to give her life a new narrative, the central theme of which is abuse. The entire process involves a redefinition of basic concepts and principles held by other members of the established mental health community. RMT rewrites the book on the nature of memory, the implications of symptomology, and the utility of specific therapeutic techniques. Moreover, there tends to be a defensiveness bordering on hostility on the part of RMT therapists toward the rest of the therapeutic community as they go their own way and are subjected to criticism for doing so. Therapeutic principles judged essential by the mainstream — including an emphasis on rational, critical, reflective assessments of all evidence in the case — are often dismissed as wrong-headed if not devious by RMT therapists.

RMT therapists routinely urge their clients to suppress their natural tendencies to rely on sterile logic and to open themselves up instead to their feelings. Rational thought can be deceptive, they say, because it may have been programmed by an unfriendly authority; feelings, on the other hand, will not lie. An initially insubstantial feeling that one may have been abused in childhood is a reliable indication that the abuse did occur, they say, and it can be clarified through the use of such techniques as guided imagery, drug-enhanced hypnotic states, and the like. RMT therapists are comfortable with the fact that memories of this sort, continually refined and elaborated over time, can become the most real things in their clients' lives, crowding out any contradictory memories and overruling any incompatible physical evidence. They are also comfortable with making such memories the basis for severing family ties and initiating criminal procedures.

Clients are willing to stay in RMT because on some important levels it supplies the sorts of answers they were looking for when they entered

5. Ofshe and Ethan Watters, *Making Monsters: False Memories, Psychotherapy, and Sexual Hysteria* (New York: Scribner's, 1994), p. 48.

therapy: it provides a compelling explanation for whatever psychological distress they may be feeling. And although in most cases people outside RMT circles perceive the clients to be getting worse the longer they stay in such therapy — increasingly distraught, fearful, haggard, alienated, and even delusional — the clients themselves are assured by their therapists that whatever new trauma they may be experiencing is necessary to achieve healing and that they can at least rest secure in the knowledge that they are now grappling with the truth instead of living a lie. Whatever the pain it may entail, the therapeutic context is seductive for many people. Recall Sherri's story in Chapter 9. "To the extent that clients regard their therapist as an understanding individual who exhibits genuine sincerity while creating an emotionally warm atmosphere, the effectiveness of psychotherapy increases," says Terence Campbell. But, he adds, a "warm and understanding atmosphere" does not constitute a specific therapy technique, and thus the effect of that client-therapist relationship "has more in common with a placebo than with any medical treatment. A placebo is defined as 'an agent of healing or change whose inherent properties do not scientifically account for such healing.' A placebo creates the appearance of a cure, but it does not genuinely heal. In medicine, placebo cures are the result of patient expectations." In other words, when clients come into therapy expecting to be helped, they develop a warm relationship with a caring person whom they really want to please. They have thus set themselves up to feel better no matter what the therapist's techniques or effectiveness. RMT therapists typically exploit patients' expectations extravagantly, submersing them in RMT literature and survivors' groups that give them very clear ideas of what sorts of memories they would be likely to recover and what sorts of resistance from friends and family they can expect. As the clients progressively alienate themselves from former friends and family, the RMT family becomes increasingly important, and the vicious circle tightens. Campbell notes that

> once a client is addicted to therapy, another remarkable decision can transpire between client and therapist. They may decide that the only remedy for the client's "addiction" is more of the same substance to which he is already addicted. Sessions may lengthen, or the number of sessions per week may increase. Consequently, the therapeutic relationship . . . remains well protected. . . . When no problems severe enough to warrant long-term therapy really exist — and often they do not — clients may respond to the influence of their therapist and invent them. Because the problems that clients invent are limited only by their imaginations,

those problems can seem particularly complex and difficult. Thus, invented problems further encourage long-term therapy . . . while continuously undermining a client's self-confidence.[6]

Darker Motives

All of the devastating effects of RMT that we have considered in this book can be forthcoming even when everyone involved has nothing but the best intentions. Therapists who are convinced that childhood abuse is pandemic, who embrace the concept of massive repression, and who accept the premise that a broad range of nonspecific symptomology constitutes reliable evidence of repressed memories of childhood abuse will naturally diagnose patients on the basis of those beliefs and promote an aggressive plan of treatment in keeping with the diagnosis. The fact that they can proceed in this fashion with a clear conscience does not excuse them for their beliefs and actions, however; I would still argue that there is no excuse for clinging to a set of beliefs that is so clearly controverted by established psychotherapeutic principles, scientific research on memory, and an overwhelming amount of anecdotal evidence, especially when the results are so demonstrably destructive. I am simply saying that I believe it is possible for clients and therapists to engage in RMT in the sincere belief that they are doing the right thing. That is one sort of tragedy. But there is also evidence of another sort of tragedy, evidence that some therapists are cynically taking advantage of vulnerable clients for profit.

Many have observed that laypeople are always at something of a disadvantage when they seek out the services of professionals. We go to them for services we cannot get anywhere else, services that derive from the special knowledge they possess. Because we don't possess that knowledge ourselves, we have no immediate way of assessing their expertise. We hope that licensing procedures and peer review will ensure a basic level of expertise, and we can seek out recommendations from community agencies, friends, and the like, but ultimately we have to place our trust in some individual and hope for the best.

When we visit a physician for a check-up or because of some ailment, we can be reasonably assured, because of mandatory training and the constraints of the Hippocratic Oath, that the doctor will have the skills to

---

6. Campbell, *Beware the Talking Cure: Psychotherapy May Be Hazardous to Your Mental Health* (Boca Raton, FL: Upton Books, 1994), pp. 21-24.

heal us if healing is possible or at least that he or she will do no harm. Medical care providers have access to a wide range of drugs, devices, and techniques that have been tested and proved effective. Things are different in the realm of psychotherapy. For one thing, licensing procedures are different. Anyone can offer counseling, regardless of education and free of any peer supervision. Moreover, professionals within the ranks of the psychotherapeutic community have acknowledged that although some of their colleagues pay lip service to the Hippocratic Oath, it is not always as clearly applicable in their profession as in the medical profession. Much psychotherapy practiced today has virtually none of the medical profession's scientific guidelines, strictures, or safeguards: no informed consent, no assurance that the techniques used are safe and effective, and no scientific demonstration that any of it will provide the cure being sought. To some extent, psychotherapy has benefited from the trust that people have had in medicine generally. Psychiatry, since it is a branch of medicine, is often viewed in the light of the considerable medical advances of the past century, even though psychiatrists often base opinions on evidence much less secure than that needed to ground most medical opinions. Few clinical therapists today keep abreast of the scientific research in their field, and many profess a greater confidence in their own intuition than in such research in any event. Given the general absence of objective standards for assessing many aspects of traditional psychotherapy, it is difficult for anyone to gainsay a therapist's diagnosis, course of treatment, or declaration of a cure.

An issue that has become a concern of insurance companies is the duration of therapy. Many therapists believe that the treatment of simple depression, for example, can take a very long time. It is commonly assumed in the profession that short-term therapy may work for comparatively well-defined and limited problems such as panic attacks but that the treatment of more serious disorders will often take years of persistent, intensive therapy. But this assumption is based less on any objective evidence than on the simple belief that short-term therapies do not work for certain problems. Some state psychological associations have requested insurance reimbursements for up to 150 sessions per year for serious problems — one session every other day, excluding weekends — without providing any empirical basis for concluding that such frequency promotes an earlier or more effective cure.

An hour with a therapist (the standard session is fifty minutes) costs an average of $125 in North America. Many insurance experts are predicting that new health-care proposals will bring an end to coverage for this sort of traditional therapy. "It's clear that classical psychoanalysis, which is four

264

to five times a week for a four-to-five-year duration, will not be covered," says Frederick Goodwin, director of the National Institute of Mental Health. "It won't be covered because there is no real evidence that it works."[7]

R. Christopher Barden, now president of the National Association for Consumer Protection in Mental Health Practices, has won several high-profile cases against RMT therapists and claims to have established that some of them were motivated principally by simple greed. Barden notes that insurance companies authorize payments for therapy under the guide-lines of the American Psychiatric Association's *Diagnostic and Statistical Manual of Mental Disorders*. This manual specifies that treatments for simple depression should be completed within two to six months, which generates an average fee of about $2,000. A course of treatment for repressed memories of childhood abuse or a dissociative disorder, on the other hand, can easily end up costing as much as $500,000. And therapists who are willing to diagnose a new disorder when payments for a given course of treatment come to an end can, over a period of years, extract millions of dollars from insurance companies for each individual patient — which was the case with Mary S. and Patti B., as we noted in Chapter 8. It should not surprise us that some unscrupulous individuals would yield to that kind of temptation, even if it entailed consigning clients to years of hellish existence.

Dr. Jack Leggett is a clinical psychologist who has reviewed mental health claims for insurance companies around the country. Beginning in the late 1980s, Leggett began to notice a startling pattern in patients who were diagnosed with multiple personality disorder: a disproportionate number had employers — or their spouses had employers — with very generous insurance policies. He noticed that the "big-coverage insurance programs were targeted, and that the incidence of MPD was far beyond anything that could be considered reasonable for a given population." According to Leggett, a great deal of money was being spent, and the patients were all getting worse instead of better. He also discovered that questioning the bills, let alone the diagnoses, of any of those MPD patients could have unpleasant consequences: "I was met with the most hostile responses that I've come across in all the years I've done any kind of case management or clinical supervision. Beginning with discounting my credibility and that of the board-certified psychiatrists and psychologists I worked with, it ex-tended to rather strange suggestions that I, or the organization I worked

---

7. Goodwin, in "The Search for Satan," PBS *Frontline* documentary produced by Ofra Bikel, originally broadcast 24 October 1995.

for, might be related to these satanic cults. I was threatened with being labeled as a co-conspirator with the cults."[8]

About the excesses of the current generation of psychotherapy, Neil Jacobson says, "Carried away with our popular acceptance, we have promised far more than we can deliver. We need to take a close look at our excesses and our often tenuous relationship to scientific principles. . . . Therapists can no longer afford to ignore the scientific foundations of their profession, for in the long run, science is all 'that presumably distinguishes [therapists] from the expanding cadre of self-proclaimed psychics, new-age healers, religious gurus, talk-show hosts, and self-help book authors.' "[9]

The Current Legal Direction

There are signs that some of the more hysterical expressions of concern about an epidemic of child abuse in our culture are now abating, though the main activists have given no quarter in their crusade. From the mid-1980s to the early 1990s, twenty-three states responded to pressure from women's groups and child advocates by creating a legal mechanism for both criminal and civil actions based on the recovery of repressed memories. In effect, these new state laws suspend the statute of limitations in recovered-memory cases, allowing the ostensible victim a period of up to three years after recovering the memories in which to file charges against the alleged perpetrators, even if the presumed crime took place decades before. Such laws have been used by many RMT clients to sue their parents for damages. Many parents have settled out of court; some have gone to jail; some remain under house arrest.

But the courts have recently turned a significant corner on this issue: across the country, judges and juries have begun to express increasing skepticism about claims based on repressed memory. One breakthrough came in a California case in which a father was awarded damages against his daughter's therapists. The father, Gary Ramona, was a winery executive living in Napa, California. His daughter Holly charged him with having abused her in childhood on the basis of memories recovered with the help of RMT therapists who used sodium amytal as part of the therapy. The scandal associated with the charges led to the loss of Ramona's job and the failure of his marriage. The court determined that Holly's therapists had implanted false memories of abuse and awarded Gary $500,000 in damages.

8. Leggett, in "The Search for Satan."
9. Jacobson, "The Overselling of Therapy," *Networker*, March/April 1995, pp. 46-47.

The victory was significant because it was the first such case in which damages were awarded against a third party: prior to this, only clients had been successful in suing therapists.

In two separate cases in Minnesota, patients who said psychiatrist Diane Humenansky coerced them into believing that they had been abused in satanic rituals as children were awarded about $2.5 million each when the court found the psychiatrist guilty of malpractice. "This verdict establishes for the rest of the country that this practice has got to stop," said Christopher Barden, the lawyer for the plaintiffs. "To have an entire treatment based on junk science is inappropriate. Implanting false memories is an extremely dangerous practice. Wherever they are in the U.S., licensing boards and professional associations should do all they can to stop it immediately."[10]

In another fairly well-known case, *State of New Hampshire v. Hungerford*, Presiding Justice William Groff concluded that repressed memory testimony is not sufficiently reliable to be admitted as evidence: "The Court finds that the testimony of the victims as to their memory of the assaults shall not be admitted at trial because the phenomenon of memory repression, and the process of therapy used in these cases to recover memories, have not gained general acceptance in the field of psychology, and are not scientifically reliable."[11]

In May 1997, the Indiana legislature passed, by a unanimous vote in both houses, a law requiring that all patients be informed of their therapists' training and credentials, that every "mental health provider shall inform each patient . . . of the reasonably forseeable risks and relative benefits of proposed treatments and alternative treatments," and that all patients have the right to withdraw consent for treatment at any time. The "mental health system will never be the same again," says Christopher Barden. "It is indeed shocking that many, if not most, forms of psychotherapy currently offered to consumers are not supported by credible scientific evidence. Consumers will now have to be told that psychotherapists who want to talk about the patient's childhood are offering them what is at best an experimental and quite possibly a harmful procedure." Barden, who drafted the legislation with help from several dozen prominent psychologists, said, "We did not expect to see passage of portions of this act for years. This is a stunning

10. Barden, quoted in "Doctor Loses False-Memory Suit," Associated Press story, 2 August 1995.
11. Groff, decree in *State of New Hampshire v. Joel Hungerford and John Morahan*, Hillborough County Superior Court, Manchester, NH, 1995.

victory for our efforts to produce badly needed reforms in the psychotherapy industry. . . . The mental health system needs an overhaul, and the Indiana law is a major step in the right direction."

As noted in Chapter 8, about ten suits are pending against SRA therapist Judith Peterson, and eight to ten are pending against Bennett Braun, hailed by many as America's leading authority on MPD/SRA. Some have argued that the courts may be the only place in which we will be able to put an end to the witch hunt, to put the brakes on the RMT juggernaut. As the courts and the public learn more about RMT, they are concluding that the methods and techniques it employs are questionable if not downright unethical. Most of the legal malpractice suits brought by parents and guardians of clients against therapists have ended in judgments against the therapists. The Salem witch trials ended when the "spectral evidence" — dreams, visions, and hallucinations — were no longer judged admissible. Three hundred years later, the courts are once again judging that the dreams and visions conjured up in RMT sessions should not be admissible as evidence on the basis of which to charge, convict, and imprison people.

Ideological Polarizations

Why have so many people in one of the most sophisticated, well-educated, and privileged societies in the world fallen prey to the hysteria associated with RMT and MPD/SRA? I agree with Stan Passy that at least part of the reason is that we have a deep-seated need to locate a source of evil in the world external to ourselves, and we have lost the concept of hell that once filled that need for the great majority of our people. Since the fall of international Communism — the "evil empire," as Ronald Reagan memorably dubbed it — Americans have been restlessly pursuing other candidates for the position. A surprising number, apparently convinced by the dramatic stories in tabloids, supermarket paperbacks, and made-for-TV movies, have bought into the notion of a vast global conspiracy of Satan worshipers who subject innocents to ritual sexual abuse and blood sacrifice. Others point their guns at evil less literally demonic but no less hellish. Kee MacFarlane, the main facilitator and therapist for the McMartin children, testified to a packed Congressional hearing that the country was in the throes of organized child-abuse "conspiracies," that the McMartin Preschool was only "a ruse for larger unthinkable networks of crimes against children," and that these conspiracy rings had "greater financial, legal, and community resources than any of the agencies trying to uncover them" —

which is presumably why the FBI, INTERPOL, and local police forces have never found any evidence of them.

The camps on either side of the repressed memory/false memory syndrome battle are so polarized (it is the single most polarized issue in the psychological and sociological professions in our generation) that it is difficult to foresee any rapprochement between them in the near future. Adherents of repressed memory syndrome, who believe that childhood sexual abuse is rampant, condemn anyone who is doubtful of their claims or critical of their agenda; they say that all who deny abuse accusations are "in denial," and they refer to falsely accused parents who have found support in the False Memory Syndrome Foundation as "perpetrators" and "pedophiles." Falsely accused parents and critics of RMT, for their part, believe that the evil lies with the therapists, radical feminists, and survivor advocates, who they feel have duped their children, rewritten their childhood narratives for them, and turned them against their parents and family — in a real sense, abducted and abused them. Because so much is at stake here — the survival of families on the one hand and the survival of a belief system on the other — and because most people seem unable to perceive the issues in anything other than black-and-white terms, the chances for a breakdown of the impasse between the two sides seem slim.

As we have learned in the other polarized conflicts of this latter part of the twentieth century — in race relations, gender wars, religious and political strife, and regional conflicts — one person's freedom fighter is another person's terrorist. Perhaps the biggest contributor to all this polarization is what I have referred to as "demonizing of the Other," a primitive response to unfamiliar people and ideas that is increasingly evident in our multicultural society today. It runs rough-shod over the concept that we all, first of all, share traits that are human, and thus traits that are bad, good, charitable, selfish, sometimes violent and sometimes nurturing, and everything in between — but undeniably and essentially human withal.

Regrettably, the shrillest special interest groups seem to be getting the upper hand in one debate (or, rather, ideological slugfest) after another. "The sucking sound (the phrase is Melville's) is that of the entire population disappearing into a communal maelstrom," says Mark Helprin. "No longer is the family supposed to be the fundamental unit of society. The wife and female children owe their allegiance to womanhood. The children's loyalties lie not with their oppressive parents but with the class interests of children. If one of them is adopted, he must cleave to his ethnic or racial group, unless she is a girl, whereupon she may be a woman first. Even the dog has a union card, and if he feels abused will summon the defenders of animal rights."[12]

In a recently published book of prayers, Marian Wright Edelman, the nation's premiere children's advocate, refers to those who disagree with her on how tax dollars ought to be spent as "Herods." That is the rhetoric not of poetry or prayer but of propaganda. With a word she dismisses those on the other side of the national policy debate to the ranks not just of child murderers but of monsters who would massacre all children; in doing so, she effectively puts an end to any reasonable discourse. Proponents of RMT indiscriminately dismiss their critics as "perpetrators." Distinguished professor of psychiatry Paul McHugh has been called a "pederast" within certain segments of the psychiatric cocktail circuit for questioning the assumptions of RMT and MPD/SRA. The same sort of vilification has been applied to a host of courageous female writers, psychologists, and educators who have bravely, defiantly, and persistently gone against the current of runaway child abuse hysteria and the excesses of radical feminism.

Postscript

F. Scott Fitzgerald wrote that "the test of a first-rate intelligence is the ability to hold two opposed ideas in the mind at the same time, and still retain the ability to function." In our fractious times, sanity itself may depend on the ability to appreciate the value of views diametrically opposed to our own — the ability to appreciate the capacity for good and evil in all of us. We need a saner alternative to shouting at each other across battle lines from walled camps. We need to develop a tolerance not only for other people and other views but also for the inherent ambiguities of life itself. There are many matters of the mind and emotions that remain mysteries to us, many questions for which we have no one right answer. Perhaps the proponents and the critics of RMT could take a first step toward genuine dialogue by stressing some points of agreement. For openers, both sides could agree that child abuse is a terrible problem and that it was underreported in this country for many years. Certainly people of good conscience could also agree that every effort should be made to prevent any false accusations of abuse. From there, perhaps it would be possible to discuss practical methods for assessing the relative validity of claims, techniques, and conclusions. True child advocates

---

12. Helprin, "Diversity Is Not a Virtue," in *Reinventing the American People: Unity and Diversity Today,* ed. Robert Royal (Grand Rapids: William B. Eerdmans, 1995), p. 73.

should be interested in preventing abuse regardless of whether the perpetrator is a pederast or a misguided therapist.

*   *   *

It took five years for the people of Massachusetts to conclude that they had presided over a terrible miscarriage of justice. When they reached that conclusion, they confessed, did penance, and made reparations to the families of those who had been falsely accused and wrongfully executed. "We walked in clouds and could not see our way," said Rev. John Hale, whose testimony had led to the execution of a "witch." Their actions stand in stark contrast to those of the leaders in the current sexual abuse witch hunt. Will those who have filed charges on the basis of recovered memories ever find the grace to recant and apologize to those they have wrongfully accused?

For my own part, I have tried to be fair in presenting the ideas and arguments of those who believe in the reality of repressed memory, multiple personality disorder, and satanic ritual abuse even though my interpretation of the evidence has convinced me that they are tragically misguided. But I do not believe that anyone can justifiably deduce from my skepticism about RMT that I am oblivious to the problem of child abuse. Let me reiterate in the plainest possible language: child abuse is a tragedy that was ignored or neglected or underreported by psychiatrists, psychologists, clergy, and police for the first three-quarters of this century, and it continues to be a significant problem today. I have no sympathy for *any* adult who would rape or torture a child, and I cannot imagine what could induce any parent to molest a son or daughter. I fully support all laws and programs that effectively reduce violence against children and punish those who commit such violence. But I also believe that therapists have an obligation to observe the medical conventions of informed consent and implement only those treatments that have been proven safe and effective. All of our efforts to reach these goals must be based on fact rather than prejudice, science rather than hysteria, and reason rather than political ideology. Our own well-being and the well-being of our children depend on it.

Select Bibliography

Several books have been invaluable to me in the preparation of this book, as I have noted in some of the footnotes. Mark Pendergrast's *Victims of Memory* is the most voluminous, best-researched, and simply best book on the whole problem of recovered memory therapy and false accusations of abuse. *Satan's Silence* by Debbie Nathan and Michael Snedeker is the boldest, most comprehensive exposé of what they call "ritual abuse and the making of a modern American witch hunt." Meticulously researched and documented, this book is essential reading for anyone interested in the shape of child abuse hysteria in this country. Lawrence Wright's *Remembering Satan* is a brilliant account and interpretation of the Paul Ingram story, in which false accusations of ritualistic abuse became a religious obsession in Olympia, Washington. Elizabeth Loftus has organized and written up invaluable memory research in numerous journal articles and her book (with Katherine Ketcham) *The Myth of Repressed Memory*. Her written testimony and court testimonies have been a great inspiration to parents accused of sexually abusing their children. This is also true of Richard Ofshe, whose book (with Ethan Watters) *Making Monsters: False Memories, Psychotherapy, and Sexual Hysteria* was very helpful to me in researching the "memory wars."

Several articles are also seminal to this discussion and were of great help to me. Debbie Nathan's "Cry Incest" was the first indication to me of the national scope of false memories and child abuse hysteria. John Taylor's "The Lost Daughter" is the best article on multiple personality disorder, the Sybil syndrome, and the "perverse ministrations of the therapy police" in popular literature. Two articles by Paul McHugh in *The American Scholar*,

"Psychiatric Misadventures" and "Psychotherapy Awry," provide essential analyses of how psychotherapy in its current theories and diagnoses has followed what he calls the "gusty winds of fashion." Michael Yapko's 1993 article "The Seductions of Memory" (in *Networker*) offers a crucial early warning to therapists about the perils of the power of suggestion in producing or implanting false memories. Christina Hoff Sommers's *Who Stole Feminism?* supplied me with a huge amount of data for my chapter on feminism; her exposure of fraudulent advocacy research and reports by gender feminists is immensely important in interpreting the radical feminist contributions to the RMT/MPD/SRA debate. Finally, Wendy Kaminer's essay "Feminism's Identity Crisis," an analysis of the marriage of "third-wave" feminism and recovery therapy, and her book *I'm Dysfunctional, You're Dysfunctional,* are not only great reads but must reads for those interested in and alarmed by the invasion of the recovery/victimization culture into psychotherapy and religion.

*   *   *

"The Amiraults Got a Trial, Not Justice." *Wall Street Journal,* 20 June 1995.

Bass, Ellen, and Laura Davis. *Beginning to Heal.* New York: HarperPaperbacks, 1993.

————. *The Courage to Heal.* 3d ed. New York: HarperPerennial, 1994.

Begley, Sharon, with Martha Brant. "You Must Remember This." *Newsweek,* 26 September 1994, pp. 68-69.

Bellow, Saul. *A Theft.* New York: Penguin Books, 1989.

Blinkhorn, Lois. "Sexual Abuse Cases on Trial." *Milwaukee Sentinel,* 10 July 1994.

Blume, E. Sue. *Secret Survivors: Uncovering Incest and Its After Effects in Women.* New York: Ballantine, 1991.

Boakes, Janet. "False Memory Syndrome." *The Lancet,* 21 October 1995, pp. 1048-49.

Boyer, Peter. "Children of Waco." *The New Yorker,* 15 May 1995, pp. 38-45.

Borch-Jacobsen, Mikkel. "Sybil — The Making of a Disease: An Interview with Dr. Herbert Spiegel." *New York Review of Books,* 24 April 1997, pp. 60-64.

Boyd, Jamie. "Six of the Best." *Globe and Mail,* 8 June 1994.

Bradshaw, John. *Bradshaw on the Family: A Revolutionary Way of Self-Discovery.* Deerfield Beach, FL: Health Communications, 1988.

Brown, Joanne Carlson, and Carole R. Bohn, eds. *Christianity, Patriarchy and Abuse.* Cleveland: Pilgrim Press, 1989.

Butler, Katy. "Caught in the Cross Fire." *Networker,* March-April 1995.

Campbell, Terence W. *Beware the Talking Cure.* Boca Raton, FL: Upton Books, 1994.

Capps, Donald. *The Depleted Self: Sin in an Age of Narcissism.* Princeton, NJ: Princeton University Press, 1992.

Carlson, Margaret. "The Sex-Crime Capital." *Time,* 13 November 1995.

Ceci, S. J., and M. Bruck. "Suggestibility of the Child Witness: A Historical Review and Synthesis." *Psychological Bulletin* 113 (1993): 403-39.

Chapman, Stephen. "Concern for Family Provokes Backlash from Some Feminists." *Chicago Tribune*, 24 July 1994.

————. "Fighting Poverty." *Chicago Tribune*, 21 September 1995.

Coleman, Lee. "Learning from the McMartin Hoax." *Issues in Child Abuse Accusations* 1 (1989): 68-71.

"Common Sense Welfare." *Wall Street Journal*, 23 August 1995.

Coughlin, Ellen. "Recollections of Childhood Abuse: Contending Research Traditions Face Off in Debate over 'Recovered Memory.'" *Chronicle of Higher Education*, 27 January 1995.

Crews, Frederick. *The Memory Wars: Freud's Legacy in Dispute*. New York: New York Review of Books, 1995.

Dawes, Robin. "Biases of Retrospection." *Issues in Child Abuse Accusations* 1 (1989): 25-28.

————. "Giving up Cherished Ideas: The Rorschach Ink Blot Test." *Issues in Child Abuse Accusations* 3 (1991). Excerpted from *Rational Choice in an Uncertain World*. New York: Harcourt Brace Jovanovich, 1988.

————. *House of Cards: Psychology and Psychotherapy Built on Myth*. New York: Free Press, 1994.

Dineen, Tana. *Manufacturing Victims: What the Psychology Industry Is Doing to People*. Montreal: Robert Davies, 1996.

Doehr, Eva. "Inside the False Memory Movement." *Treating Abuse Today* 4 (1994).

Dowd, Maureen. "Please, Don't Hold up Boorish Roseanne as the Feminist Ideal." *Chicago Tribune*, 4 September 1995.

Drell, Adrienne. "Bible Scholar Sues to Fight Taint of Sex Harrassment." *Chicago Sun-Times*, 25 March 1994.

Dworkin, Andrea. *Intercourse*. New York: Free Press, 1987.

————. *Pornography: Men Possessing Women*. New York: E. P. Dutton, 1989.

————. *Woman Hating*. New York: E. P. Dutton, 1974.

Elshtain, Jean Bethke. "Suffer the Little Children." *New Republic*, 4 March 1996, pp. 33-38.

Erickson, Erik H. *Childhood and Society*. New York: W. W. Norton, 1964.

False Memory Syndrome Foundation. *FMS Foundation Newsletter*, all issues.

Faludi, Susan. "I'm Not a Feminist, but I Play One on TV," *Ms.*, March/April 1995, pp. 31-39.

Fox-Genovese, Elizabeth. *Feminism without Illusions: A Critique of Individualism*. Chapel Hill, NC: University of North Carolina Press, 1991.

Frazer, Elizabeth, Jennifer Hornsby, and Sabina Lovibond, eds. *Ethics: A Feminist Reader*. Cambridge: Blackwell, 1992.

Fredrickson, Renee. *Repressed Memories: A Journey to Recovery from Sexual Abuse*. New York: Fireside/Parkside, 1992.

French, Marilyn. *The War against Women*. New York: Summit Books, 1992.

Gardner, Martin. "Notes of a Fringe-Watcher." *Skeptical Inquirer* 17 (Summer 1993).

Gardner, Richard. "Modern Witch Hunt — Child Abuse Charges." *Wall Street Journal*, 22 February 1993.

————. *Sex Abuse Hysteria: Salem Witch Trials Revisited.* Cresskill, NJ: Creative Therapeutics, 1991.

————. *True and False Accusations of Child Sex Abuse: A Guide for Legal and Mental Health Professionals.* Cresskill, NJ: Creative Therapeutics, 1992.

Goldstein, Eleanor, with Kevin Farmer. *Confabulations: Creating False Memories — Destroying Families.* Boca Raton, FL: Upton Books, 1994.

————. *True Stories of False Memories.* Boca Raton, FL: Upton Books, 1993.

Goleman, Daniel. "Childhood Trauma: Memory or Invention?" *New York Times,* 21 July 1992.

————. "Miscoding Is Seen as the Root of False Memories." *New York Times,* 31 May 1994.

————. "Studies Reveal Suggestibility of Very Young as Witnesses." *New York Times,* 11 June 1993.

Gray, Paul. "The Assault on Freud." *Time,* 29 November 1993, pp. 47-51.

Greven, Philip. *Spare the Child: The Religious Roots of Punishment and the Psychological Impact of Physical Abuse.* New York: Vintage Books, 1992.

Gross, Andrea. "Who's Telling the Truth?" *Ladies Home Journal,* June 1994, pp. 72-76.

Hacking, Ian. "Multiple Personality Disorder and Its Hosts." *History of the Human Sciences* 5 (1992).

Hagen, Margaret. *Whores of the Court.* New York: Regan Books, 1997.

Hamill, Pete. "Woman on the Verge of a Legal Breakdown." *Playboy,* January 1993, pp. 138-40, 184-89.

Herman, Ellen. *The Romance of American Psychology: Political Culture in the Age of Experts.* Berkeley and Los Angeles: University of California Press, 1995.

Hillman, James, and Michael Ventura. *We've Had a Hundred Years of Psychotherapy — and the World's Getting Worse.* San Francisco: HarperSanFrancisco, 1993.

Holmes, David. "The Evidence for Repression: An Examination of Sixty Years of Research." In *Repression and Dissociation: Implications for Personality Theory, Psychopathology, and Health,* edited by Jerome Singer. Chicago: University of Chicago Press, 1990.

————. "Is There Evidence for Repression? Doubtful." *Harvard Mental Health Letter,* June 1994.

Hughes, Robert. *Culture of Complaint: The Fraying of America.* New York: Warner Books, 1994.

Jacobson, Neil. "The Overselling of Therapy." *Networker,* March-April 1995.

Jaroff, Leon. "Lies of the Mind." *Time,* 29 November 1993, pp. 52-59.

Johnson, Sonia. *Going Out of Our Minds: The Metaphysics of Liberation.* Freedom, CA: Crossing Press, 1987.

Kaminer, Wendy. "Feminism's Identity Crisis." *Atlantic Monthly,* October 1993, pp. 51-68.

————. *I'm Dysfunctional, You're Dysfunctional: The Recovery Movement and Other Self-Help Fashions.* New York: Vintage Books, 1993.

Koocher, Gerald P., et al. "Psychological Science and the Use of Anatomically

Detailed Dolls in Child Sexual-Abuse Assessments." *Psychological Bulletin* 118 (September 1995): 199-222.

Lalich, Janja, and Madeleine Landau Tobias. *Captive Hearts, Captive Minds: Freedom and Recovery from Cults and Abusive Relationships.* Alameda, CA: Hunter House, 1994.

Lamb, Sandra E. "Tragic Delusions: How 'Recovered' Memories Tear Families Apart." *Family Circle,* 18 July 1995.

Landes, Alison, et al., eds. *Child Abuse — Betraying a Trust.* Wylie, TX: Information Plus, 1995.

Legrand, Ross, Hollida Wakefield, and Ralph Underwager. "Alleged Behavioral Indicators of Sexual Abuse." *Issues in Child Abuse Accusations* 1 (Spring 1990): 1-5.

Levin, Michael. *Feminism and Freedom.* New Brunswick, NJ: Transaction Books, 1987.

Loftus, Elizabeth. "Therapeutic Recollection of Childhood Abuse: When a Memory May Not Be a Memory." *Champion,* March 1994.

Loftus, Elizabeth, and Katherine Ketcham. *The Myth of Repressed Memory: False Memories and Allegations of Sexual Abuse.* New York: St. Martin's Press, 1994.

Loftus, Elizabeth, and Maryanne Garry. "Pseudomemories without Hypnosis." *The International Journal of Clinical and Experimental Hypnosis* 42 (October 1994).

Luza, Sabrina, and Enrique Ortiz. "The Dynamic of Shame in Interactions between Child Protective Services and Families Falsely Accused of Child Abuse." *Issues in Child Abuse Accusations* 3 (Spring 1991).

MacKinnon, Catharine A. *Toward a Feminist Theory of the State.* Cambridge: Harvard University Press, 1989.

Manshel, Lisa. *Nap Time: The True Story of Sexual Abuse at a Suburban Day-Care Center.* New York: William Morrow, 1990.

Marty, Martin. "Feminism in Religion." *Context,* 6 March 1993.

————. "Watch for Freudian Memory Slips." *Context,* 1 February 1994.

Matalin, Mary. "Stop Whining." *Newsweek,* 25 October 1993, p. 62.

Matzek, Virginia. "A Conversation with Richard Ofshe." *California Monthly,* March-April 1993.

Maxson, Jane. "Crisis in Education: False Allegations of Child Abuse." *Issues in Child Abuse Accusations* 3 (Spring 1991).

McHugh, Paul R. "Multiple Personality Disorder." *Harvard Mental Health Letter* 10 (September 1993).

————. "Psychiatric Misadventures." *American Scholar* 61 (Autumn 1992): 497-510.

————. "Psychotherapy Awry." *American Scholar* 63 (Winter 1994): 17-30.

Meacham, Andrew. "Study Disputes Link between Eating Disorders, Sexual Abuse." *Chances,* April 1993.

"Memory and Reality: Reconciliation; Scientific, Clinical and Legal Issues of False Memory Syndrome." Conference publication of the FMS Foundation and Johns Hopkins Medical Institutions, 9-11 December 1994.

Missildine, W. Hugh. *Your Inner Child of the Past*. New York: Simon & Schuster, 1963.

Mockaitis, Caia. "Beijing Conference Is Hostile to Women and Families." *Chicago Tribune*, 30 August 1995.

Morrow, Lance. "Men: Are They Really That Bad?" *Time*, 14 February 1994, pp. 53-59.

Myers, John E. B. *The Backlash: Child Protection under Fire*. Thousand Oaks, CA: Sage Publications, 1994.

Nathan, Debbie. "Cry Incest." *Playboy*, October 1992, pp. 84-88, 162-64.

Nathan, Debbie, and Michael Snedeker. *Satan's Silence: Ritual Abuse and the Making of a Modern American Witch Hunt*. New York: BasicBooks, 1995.

Neimark, Jill. "It's Magical, It's Malleable, It's . . . Memory." *Psychology Today*, January/February 1995, pp. 44-49, 80, 85.

Ofshe, Richard, and Ethan Watters. *Making Monsters: False Memories, Psychotherapy, and Sexual Hysteria*. New York: Scribner's, 1994.

————. "Making Monsters." *Society*, March-April, 1993, pp. 4-16.

Paglia, Camille. *Sexual Personae: Art and Decadence from Nefertiti to Emily Dickinson*. New York: Vintage Books, 1991.

Pasley, Laura. "Misplaced Trust: A First-Person Account of How My Therapist Created False Memories." *Skeptic* 2 (1994).

Pauser, Fred. "A Response to *Treating Abuse Today*." Unpublished paper, March 1995.

Pendergrast, Mark. *Victims of Memory: Incest Accusations and Shattered Lives*. 2d ed. Hinesburg, VT: Upper Access Books, 1996.

Pendergrast, Mark, and Eleanor Goldstein. "Is This Justice?" Boca Raton, FL: Upton Syndication, 1995.

Penhaie, Ed. "Father Torn by Incest Accusation." *Seattle Post-Intelligencer*, 11 December 1992.

Piper, August, Jr. *Hoax and Reality: The Bizarre World of Multiple Personality Disorder*. Northvale, NJ: Jason Aronson, 1997.

Plantinga, Cornelius, Jr. *Not the Way It's Supposed to Be: A Breviary of Sin*. Grand Rapids: William B. Eerdmans, 1995.

Pope, Harrison G., Jr. *Psychology Astray: Fallacies in Studies of "Repressed Memory" and Childhood Trauma*. Boca Raton, FL: Upton Books, 1997.

Procter-Smith, Marjorie. *Praying with Our Eyes Open: Engendering Feminist Liturgical Prayer*. Nashville: Abingdon Press, 1995.

Prose, Francine. "Bad Behavior." *New York Times Magazine*, 26 November 1995, pp. 34-36.

Rabinowitz, Dorothy. "A Darkness in Massachusetts." *Wall Street Journal*, 30 January 1995.

————. "Wenatchee, A True Story — III," *Wall Street Journal*, 8 November 1995.

Reiff, Philip. *The Triumph of the Therapeutic: Uses of Faith after Freud*. New York: Harper & Row, 1968.

Roberts, Robert C. *Taking the Word to Heart: Self and Others in an Age of Therapies*. Grand Rapids: William B. Eerdmans, 1993.

Rose, Elizabeth S. "Surviving the Unbelievable." *Ms.*, January-February 1993, pp. 40-45.

Royal, Robert, ed. *Reinventing the American People: Unity and Diversity Today.* Grand Rapids: William B. Eerdmans, 1995.

Rubin, Bonnie Miller. "Presumed Guilty." *Chicago Tribune,* 30 May 1993.

Samuelson, Robert J. *The Good Life and Its Discontents: The American Dream in the Age of Entitlement, 1945-1995.* New York: Times Books, 1996.

Saulter, Stephanie, and Carol Ness. "Buried Memories, Broken Families." *San Francisco Examiner,* 4-9 April 1993.

Schaef, Anne Wilson. *When Society Becomes an Addict.* San Francisco: Harper & Row Perennial Library, 1987.

Schmitz, Jon. "Jury Finds Psychiatrist Negligent in Treatment." *Pittsburgh Post-Gazette,* 17 December 1994.

Shapiro, Laura. "Rush to Judgment." *Newsweek,* 19 April 1993, pp. 54-60.

Sifford, Darrell. "Accusations of Sex Abuse, Years Later." *Philadelphia Inquirer,* 24 November 1991.

Simpson, Paul. *Second Thoughts: Understanding the False Memory Crisis and How It Could Affect You.* Nashville: Thomas Nelson, 1996.

Sjoo, Monica, and Barbara Mor. *The Great Cosmic Mother: Rediscovering the Religion of the Earth.* San Francisco: Harper & Row, 1987.

Smith, Susan. *Survival Psychology: The Dark Side of a Mental Health Mission.* Boca Raton, FL: Upton Books, 1995.

Sommers, Christina Hoff. *Who Stole Feminism? How Women Have Betrayed Women.* New York: Simon & Schuster, 1994.

Strossen, Nadine. *Defending Pornography.* New York: Charles Scribner's Sons, 1995.

Swagman, Beth A. *Too Close for Comfort: Understanding and Responding to the Reality of Abuse.* Grand Rapids: CRC Publications, 1994.

Sykes, Charles J. *A Nation of Victims: The Decay of the American Character.* New York: St. Martin's Press, 1992.

Tavris, Carol. "Beware the Incest-Survivor Machine." *New York Times Book Review,* 3 January 1993, pp. 1, 16-17.

Taylor, Bill. "Therapist Turned Patient's World Upside Down." *Toronto Star,* 19 May 1992.

Taylor, John. "The Lost Daughter." *Esquire,* March 1994.

Toufexis, Anastasia. "When Can Memories Be Trusted?" *Time,* 28 October 1991, pp. 86-88.

Updike, John. "Elusive Evil." *The New Yorker,* 22 July 1996, pp. 62-70.

Vitz, Paul C. *Psychology as Religion: The Cult of Self-Worship.* 2d ed. Grand Rapids: William B. Eerdmans, 1994.

Vos, Mirth. "A Minister's Adultery Is Sexual Abuse." *The Banner,* 30 May 1994, pp. 20-23.

Wakefield, Hollida. "The Confrontation Clause and the Child Witness." *Issues in Child Abuse Accusations* 2 (Spring 1990).

Wassil-Grimm, Claudette. *Diagnosis for Disaster: The Devastating Truth about False Memory Syndrome and Its Impact on Accusers and Families.* Woodstock, NY: Overlook Press, 1995.

Whitfield, Charles. "Guidelines for Assisting with Memories of Trauma." Handout at conference, Holy Family Hospital, Des Plaines, IL, 25 February 1994.

————. *Healing the Child Within.* Pompano Beach, FL: Health Communications, 1987.

Wright, Lawrence. *Remembering Satan: A Case of Recovered Memory and the Shattering of an American Family.* New York: Alfred A. Knopf, 1994.

Yapko, Michael. "The Seduction of Memory." *Networker,* September-October 1993, pp. 31-37.

————. *Suggestions of Abuse.* New York: Simon & Schuster, 1994.

Index